Basics of Oncology

Frederick O. Stephens · Karl R. Aigner

Basics of Oncology

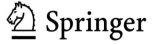 Springer

**Frederick O. Stephens, AM, MD,
MS, FRCS (Ed), FACS, FRACS**
Emeritus Professor and
former Head of Department of Surgery
The University of Sydney
Former Head of Surgical Oncology
The Royal Prince Alfred and Sydney Hospitals
16 Inkerman Street
Mosman NSW 2088
Australia
fredstephens@optusnet.com.au

Karl R. Aigner, MD
Professor of Surgery
Department of Surgical Oncology
Medias Klinikum GmbH & Co. KG
Abt. Onkologische Chirurgie
Krankenhausstr. 1
84489 Burghausen
Germany
Prof-aigner@medias-klinikum.de

ISBN: 978-3-540-92924-6   e-ISBN: 978-3-540-92925-3
DOI: 10.1007/978-3-540-92925-3
Springer Dordrecht Heidelberg London New York

Library of Congress Control Number: 2008944024

Cover design: Frido Steinen-Broo, eStudio Calamar, Spain

Printed on acid-free paper

Springer is part of Springer Science+Business Media (www.springer.com)

Contributing Authors

Tim Allen-Mersh, MD, FRCS
Professor, Division of Surgery,
Oncology Reproductive
Biology and Anaesthetics
Imperial College School of Medicine
Chelsea and Westminster Hospitals
London

Gabriel Hortobagyi, MD, FACP
Professor, Department of Breast
Medical Oncology
The University of Texas,
MD Anderson Cancer Center
Houston, TX, USA

David Khayat, MD, PhD
Professor, Department of Medical
Oncology Salpetrière Hospital
Paris, France

Steven M. Picksley, BSc, PhD
Department of Biomedical Sciences
University of Bradford
Bradford, England

Paul Sugarbaker, MD, FACS, FRCS
Professor, The Center for Surgical
Oncology, Washington Hospital Center
and Washington Cancer Institute
Washington, DC
USA

Tetsuo Taguchi, MD, PhD
Professor, Department of
Oncologic Surgery
Research Institute for Microbial
Disease, Osaka University
Japan Society for Cancer
Chemotherapy
Osaka
Japan

John F. Thompson, MD, FRACS, FACS
Professor, The University of Sydney,
Departments of Melanoma and
Surgical Oncology, The Royal Prince
Alfred Hospital, Sydney,
Melanoma Institute Australia
& The Sydney Melanoma Unit,
The Royal Prince Alfred Hospital,
The Mater, Royal North Shore,
Westmead Hospitals, Sydney,
Australia

Dedication

Working in oncology is a very satisfying career. It is particularly satisfying to be able to help people with this most distressing and worrying health problem. Most patients are cured but for some cure is not a possibility with our present state of knowledge. All can be helped.

In most cases our patients become our friends and some become very special friends. They honour us with their friendship and trust and this makes our work feel more than worthwhile, indeed a special reward.

We are also grateful for our teachers of the past and for our present colleagues without whose cooperation our work would be of limited value and progress would be difficult.

Like all teachers, we are inspired by our students. We not only pass on knowledge to them, we also learn from them. To have interested and enthusiastic students is a real stimulus and privilege.

As is obvious from the authorship of this book we have been privileged to make close and lasting friendships across national borders and across borders of traditional disciplines. We treasure these friendships dearly from their personal aspects as well as being able to learn from each other and to stimulate each other in clinical work and research. It is sad that so much cancer is still with us, but the constant mutual commitment to improving methods of care and discovering new information on prevention and treatment for the betterment of people everywhere is itself a reward, which we all share with respect and gratitude.

Finally we acknowledge that our work is demanding of time and energy. This is time and energy in which our wives, families and friends have so often had to make allowances for our absence. Without their love, support and acceptance of the conditions of our work, this work and our efficiency would be severely compromised. They have often joined us and at other times have had to stand by without us when we were concentrating on other things we could not always share with them. We especially owe our loved ones a debt of thanks and gratitude.

We proudly dedicate this book to all of these people.

Preface

Who Should Read This Book

In Western societies and other developed countries, cancer is the leading cause of death, after cardiovascular disease. It is therefore a major component of medical undergraduate curricula and of primary concern to nurses and allied health-workers.

Presently most undergraduate students learn about cancer from a broad range of general and specialist books and journals. Medical students read about cancer in textbooks of surgery, pathology and cancer medicine as well as in general and specialist journals and from time to time in newspaper reports, magazines and from various other sources.

We the authors teach, practise and conduct research in different specialty areas in different parts of the world. We agreed that we should write this book as an easily understood and general overview of cancer for students of medicine, nurse oncologists, students of medical sciences and other health professionals in all parts of the world. It is intended to serve as a basis for more detailed or specialised studies that will be needed in different areas of practice and in different countries. Different countries will emphasise different aspects according to their more specific community needs, incidence, traditions and available health-care facilities and systems.

What This Book Is About

This book is intended to give an introduction to the scientific and clinical aspects of cancer, that is the broad range of concepts of causes, pathology, clinical features, possible investigations, treatments and outcomes both for cancers in general and for the common cancers in different countries. It should be a basis for further study as appropriate for all areas of oncology no matter where it is practised or in what particular professional discipline. The purpose of this book is not to cover all social, personal, environmental or financial aspects of cancer nor to discuss details of supportive services available. These important aspects will differ in different countries with different social, medical and administrative services and facilities as well as different traditional practices and requirements.

Ideal comprehensive facilities and services may or may not be available. Other books, specifically written for students and practitioners in different countries with different curriculum requirements, may be needed to cover these aspects.

Objective of This Book

The objective of this book is to develop graded information from very basic to more sophisticated understanding of present knowledge about cancer. For some students this may well meet all their needs, but for students wishing to undertake further studies in cancer this book will serve as a sound basis for more detailed or specific studies.
To achieve this, the book will

- Cover basic medical, scientific and clinical aspects of cancer
- Explain how and why people develop cancer
- Indicate how the body reacts to cancer
- Describe how cancer presents
- Outline principles of cancer prevention, investigation, diagnosis and management

This information applies in all countries. It is the essential requirement for understanding cancer no matter where studied or practised. We believe this basic information about cancer is best introduced early in a student's career before other details of personal, psychological, social, management practices and traditions are studied in detail in different communities.

More detailed and comprehensive information on specialised areas of knowledge, research and practice is expanded in more specialised books and publications, some of which are listed in the final section of this book.

Sydney, Australia   **Frederick O. Stephens**
Burghausen, Germany   **Karl R. Aigner**

Acknowledgements

The authors wish to acknowledge the help of a number of friends and colleagues.

Under the direction of Mr Ray Barbour all members of the audio-visual department of the Royal Prince Alfred Hospital, Sydney, were most generous and skilled in helping provide the illustrations. In particular we want to thank Mr Anthony Butler for preparing the clinical illustrations and artist, Mr Bob Haynes, who converted our rough diagrams into meaningful illustrations.

We are grateful to Oxford University Press for permission to reproduce illustrations first published in *All About Prostate Cancer, All About Breast Cancer* and *The Cancer Prevention Manual* written by one of us (FOS).

Dr Jean Philippe Spano, assistant to Professor Khayat in Paris, kindly read the manuscript and made a number of helpful suggestions.

Dr Murray Brennan, Professor and Chairman of the Department of Surgery at the Memorial Sloan-Kettering Cancer Center, New York, read the original manuscript and kindly made a number of helpful suggestions.

Dr David Pennington, Senior Surgeon in Plastic and Reconstructive Surgery at the Royal Prince Alfred Hospital, Sydney, provided the illustrations of breast reconstruction of one of his patients.

Professor Graham Young, Director of The Kanematsu Institute at the Royal Prince Alfred Hospital, gave helpful advice with regard to Chap. 19.

Some of the case reports were provided by distinguished friends and colleagues. For these we are especially grateful to Professor Graham Young, Dr Jean-Philippe Spano, Professor Jonathan Carter, Dr Michael Stevens, Dr Robin Saw, Dr Robert Stephens, Dr Chris Hughes, Dr Ian Kalnins, Dr Andrew Parasyn, Professor John Watson, Professor Bruce Barraclough and Dr Graeme Brazenor.

The authors are indebted to Belinda Bonham for editorial help in preparing the manuscript and Renata Atkins for help in design and presentation.

Contents

Part III   Most Common Cancers

Part I
The Cancer Problem

What Is Malignancy?

1

In this chapter you will learn about:

> *Prevalence of cancer*
> *Benign and malignant tumours*
> *Dangers of malignant tumours*
> *What causes malignancy*

A malignant growth is characterised by a continuing, purposeless, unwanted, uncontrolled and damaging growth of cells that differ structurally and functionally from the normal cells from which they developed.

The commonly used term for a malignant growth is a cancer – *cancer* is Latin for crab. The condition was called cancer in ancient times because an advanced cancer was thought to resemble a crab, with "claws" reaching out into surrounding tissues.

All living plants and animals are composed of living cells that often need to divide to produce more cells for growth and development, and also to replace cells that have been damaged or have died. The process of cell proliferation (cell division and cell growth) is controlled by genes in the DNA of the cell nucleus. The genes are inherited from parents and bestow particular features in the offspring, including height, colour, weight and countless other distinctive features and functions of the tissues. The process is normally under remarkably well-balanced control. A cancer forms when this genetic control is damaged or lost in one or more cells, which then continue to divide and divide again producing more abnormal cells that continue to divide and increase in number when and where they should not. The masses of unwanted dividing cells cause damage to other cells and tissues in the body. They are no longer controlled by normal genes that stop division after normal body needs have been met. They just go on dividing in spite of causing damage to other tissues and body functions. This is a cancer. All the causes of cancer are now known to directly, or indirectly, damage these normal genes that regulate cell division.

Cancer is Latin for crab.

F. O. Stephens and K. R. Aigner, *Basics of Oncology,*
DOI: 10.1007/978-3-540-92925-3_1, © Springer-Verlag Berlin Heidelberg 2009

One obvious factor is that the longer we live the more chance there is for the genes that regulate cell proliferation to become damaged by exposure to agents that damage the genetic blueprint, DNA. So most cancers become more common the longer we live; most cancers are more common in old age. Another factor is the rate of division for growth and replacement of tissues. Tissues like skin, bowel lining or lining of air passages (especially in the lungs), and blood cells are constantly being shed and replenished. Breast cells are constantly changing due to hormone activity over a woman's years of fertile life. With all this constant cell proliferation there is more likelihood of mistakes being made in the process of copying the genetic blueprint to daughter cells, especially as the process becomes less accurate as we get older. A mistake or error in copying the genetic blueprint is called a genetic mutation. These then are the tissues most likely to undergo malignant change. Bone growth is greatest in growing young people and testicular activity is greatest in young adult males and these are the periods of life most prone to cancers of these tissues. As men grow old the slow but constant changes in the prostate gland make it more likely that factors causing a change in cells might go wrong after years of exposure to the driving force of male hormones. So prostate cancer becomes increasingly common in old age.

The remarkable thing is not that something goes wrong from time to time in the delicate process of cell division but that things don't go wrong more often. In all life there is a continuous delicate living process involving countless generations of cell division. The better we care for our bodies with good living practices the greater the likelihood of preventing something, possibly uncontrollable, from seriously going wrong.

These good living practices include having good nutrition, healthy exercise, safe sex and avoiding exposure to potentially damaging agents in our environment. All of these practices serve to reduce the exposure of the genetic material in cells to agents that could cause changes in the genetic blueprint.

In the normal genetic make-up there is a braking mechanism to stop cell division when the need for more cells has been satisfied.

Whilst most normal body tissues are composed of cells that have the ability to grow or reproduce, they normally only do so when there is a need. When this need has been satisfied they stop reproducing. In the normal cell there is a braking mechanism to stop cell division when the need for more cells has been satisfied. Cells in such tissues as the skin or blood or the lining of the mouth, throat or alimentary tract, wear out quickly and are constantly being replaced. They are normally replaced only to meet the immediate need of the body, after which reproduction stops. Also, after injury or cell death, surrounding cells reproduce to replace and repair damaged tissues but there is an in-built mechanism that stops the cell reproduction once the injury has been repaired and the wound has healed. The "switch on" and "switch off" mechanisms are governed by two different types of genes, whose functions are either to promote or to suppress cell division and cell growth. These are called proto-oncogenes and tumour suppressors. Proto-oncogenes respond to growth signals and are positive regulators of cell proliferation, only in the presence of appropriate growth signals. Tumour suppressor genes conversely act as negative regulators of cell growth and suppress or check the unregulated growth of cells. So in the normal cell the "switch-off" mechanism is the response to the absence of specific growth signals.

Some, but not all, body tissues retain a lifelong ability to replicate themselves to meet the body needs. For example, after surgical removal of as much as three quarters of a normal liver, the remaining liver will grow back to its original size within about 6 weeks and then stop. The nature of the "switch off" mechanism is not fully understood – but it is clearly a critically important process that is normally under genetic control.

In the case of a malignancy there is no "switching off" mechanism. Some of the proto-oncogenes have now acquired mutations that mean they promote cell growth even in the absence of appropriate growth signals, i.e. they become oncogenes (cancer promoting genes) and some of the tumour suppressor genes are inactivated, such that abnormal growth goes unchecked. Abnormal and unwanted cells then invade into surrounding tissues and possibly blood and lymph vessels, or body cavities, thereby spreading to other parts of the body, where they establish new damaging colonies of unwanted growing cells. These colonies are called secondary or metastatic cancers, known as *secondaries* or *metastases.*

1.1 Nature of a Malignancy

A malignancy is therefore totally different from an infection, which is caused by organisms from outside the body invading body tissues and causing damage. The body defences recognise invading organisms as foreign and protective measures are set in train to destroy them. Invading cancer cells, on the other hand, are abnormal cells that have developed from the body's own cells and are therefore allowed to further develop and infiltrate other tissues without the control normally provided by natural body defences.

Cancer cells also have different features and take on a different microscopic appearance from the cells from which they developed. Cancer cells become bizarre in size, shape and other features. As a rule, the more bizarre they become, the more aggressive and malignant is their behaviour. Cancer cells are usually derived from a single original cell, and are said to show a clonal origin. The nucleus is often irregular, larger and darker in colour and may even be duplicated in the one cell. The cytoplasm is often relatively smaller, irregular in size and shape and without the special features of the cell of origin. There may be cells not only of different sizes and shapes but also with different staining properties (pleomorphic). These changes are brought about by changes in the tumour suppressor genes and oncogenes that are responsible for the control of cell division.

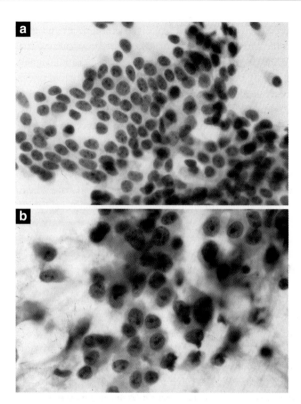

Fig. 1.1. Photomicrographs showing (**a**) breast cells of normal appearance aspirated from a benign breast lump and (**b**) highly malignant anaplastic breast cancer cells aspirated from a breast cancer (400×)

EXERCISE

Study the cells in Fig. 1.1. In what ways do cells differ in Fig. 1.1a, b?

1.2   What is the Prevalence of Cancer?

Cancer is known to occur in all societies and in all parts of the world. It affects animals as well as man. In humans, cancer is known to have been present in ancient times as well as in modern communities. However, the types of cancer most prevalent in a community will vary with the age, sex distribution and race of people in the community, as well as the geographical situation, the economic and environmental situation and habits of the people including their diets. (See Appendix showing incidence of different cancers in different countries.)

In developed countries cancer is responsible for about 25–30% of deaths. It is second to cardiovascular disease as a cause of death. Young people in developed societies are much more at risk of dying from causes other than cancer such as infectious diseases (including AIDS) or as a result of trauma (especially accidents in homes or on the roads, gunshot wounds or suicide), than from cancer. Although cancer can occur at any age it is relatively uncommon before the age of 40 years but as people grow older the risk of cancer progressively increases.

1.3   Tumours Benign and Malignant?

Non-malignant or *benign* tumours are much more common than malignant tumours. A benign tumour is a limited growth of cells that seems to be under some sort of control. Although there is no apparent purpose in the growth, the cells are more mature and closely resemble the cells from which they developed. Once the growth reaches a certain size, it usually slows or stops, such as a mole on the skin. All the cells of a benign tumour stay together as a lump or swelling that is usually confined by a capsule or lining of fibrous tissue. They do not spread to other parts of the body and are generally easily removed by surgery.

There are two broad groups of solid tissue malignant tumours, commonly called cancers. They are *carcinomas* and *sarcomas*. Carcinomas are malignant tumours of epithelial origin, such as lining cells of skin, the alimentary tract, respiratory tract, bladder or glands such as pancreas, thyroid or salivary glands. Sarcomas are malignant tumours of connective tissue such as bone, cartilage, muscle, fat, fascia, nerve or blood vessel. Carcinomas are much more common than sarcomas.

In a malignant tumour the cells look less like the cells from which they developed. The term *anaplasia* is used to describe cells that have lost their distinctive features. The multiplication of cells also continues without control (Fig. 1.2).

Very occasionally benign tumours can be life-threatening simply because of their size and location. An example is meningioma, which is a benign, slowly growing tumour that arises from the meninges covering the brain. It can eventually prove fatal if not removed because it compresses the surrounding normal brain tissue and eventually interferes with vital brain functions. A meningioma is nevertheless classified as a benign tumour because its cells do not invade surrounding tissues or spread to other parts of the body via the bloodstream or the lymphatic system and its removal by surgery should result in cure.

Fig. 1.2. Illustrations of degrees of cell degeneration into cancer

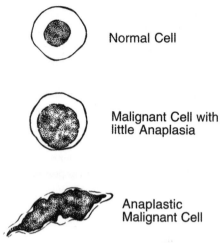

Normal Cell

Malignant Cell with little Anaplasia

Anaplastic Malignant Cell

1.4   Dangers of Malignant Tumours

If a malignant tumour is detected while it is still small and before it has metastasised, it can usually be completely removed surgically or destroyed by radiotherapy or other means, before any serious damage has been done. The danger it poses will have been eliminated and the patient will have been cured.

Malignant tumours become dangerous when they damage surrounding tissues and when they establish metastases in other organs and tissues. To metastasise cancer cells have an ability to break away from where they arose and penetrate or spread into other tissues including blood and lymph vessels. Some cancers, like basal cell cancers (BCCs) of skin have a low grade of malignancy. They almost never metastasise but others, like some melanomas, produce malignant cells with much greater ability to invade, break free and penetrate into blood and lymph vessels relatively early in the disease. Such cancers become highly aggressive and high grade and may establish early metastases. The ability of some cancers to metastasise is not completely understood. It appears to be related to imperfect intercellular cementing substances and is acquired through alterations in genes that cause proteases, angiogenic factors and dysregulation of adhesion factors. Proteases allow penetration of cells through tissues, angiogenic factors promote development of new cancer capillaries for nutrition of the malignant cells and dysregulation of adhesion factors "set cells free" to allow individual cell penetration rather than being held together as one tissue. The more of these factors associated with a cancer, the greater will be its malignancy and degree of spread.

Cancer cells have been likened to seeds of a weed growing in a garden. Just as some seeds will grow in some soils and some need special soil conditions, so too, some cancer cells tend to grow more readily in some tissues as opposed to other tissues. Some tissues seem to be disposed to different types of metastatic cell growth. For example breast and prostate cancer cells are very likely to form metastases in bone; sarcoma cells and kidney cancers seem to grow preferentially in lung; and alimentary tract cancer cells are most likely to grow as metastases in the liver. Lymph nodes are the most common sites for metastatic spread of most cancers but are not often the site of metastases of sarcomas. Other tissues appear to have general resistance to metastases. The spleen and muscles are rarely the site of metastatic cell growth except for melanoma cells, which seem to grow readily in virtually any tissue including lung, liver, brain and bone as well as lymph nodes. Squamous cancers from skin and other tissues spread most often to nearby lymph nodes, then to more distant lymph nodes but further spread seems to be delayed. However sooner or later they will metastasise further to lungs or other organs or tissues.

Metastatic growths damage and destroy the organ or tissue in which they are growing. For example, metastases in the liver interfere with the function of the liver, metastases in the lung block air passages leading to lung infection or pneumonia and metastases in the brain often result in headaches first and eventually convulsions or coma. Bone metastases often cause pain and weakness of the bones that may then collapse or break.

1.5   What Causes Cancer

1.5.1   Is There a Single Cause Or a Single Common Pathway?

For generations doctors, researchers, other health workers, philosophers, unconventional practitioners and sometimes "quacks" have been trying to find a single cause for all cancers, and consequently a single cure. No such cause has been found and probably none exists. Many different factors initiate changes in cells that lead to cancer. Current evidence would suggest that all causes of cancer act by generating damage to the genetic blueprint of cells, specifically causing mutations in proto-oncogenes and tumour suppressor genes. In many cases the mutations in such genes can be linked directly to the types of DNA damage associated with the agents that cause cancer e.g. UV-light and tobacco tar, and each has its own signature form of DNA damage, providing evidence of "direct cause and effect". Even tumour viruses cause cancer by altering the cell's genetic blueprint, either by directly altering the expression of proto-oncogenes, or indirectly, through the inactivation of tumour suppressor proteins, in effect, over-riding the genetic blueprint. Today it is believed that cancer arises from a single cell that has acquired 6–12 genetic changes (mutations) in key tumour suppressor and proto-oncogenes. This explains the clonal origin of cancers, and why cancer incidence increases with age, due to the sequential accumulation of these mutations; and also why some familial cancers are inherited at an earlier age, as such individuals would already have one of these pre-disposing mutations at birth. While we can minimise our own risk of cancer by adopting a healthy life-style, we cannot completely eliminate the risk, as within all our cells are natural metabolites that can potentially cause such mutations.

Smoking is a major cause of many health problems and in modern societies it is the foremost preventable cause of cancers.

1.5.2   Apoptosis

While so far cancer has been discussed simply in relation to uncontrolled cell proliferation, there is another important counter-balance to cell growth, namely that of cell death. Cell death is a natural feature of cells that occurs in damaged cells, and also during development, for example, in the foetus the development of our fingers arises from the death of the web of cells between the fingers. This process of cell death is known as apoptosis. It is a highly regulated and biochemically defined process, distinct from simple necrosis (where cells simply spill out their contents). Cells that have extensive genetic damage often spontaneously undergo apoptosis, and in effect "commit suicide" for the greater good of the host. This is an important mechanism for suppressing tumour development. Indeed, the main aim of chemotherapy and radiotherapy is to induce such extensive genetic damage in tumours that the cancer cells undergo apoptosis. Cells that escape, or evade, this apoptotic process form tumours that are more resistant to chemotherapy and radiotherapy, and are associated with poor prognosis.

1.5.3   Carcinogens

There are many known cancer causing agents (carcinogens) but whatever the end result of their actions they all cause genetic mutations resulting in different types of cancers.

1.5.4   Tobacco Smoking

Smoking is a major cause of many health problems and in modern societies it is the foremost preventable cause of cancers. Tobacco smoking is responsible for an increased incidence of cancers of the lung, mouth, throat and larynx as well as cancers of the oesophagus, stomach, pancreas, kidney, bladder, cervix uteri and in the long term even the breast.

EXERCISE

Study Fig. 1.3 and list the potential long-term effects of cigarette smoking.

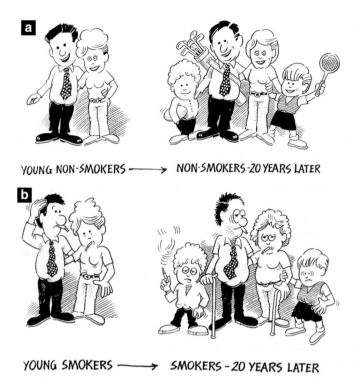

YOUNG NON-SMOKERS ———→ NON-SMOKERS -20 YEARS LATER

YOUNG SMOKERS ———→ SMOKERS - 20 YEARS LATER

Fig. 1.3. (**a**, **b**) Tobacco smoking is responsible for many health problems including many cancers

1.5.5 Alcohol

The association between alcohol and cancer is not so clear. There is an obvious association in heavy drinkers, especially of strong spirits, with cancers in the oesophagus. The incidence of oesophageal cancer is significantly increased in both heavy drinkers and tobacco smokers in any of its forms (whether it be cigarettes, pipes or cigars). However people (especially males) who are both heavy drinkers and heavy smokers have a much higher incidence than with just alcohol alone or tobacco alone. Such an increased risk association is seen in cancers of the alimentary tract from pharynx to colon and including the pancreas.

There is a secondary association between alcohol and primary liver cancer. Alcohol causes cirrhosis of the liver and cirrhosis sometimes predisposes the patient to primary liver cancer.

1.5.6 Betel Nut

In some countries a locally grown nut, betel nut, is cheaply produced and is often chewed. It may become habit forming rather like chewing gum rather than in itself being addictive. When not being chewed, betel nut is often held in the cheek area of the mouth, lined by buccal mucosa. It has carcinogenic properties that commonly cause cancers of the mucous membrane lining the mouth, especially in the buccal mucosa. When mixed with tobacco leaf or lime, or both, the *carcinogenic* properties are increased.

The habits of chewing betel nut or tobacco leaf are responsible for a considerably increased incidence of cancer in the mouth of people who live in India, Pakistan, South East Asia and New Guinea, where these habits are common.

1.5.7   Sunshine

Excessive ultra-violet light from sunshine is predominantly responsible for a greatly increased incidence of skin cancers, especially in fair-skinned people who live in sunny tropical or sub-tropical climates. UV light of solariums can be equally damaging in even shorter periods of time (Figs. 1.4 and 1.5).

1.5.8   Other Forms of Irradiation: X-rays and Atomic Irradiation

Increased incidence of cancers in the skin of the hands in people who held X-ray plates in their hands during the early use of X-ray machines was the first evidence that irradiation with X-rays would cause certain cancers. An increased incidence of other cancers, including thyroid cancer and leukaemias, followed the atomic irradiation exposure after the World War 2 atomic bomb explosions at Hiroshima and Nagasaki and the atomic energy plant accident in Chernobyl (Russia) in 1986. This confirmed the risk of these forms of irradiation in causing cancer.

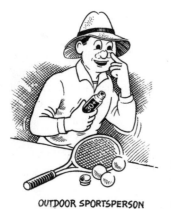

OUTDOOR SPORTSPERSON

Fig. 1.4. Diagram illustrating simple preventive measures to protect against skin cancers. People and communities should be encouraged to adopt such lifestyle practices as a routine. Note the hat, protective-cream and long sleeved shirt

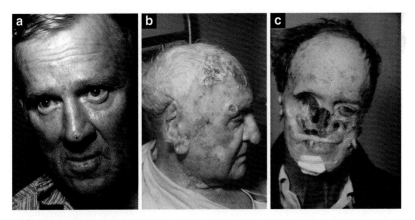

Fig. 1.5. (**a–c**) Photographs showing early, late and extremely late effects of sun damage with increasing hyperkeratoses, BCCs and SCCs

1.5.9   Industrial Irritants and Carcinogens

The first cancer in Western countries found to be caused by a chemical agent was cancer of the scrotum. This cancer commonly developed in chimney sweeps in Britain in the eighteenth century. The cause was found to be soot that collected in the scrotal area. Later, certain dyes used by German workers in chemical factories and excreted in the urine were found to be associated with an increased incidence of bladder cancer. People using phosphorus to paint luminous dials on clocks and watches were also found to have a high incidence of bone cancer (osteosarcoma). The phosphorus was absorbed from the habit of the workers wetting the tips of their paintbrushes with saliva by putting the brushes in their mouths.

1.5.10   Chemical Carcinogens

A number of chemical agents can cause cancer in experimental animals. Similarly chemical agents are known to be present in tobacco tars and in products of the petroleum and other industries.

1.5.11   Hormones

Increased hormones or prolonged hormone exposure can be associated with increased risk of some cancers. There is an increased risk of breast cancer in women having hormone replacement therapy (HRT) for postmenopausal symptoms. Prostate cancer in men is known to be an androgen dependent tumour. Without androgens prostate cancer will not grow. Other cancers that are sometimes linked to hormones include cancer of the body of the uterus.

1.5.12   Viruses

Viruses have been extensively studied as possible causes of human cancers. These investigations have been stimulated by evidence that certain viruses cause cancers in animals and that human warts, which are benign tumours, are known to be caused by a virus. A *"human papilloma virus"* (HPV) may also sometimes cause wart-like papillomas in the skin of people and these can become malignant. One form of HPV is sexually transmitted and can cause cancer of the uterus, vagina or vulva in women or cancer of the penis in men. HPV is now known to be the most common cause of cancer of the cervix.

There is now evidence that some other viruses appear to be responsible for some other human cancers. For example, there is cancer that arises in the back of the nose, most common in Chinese who live in or near the Quantong province of China near Hong Kong. In these people there is a high incidence of infection with the *Epstein-Barr virus* that probably plays a part in the development of this cancer. The malignant tumour *Burkitt's lymphoma*, most common in certain parts of Africa and New Guinea, is also associated with a high incidence of infection with the Epstein-Barr or a similar virus.

Convincing evidence that viruses play a role in the development of some cancers comes from analysis of the incidence of cancer in patients who have received solid organ transplants (e.g. kidney, heart, liver). These patients receive lifelong immunosuppression to prevent rejection of their transplanted organ, and apparently as a result of this have an increased incidence of cancers but especially of those cancers known to be associated with viral infections. In Australian renal transplant recipients, for example, the incidence of squamous cell carcinoma is 100 times that in the rest of the population – and a clear association with HPV has been demonstrated. Similarly increased is the incidence of carcinoma of the cervix (also known to be associated with HPV), hepatoma (associated with the hepatitis B and hepatitis C viruses), non-Hodgkin lymphoma (sometimes associated with the Epstein-Barr Virus) and Kaposi's sarcoma (associated with Cytomegalovirus infection). Similar tumours are seen in patients with AIDS whose immune systems are damaged, not by drugs, but by the virus that causes immune-deficiency.

1.5.12.1   *Recent studies of viruses at a molecular level*

At a molecular level viruses have been shown to cause cancer in a number of ways. Firstly, many viruses encode proteins that directly target and inactivate host tumour suppressor genes such as the p53 and retinoblastoma (RB) tumour suppressors. This allows the virus to kick start cells into dividing so they can replicate their genetic material using the host replication machinery in S-phase of the cell cycle. Viruses through having to compete with the host cell have strongly expressed genes to assist their propagation, and sometimes they inappropriately activate the expression of host proto-oncogenes, or are indirectly associated with chromosomal re-arrangements that place the host proto-oncogenes under the genetic regulation of the virus.

1.5.13 Bacteria

Evidence of a direct link between bacteria and cancer is unclear although prolonged inflammation of ulcers caused by prolonged bacterial activity can predispose to malignant change. Perhaps the most apparent association of a link between bacteria and cancer is the common finding of *helicobacter* organisms in gastric cancer.

1.5.14 Pre-Existing Abnormalities

It is a common observation that congenitally abnormal tissues, chronically irritated tissues, chronically atrophic or degenerate tissues, chronically inflamed or ulcerated tissues, or severely scarred tissues are more likely to develop malignant cells than are normal tissues. Examples include cancer that develops in an undescended testis, and squamous cell cancer that develops in a chronic ulcer resulting from a severe burn. Also, pre-existing benign tumours such as *polyps*, *papillomas* and *adenomas* have a propensity to undergo malignant change; some types more than others.

1.5.15 Nutritional Deficiencies and Food Habits

Deficiencies of certain vitamins, trace elements, anti-oxidants, naturally occurring plant hormones and other plant products including natural fibre have been linked to increased risk of several cancers of different types, in different body systems and in different communities and racial groups often living in different parts of the world. High animal fat content of food appears to be associated with increased risk of some cancers; whilst a diet rich in fresh fruit and vegetables appears to be protective. Details of these associations are discussed later in this chapter under the heading *diet* and in the chapters of the various cancers concerned, especially Chaps. 12, 13 and 16.

1.5.16 Estimate of Known Risk Factors and Associations with Cancer

The association of the most common skin cancers with ultraviolet light is clear. Of the other known and potentially avoidable cancer risk factors it has been variously estimated that food, alcohol and tobacco might be associated with about 70%, viruses and bacteria about 10%, heredity about 10%, physical factors (e.g. chemicals, irradiation, chronic trauma) about 5% and other factors about 5%.

1

The largely unknown factor is of inevitable degeneration especially associated with old age. If all the known factors could be avoided how many people would eventually develop a cancer, as part of the inevitable degeneration of tissues associated with old age, is quite unknown. However, it is certain that with less cancer in younger people many more people would be living longer and healthier lives, but malignant cells would eventually develop in most old people after so many years of repeated cell reproduction in so many tissues.

EXERCISE

What genes might contribute to an increased risk of breast cancer?

Epidemiology

2

In this chapter you will learn about:

> *Comparative cancer incidence*
> *People most at risk*
> *Viral and other infection associations*
> *Heredity and genetic factors*
> *Age*
> *Predisposing and pre-malignant risk factors*
> *Gender*
> *Diet*
> *Race*
> *Geographic associations*
> *Environment*
> *Occupation and cancer*
> *Habits and lifestyle*
> *Possible psychological factors*
> *Cancer registries*

2.1   Comparative Cancer Incidence

The incidence of cancers is very different in different countries (see Appendix). The most obvious differences are between developed and developing countries. Cancers of the lung, prostate, breast, colo-rectum and pancreas are all much more common in developed countries and cancers of oesophagus and liver are much more common in developing countries. Other cancers that are at least twice as common in developed countries are cancers of skin, uterus, ovary, bladder, kidney, testis, brain, the lymphomas, leukaemias and multiple myeloma. Nasopharyngeal cancers are more than twice as common in developing countries.

Table 2.1 shows the year 2001 incidence of the most common internal cancers in the United States and the incidence of death rates from these cancers.

The incidence of cancers is very different in different countries (see Appendix). The most obvious differences are between developed and developing countries.

F. O. Stephens and K. R. Aigner, *Basics of Oncology,*
DOI: 10.1007/978-3-540-92925-3_2, © Springer-Verlag Berlin Heidelberg 2009

2

Table 2.1 The year 2001 incidence of the most common internal cancers in the United States and the incidence of death rates from these cancers

Cancer	Incidence	Deaths
Prostate	198,100	31,500
Breast	193,700	40,600
Lung	169,500	157,400
Colon and rectum	135,400	56,700

2.2 People Most at Risk

Although the risk of developing cancer is much lower in young people cancer can affect people of any age, race or occupation in any part of the world. People who have been cured of one cancer often ask about the risk of developing a second cancer. Whilst it is true that some people have an increased predisposition towards developing cancer, in most cases people who have already had one cancer cured have only a slightly greater risk of developing a second cancer than do people who have never had a cancer. For example, a woman who has been cured of breast cancer has an increased risk of developing cancer in the other breast and a somewhat increased risk of developing cancer of the uterus or ovary, but the majority of these people never develop any other serious cancer. Again, people who have been treated and apparently cured of one bowel cancer do have an increased risk of developing a second cancer elsewhere in the bowel but most do not. It is also true that people who have been cured of one type of cancer have a slightly increased risk of developing a second cancer, not only of the same system but of another system of the body, but the increased risk is small. However, the risk of developing a second cancer is increased if they continue to indulge in an obviously cancer-causing habit such as cigarette smoking or if they inherit a mutation in a tumour suppressor or proto-oncogene. There is also an increased risk of developing a leukaemia in some people 20 years or so after treatment of another cancer with a prolonged chemotherapy program.

2.3 Viral and Other Infection Associations

In the normal course of events cancer cannot be passed directly from one individual to another.

In the normal course of events cancer cannot be passed directly from one individual to another. The present day worldwide scourge of acquired immune deficiency syndrome (AIDS) is caused by a virus infection that can predispose to cancer but AIDS is not itself a cancer. In this disease the sufferer's natural immune defences against infection and cancer are damaged, resulting in a higher incidence of cancer developing in affected people. Several cancers are now commonly associated with HIV infection or AIDS. These include a sarcoma of soft tissues called Kaposi's sarcoma, lymphomas of the central nervous system, non-Hodgkin lymphoma and cancer of the cervix. Each of these is described and discussed in Part 3 of this book.

Similarly, liver cancer is not infectious but a common precursor of liver cancer is the chronic inflammatory changes in the liver due to hepatitis B or hepatitis C infection. These hepatitis infections do spread easily from person to person, mainly from food or intimate contact. In the case of hepatitis C, blood transfusion or sharing of intravenous needles is also a common method of spread. Liver cancer therefore develops more commonly in people who have been infected. However in many cases the liver cancer doesn't develop until at least 20 years after infection. This is known as "the latency period" and is consistent with the clonal origin of cancers and that five to eleven other genetic alterations are required for cancer to develop.

The human papilloma virus is sometimes responsible for papillomas or squamous cell carcinomas of skin or genitals of either sex. It is often transmitted during the sexual intercourse and is particularly associated with cancer of the cervix. The latency period for the development of cervical cancer from human papilloma virus is 5–30 years.

Viruses can act by modulating the function of proto-oncogenes and tumour suppressors. These original findings provided initial molecular insights into the genetic basis of cancer.

2.4   Heredity and Genetic Factors

Molecular biology and studies of association of genes with cancer is one of the most stimulating, challenging and exciting fields of cancer research.

At this stage information about three genetic concepts is important. These still evolving concepts are about cancer *proto-oncogenes, tumour suppressor genes* and *cell cycle regulation genes.* It is certain that these concepts will be modified, changed or added to fairly rapidly as more information is gathered in this relatively new but exciting area of study being carried out in many laboratories in many parts of the world. It is not known whether all the different carcinogenic factors already described all activate "biological triggers" in cells. Whatever the mechanism or combination of mechanisms, it seems that cancers are ultimately caused by changes in tumour suppressor genes or *proto-oncogenes* that convert them into *oncogenes*, i.e. genes that can cause cancer.

About 10% of breast cancers result from breast tissue changes due to one of several specific genes that have been inherited from a parent.

2.4.1   Tumour Suppressors, Proto-Oncogenes and Cancer-Oncogenes

The many functions of our body cells are controlled by genes. Genes are coded in the DNA that makes up the chromosomes or genetic library of our cells. Like the genes that determine features like eye colour and blood group, we inherit these controlling genes from our parents. There is a link between genetic make-up and some cancers.

Different genes are associated with different cancers for example the *BRCA1* gene is often associated with either breast cancer or ovarian cancer. The *BRCA2* gene can be associated with either breast cancer or pancreas cancer. Recent studies have also shown a link between the BRCA2 gene and prostate cancer, particularly prostate cancer in younger men.

The *p53* gene is the gene most commonly associated with a broad spectrum of cancers. This gene is responsible for coordinating the cellular response to DNA damage, be it a transient growth arrest to allow the cell to repair the DNA damage, or to instruct the cell to commit suicide via apoptosis if the damage was too great. p53 protein is a transcription factor that switches on expression of genes that regulate the cell cycle and cause growth arrest and apoptosis. Accordingly, it has been called the guardian of the genome because of its role in indirectly maintaining the coding integrity of the genetic blueprint. Approximately half of all cancers carry an abnormal (mutated) *p53* gene, and have lost the other normal copy. Every normal cell has two copies of every gene (except some genes of the Y chromosome in males). The mutation of one *p53* gene, leaves the other one potentially active and able to regulate cell growth and apoptosis. However, the mutant *p53* gene makes a protein that inactivates the normal *p53* by binding to the normal protein and inactivating the normal p53 protein. Since the protective role of normal p53 protein is now overcome the genetic material is unstable and the remaining normal *p53* gene is deleted from its position on chromosome 17. The mutation of one gene followed by the loss of the remaining normal gene is a common feature of tumour suppressor genes. The mutant *p53* gene by indirectly promoting cancer behaves as an oncogene, so the *p53* gene, can behave as both a tumour suppressor or an oncogene depending on whether or not it is mutated.

BRCA1 and *BRCA2* are also tumour suppressor genes and like the *p53* gene make a protein that has a role in switching on gene expression, and is involved with DNA repair and regulation of the cell cycle.

All tumour suppressor genes, play a modulating or inhibitory role in cell growth and differentiation. Factors that impair or damage these genes can therefore be carcinogenic.

Cells also contain special genes called *proto-oncogenes*. These proto-oncogenes are responsible for programmed growth in development or repair. They play a major role in co-ordinating our growth from a single fertilized egg cell into an adult with 10^{13} cells. When development or tissue repair is complete, the cell growth is switched off. Cancer-causing agents or *spontaneous genetic mutation* change the proto-oncogenes into potentially cancer-causing oncogenes, as they promote growth where and when they should not. Spontaneous genetic mutation increases as we get older as our DNA repair processes become less efficient. When an oncogene is active in a cell, the cell doesn't require growth signals to grow so that the "switched-on" mechanism of growth and repair continues instead of being "switched off" as it should be, and the cells that are produced do not later undergo apoptosis (self destruction) when they are not wanted. Unlike tumour suppressors only one genetic change is associated with these genes becoming oncogenes, as a mutation leads to the activation of the gene function in the absence of the appropriate cell growth signal. Proto-oncogenes or oncogenes are genes that encode proteins involved in all aspects of the cell signalling pathway that promote the social behaviour of cells and their growth.

Cancer causing oncogenes or defective tumour suppressors may be inherited; or result from cancer-causing agents changing proto-oncogenes into oncogenes; or result from accidental genetic mutation caused by errors in copying the genetic material in dividing cells or by genetic damaging agents within the cell (e.g. oxygen free radicals) or by external agents such as UV irradiation of sunlight. Occasionally, these errors allow cells to divide without correctly partitioning the genetic complement of cells equally between the daughter cells, such that cells now have multiple copies of the genetic material contributed by both parents, and become polyploid (have more DNA content per cell). This is a typical feature of cancer cells at times of rapid cell growth in some tissues or after the many years of cell division during the course of a normal life.

In colon cancer, molecular oncologists have identified the sequential genetic changes in specific oncogenes and tumour suppressors that lead a normal cell into becoming a cancer cell.

From breast cancer studies it has been shown that about 10% of breast cancers result from breast tissue changes due to one of several specific genes that have been inherited from a parent. Most of the remaining 90% are probably the result of an accidental genetic mutation after constant and repeated changes in breast tissue over many years during cyclical hormonal stimulation.

2.4.2 Tumour Suppressor Genes

As opposed to proto-oncogenes or cancer-oncogenes these inherited genes, tumour suppressor genes, play a modulating or inhibitory role in cell growth and differentiation. Factors that impair or damage these genes can therefore be carcinogenic.

2.4.3 Cell Cycle Regulatory Genes

In laboratory culture cancer cells can grow and divide every 24 h, however, in patients regulatory processes restrict cell doubling times to between 5 and 700 days depending on the cell type and tumour stage. The control of cell growth and division has been well studied. The cell growth cycle consists of five stages. Stage 1 starts at the end of mitosis (M) and ends at the point the genetic material is copied, and is called the G_1 phase (G = gap). This copying of the genetic material defines the next phase, known as the S phase (S = synthesis). The next stage starts at the end of DNA synthesis and ends with the cell starting mitotic division into daughter cells. The gap between the S phase and mitosis (M) is

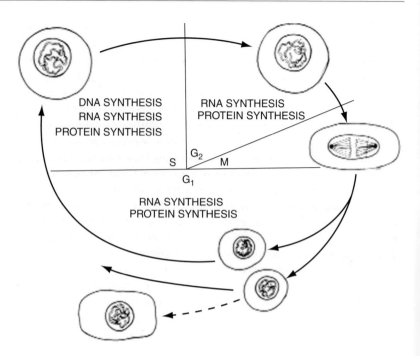

Fig. 2.1. Diagram illustrating the cycle of cell division and the sites of controlling genetic and molecular biological activity. Normal cells and cancer cells divide in a similar way but normal cells stop dividing when sufficient new cells have been made. Cancer cells keep dividing uncontrollably. The new abnormal and unwanted cells become invasive and dangerous, damaging other cells and tissues. Because they are constantly dividing, they are therefore more constantly exposed to anti-cancer drugs that predominantly affect dividing cells when they are in one or more of the stages of cell division (see Sect. 8.3.4 in Chap. 8)

known as G_2. Cells not in cycle or undergoing differentiation, are said to be in G_0, as they are no longer in cycle.

The cycle cannot proceed without a series of successive events occurring. If an event fails, then the cell arrests at defined checkpoints to allow adjustments to be made. The most notable checkpoints occur at the G_{1-S} and G_{2-M} transition points. The G_{1-S} checkpoint allows the cell to repair any DNA damage before it is copied in the S-phase, to prevent mutations becoming fixed in the genetic material. The second, G_{2-M} checkpoint allows the cell to ensure that the chromosomes are arranged correctly prior to segregation to the daughter cells (Fig. 2.1).

2.5   Molecular Biological Changes in Controlling Cell Division

The cell cycle control system is based on two partners, cyclins and cyclin-dependent kinases. Cyclins, are regulatory proteins expressed at specific stages of the cell cycle, that interact with specific cyclin-dependent kinases.

The partnerships between the cyclins and the kinases they specifically activate, ensure that environmental factors and the cell's readiness to divide directly influence progress through the cell cycle. The basis of the G_{1-S} checkpoint is well understood. Cells can enter S phase only if a certain protein (called the retinoblastoma protein after the eye cancer it is associated with) is phosphorylated by a specific cyclin activated kinase. The multiply phosphorylated RB protein then releases specific transcription factors, previously bound in an inactive form to itself, to allow them to switch-on genes involved in DNA synthesis.

In times of genetic damage, p53 tumour suppressor protein blocks the G_{1-S} transition by switching on expression of a protein, p21, that inhibits this kinase to block DNA synthesis, and stop the cells entering the S phase.

Since cancer cells exhibit unregulated growth it is not surprising that they have been shown to have genetic changes in cyclins, cyclin-dependent kinases, p53 and RB protein, to allow the cancer cells to proliferate. The nature of the genetic changes varies from cancer to cancer, which is why it has been difficult to identify the mechanisms of how cells become cancer cells.

More recently discovered are genes that inhibit or stimulate cell reproduction according to need. Impairment of these genes and their active roles in cell reproduction management can also lead to cancer.

2.5.1 Inherited Cancer Genes: Inherited and Familial Cancers

From an immediate practical and clinical point of view in some relatively uncommon cancers there is a strong hereditary factor while in other cancers, there is a less obvious hereditary factor, but for most there is no evidence of an hereditary factor at all. Among the most obvious cancers with a strong hereditary factor as a condition called *familial polyposis coli* in which, by transmission of a responsible oncogene, half the children of an affected parent are likely to develop the condition of multiple polyps in the large bowel. All those affected who do develop these particular polyps will eventually develop cancer in the bowel, usually by the age of 40.

With a rare but inherited familial condition called *Xeroderma pigmentosa* there is a high incidence of development of skin cancer.

Another rare but most often inherited condition is called the *Li-Fraumeni* syndrome. This syndrome is caused by germ-line mutations in the *p53* gene. This condition has provided a model to understand further the pathogenesis of genetic cancers. Patients with this syndrome are defective in one *allele* of the *p53* ("the guardian of the genome") or were born with one non-functional allele of it. Therefore if the other *p53* allele is affected during their life, cancer will develop.

Among the more common cancers with an increased familial incidence are cancers of the breast, stomach and bowel. Although the increased risk for relatives of sufferers is not great in most families, occasionally it may be considerable. For example there have been rare reports of families in which about half the female blood relatives have developed breast cancer. What is responsible for this apparent increased risk in a few families was largely unknown until recent discoveries of inherited genes called *BRCA1 and BRCA2* (the names are derived from BR of Breast and CA of cancer). The *BRCA1* gene is on chromosome 17 and the *BRCA2* gene is on chromosome 13. These genes behave as oncogenes on breast cells (see hereditary and genetic factors). Families with a high incidence of breast cancer may carry one or both of these genes, alternatively it may be simply that members of these families have similar lifestyle habits and have been affected by similar environmental factors.

Cancers of the stomach, colon or rectum have a significantly increased risk of developing in relatives of sufferers from these conditions, but this risk is very high only in patients with an obvious genetic predisposing cause such as familial polyposis coli. In most cases it is likely that members of these families had similar diets and other environmental factors.

Another indication of the genetic influence in association with stomach cancer is the fact there have been reports of a slightly higher risk of people with blood Group A developing cancer of the stomach than there is of people of other blood groups. Such information is well documented but the risk is so small that it is of little practical value to anyone other than statisticians and scientists studying cancer. The fact is that thousands of people of different blood groups had to be studied before any difference in cancer incidence could be substantiated and some studies have indeed not detected any difference. For the individual with blood group A the risk of being any more likely to develop stomach cancer is almost negligible.

2.6   Age

In general, the risk of developing most cancers increases with age but there are exceptions. For example it is a feature of familial cancers that they usually present at an earlier age and are more likely to be bilateral or multiple than cancers without a familial association. Also, although cancer in young people is uncommon, no age group is entirely free from risk.

2.6.1   Infants

Cancers that occur in younger age groups are often in those tissues that tend to divide and grow more in early life.

An uncommon cancer of the kidney, known as a *Wilm's tumour (or nephroblastoma)* occurs almost exclusively in infants less than 5 years of age, and may, in fact, even be present at birth. Other malignant tumours, which although uncommon, are more likely to occur in infants and young children, are *retinoblastomas* (eye), *neuroblastomas* (nerve tissue), *rhabdomyosarcomas* (voluntary muscle) and *medulloblastomas* (brain).

2.6.2   Children, Adolescents and Young Adults

The acute leukaemias, especially acute lymphoblastic leukaemia, are more likely to occur in children and adolescents than adults. Teenagers and young adults have the highest incidence of osteosarcomas as well as the highest incidence of the lymphoma known as Hodgkin lymphoma or Hodgkin disease. Burkitt's lymphoma is a tumour that predominantly affects the jaw of children most commonly in tropical Africa and New Guinea.

2.6.3   Increasing Age

Malignant tumours of the testis are not common but when they do occur it is most often in men younger than 40 years with a peak incidence at about 25 years for germ-cell testicular cancers of the *teratoma* (or non-seminoma) type. For *seminoma* type germ-cell cancers of the testis the peak incidence is at about 35 years of age. Ovarian cancer and cancer of the cervix most commonly affect women between the ages of 40 and 60 years, but cancer in the endometrial lining of the uterus, is more likely to occur in women over 60 years.

Lung cancer has become increasingly common in communities where cigarette smoking is prevalent. It most frequently occurs between the ages of 40 and 60, because it takes some years for the damaging effects of tobacco carcinogens to cause changes in the air passages that lead to cancer.

Breast cancer may affect women of any age but it is uncommon in women under the age of 30. Thereafter it increases in incidence with increasing age, having a mean of about 60 years.

The incidence of stomach and colo-rectal cancers increases with age, reaching a peak between 60 and 75 years.

Cancer of the prostate gland is essentially a disease of increasing age. It is not often seen before the age of 50 but other than skin cancer it is the most common cancer affecting men over the age of 65 and almost all men who reach the age of 90 years will have at least some low-grade prostate cancer cells.

Skin cancers and head and neck (mouth and throat) cancers become more common with increasing age. Although the sun damage to skin may have occurred many years previously and, in the case of mouth and throat cancers, the most common association is with smoking that began many years before. Melanoma is rare before puberty but after puberty it affects all age groups. It then becomes a little more common with increasing age. Unlike other skin cancers that most often occur in the skin of the face (because that skin is most constantly exposed to the sun), melanoma is not so directly related to prolonged sunlight exposure. Melanoma occurs most commonly on the trunk, thighs and lower limbs; sites not constantly exposed to the sun but areas more likely to be acutely damaged by intermittent episodes of sunburn, especially sunburn in childhood.

The strongest association with age is that for most cancers the risk of developing a cancer is greater in the older age groups. More than 70% of cancers are first detected in people over 65 years. This is probably because of the potential for more genetic mutation mistakes to be made with increasing age and because these may be made more frequently after years of exposure to toxins like tobacco.

Cancers that occur in younger age groups are often in those tissues that tend to divide and grow more in early life including brain, nerve and blood-forming cells and growing bone. In young adults during the most active reproductive age groups, the testis and ovary are at increased risk.

2.7   Predisposing and Pre-Malignant Risk Factors

Abnormal tissues in general have an increased risk of malignant change.

2.7.1   Skin

The UV-A and B wavelengths are the major carcinogenic factors of sunlight. Repeated sun damage to skin is often followed by thickening and crustiness of the surface layers of the skin called "*hyperkeratosis*". This can be a pre-malignant condition and usually precedes the development of skin cancer. Hyperkeratosis of the lips also predisposes to cancer on the lips, most commonly the lower lip (see Figs. 14.1 and 14.2).

Melanoma commonly develops in a pre-existing pigmented naevus, or mole, although sometimes a melanoma develops in skin where there has not been a mole. Fair-skinned and redheaded people have a greater risk of skin cancers including melanoma because of lack of protective pigment in their skin.

2.7.2   Oesophagus

Cancer of the oesophagus is more common in developing countries where food contamination is common. However the incidence of cancer of the lower oesophagus is now increasing in Western countries. This is often associated with a "*Barret's ulcer*", an ulcer in the lower oesophagus likely to be associated with persistent gastric reflux.

2.7.3   Stomach

People who have pernicious anaemia or chronic atrophic gastritis are six times more likely to develop stomach cancer than other people. People with gastric-ulcer disease do have an increased risk of stomach cancer although this was long disputed by some gastroenterologists who believed that gastric lesions were either benign or malignant from their onset. Most agree, however, that the *Helicobacter pylori* bacterium does sometimes cause gastric cancer as well as gastric ulcers and that effective eradication of this bacillus with antibiotics may well reduce the incidence of gastric cancer. The more common duodenal ulcer does not show an increased tendency to develop into cancer.

2.7.4   Bowel

Polyps in the large bowel (colon or rectum) predispose to an increased incidence of bowel cancer. A chronically inflamed bowel, such as in *ulcerative colitis*, has an increased risk of developing cancer. The younger the patient at the onset of the disease, the longer the disease has been present, and the greater the extent of the disease in the colon, the greater will be the risk of cancer developing. In general about 10% of people with ulcerative colitis will develop a colon cancer after about 10 years. The risk of cancer developing in *Crohn's disease*, another chronic inflammatory condition of bowel, sometimes called granular colitis, is also increased but not to the same degree.

2.7.5   Mouth and Throat

Chronic irritation of the lining of the mouth and throat, as especially seen in smokers and sometimes in diabetics, may lead to a thickening of the surface cell layer that shows as white patches called *leukoplakia*. These white patches also have a predisposition towards the development of cancer (see Figs. 14.4a).

2.7.6   Stones: Gallstones, Kidney and Bladder Stones

Cancer of the gall bladder is not common particularly in Western countries, but when it does occur it is almost always in a gall bladder containing stones, with chronic irritation and inflammation in the wall of the gall bladder. Irritating stones may also cause cancer of the pelvis of the kidney and cancer in the bladder.

2.7.7   Chronic Inflammation

Any chronically inflamed, chronically irritated or injured, or chronically degenerate (atrophic) tissue has a somewhat increased risk of developing cancer after some years. Examples include chronically discharging wounds, burn scars, and varicose ulcers of the lower legs, which occasionally develop malignant change, as well as the chronically irritated lining of the mouth, throat, and air passages of smokers in which malignant change is relatively common.

2

2.7.8   Acute Injury

Whether malignancy follows acute trauma is not clear. There are a number of incidences where tumours, especially sarcomas, have been found in tissues after some
well-documented injury such as a kick in the thigh or calf, or a blow to a bone at
football. Whether the tumour followed the injury or whether the injury simply drew
attention to a tumour that was already present is often impossible to determine.
Certainly, it must be very rare indeed for a malignant tumour to follow such an injury,
as these types of injury are very common and sarcomas of this type are rare.

2.7.9   Pre-Existing Lumps and Benign Tumours

In the case of benign tumours, there is sometimes a risk that a benign tumour
may become malignant. With some types of benign tumours, such as warts, the
risk is negligible. With the common fatty tumour, lipoma, the risk is so small
that removal of the lipoma is usually not justified. However, with others there is a
somewhat greater (but still small) risk of malignant change and surgical removal
is usually recommended. Such lesions include papilloma in the mouth or papilloma in a duct of a breast, or some soft tissue tumours, or adenomas of glands, or
some benign tumours of bone or cartilage. With still other benign tumours, such
as polyps of stomach or colon, papillomas in the bladder or especially papilloma
of the rectum, the risk of malignant change is of real significance and surgical
removal of these tumours is virtually always indicated.

2.7.10   Congenitally Abnormal Tissues

Congenitally abnormal tissues all have a greater risk of developing cancer than
do normally developed tissues. These include, a *thyroglossal cyst* (a congenital remnant of thyroid tissue high in the neck or in the back of the tongue), a
branchial cyst (a cyst resulting from a congenital developmental abnormality
in the neck) and an undescended testis (a testis that has not descended into the
scrotum at birth). The increased risks of these tissues developing a cancer are
of varying degrees. The risk is very small in the case of branchial cysts but in
the case of an *undescended testis* the risk is relatively high.

2.7.11   Gender

The incidence of
lung cancer in
women is now
approaching
that in men.

Obviously, cancers that occur in organs unique to one gender occur only in that
gender For example, cancers of the uterus, vagina or ovary are unique to females,
and cancers of the prostate or testes are unique to males, however breast cancer,
often assumed to be associated with female breasts only, does sometimes occur
in males. About 1% of breast cancers are in men.

The incidence of lung cancer has increased some ten times over the past 60 or 70 years. This increase, initially in men, has been due to increased use of tobacco products. Thirty years ago, lung cancer was ten times more common in men than in women. However, following the trend in recent years for increased use of cigarettes by women, the incidence of lung cancer in women is now approaching that in men. In most Western countries, after skin cancer, breast cancer is the most common cancer in women. However recent statistics show that in some countries, including the US, the incidence of lung cancer in women is approaching that of breast cancer and may become more common within a few years.

Skin cancers are more prevalent in men than in women because of the increased exposure to the sun of men working and playing out of doors, often without a hat or a shirt (see Figs. 10.2–10.7]. On the other hand, many cancers have a significantly different incidence in the sexes for no apparent reason. For example in most Western countries, but not all, cancer of the stomach is three times more likely to occur in men than in women and cancers of the colon and rectum are more common in males. Cancer of the oesophagus is more common in men, especially cancer of the middle and lower oesophagus; however, cancer of the upper oesophagus is more likely to occur in women. Primary liver cancer is four times more common in men than women. For some unknown reason, the incidence of cancer of the pancreas has increased in the US and in other Western countries, especially in men and mostly in men who smoke cigarettes. It is now also being seen more frequently in women, especially in women who are smokers.

2.8   Diet and Cancer: Special Dietary Preventive Ingredients

There is an association between diet and some cancers A high fibre diet is protective against bowel cancer. Whether this is a mechanical effect of the bulk of high fibre alone or some other factor is uncertain. The widely accepted theory is that diets high in meat, animal fats and highly refined foods as in Westernised, industrialised countries, can produce cancer-inducing substances (carcinogens). The absence of fibre from the diet results in a relative constipation that is thought to allow these carcinogens to stay in contact with the bowel wall for prolonged periods.

A high fibre diet is protective against bowel cancer.

In developing countries, the diet generally contains a great deal more roughage and fibre with less meat, animal fat and refined foods. The already low carcinogen content of the stool is further diluted by the bulky quantity of stool and rapidly passed by the frequent bowel motions, resulting in a low incidence of large-bowel cancer.

More recent studies have shown that the effect of fibre may be more than just increasing bulk and rapid passage of bowel contents. Fibre is basically composed of a complex carbohydrate *glucan* that can stimulate macrophages in healing wounds and may stimulate immune protective *macrophages* in the bowel wall. Glucan is found in high-fibre foods such as grains, fruit and vegetables but is not present in meat, dairy products or fatty foods (Fig. 2.2).

Fig. 2.2. Asian diets
are protective against
certain cancers

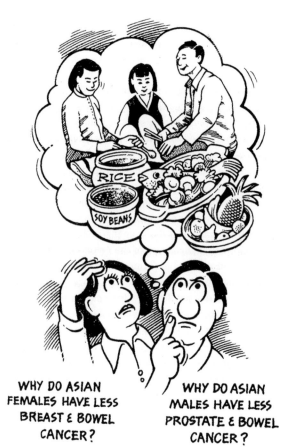

WHY DO ASIAN
FEMALES HAVE LESS
BREAST & BOWEL
CANCER?

WHY DO ASIAN
MALES HAVE LESS
PROSTATE & BOWEL
CANCER?

In addition to lower rates of bowel cancer associated with high fibre diets, Asians and others who eat predominantly plant products, also have a lower incidence of a number of other health problems that are common in Western societies. Particularly if these diets are high in legumes like peas, beans and soy, they contain abundant quantities of naturally occurring plant hormones called *phytoestrogens*. Communities having such diets have not only less bowel cancer but also a lower incidence of both breast cancer and prostate cancer. They also have a low incidence of a number of other health problems in women including osteoporosis, pre-menstrual tension and postmenopausal syndrome.

Although the evidence of a direct association between diet and cancer is strong for cancer of the large bowel, for other cancers statistical proof that diet is a major factor is highly suggestive but has not yet been confirmed. There are so many variable factors between people of different population groups that it is always difficult to prove which particular factor or factors were responsible for any difference in the incidence of cancer. For example, as well as differences in

diet there may be genetic differences, racial differences, environmental differences, or differences in social habits or customs such as smoking, differences
in the incidence of parasites or infections or even in occupational stress or
psychological factors.

However the different incidences of cancer of some tissues, such as breast
and prostate, between Asians and Caucasians appear to be related to diet.
Traditionally Asians have a diet with a high content of legumes, especially peas
and soybeans. Legumes have a high content of phytoestrogens. Several studies
suggest that this may a significant factor in the relatively low incidence of breast
diseases (including cancer) in Asian females and the relatively low incidence of
prostate cancer in Asian males. This belief is supported by evidence that before
Europeans, with increasing affluence, changed from diets high in plant foods,
including legumes, to present diets high in animal products, the incidence of
breast and prostate cancer was lower than at present and that Asians who change
their diets after migrating to the US acquire an incidence of breast and prostate
cancer, approaching that of other US citizens.

Dietary phytoestrogens may also play a protective role against colon cancer
and pancreas cancer but evidence for this is less clear.

Studies especially from France, Italy and Greece have shown that anti-oxidant
properties of red wine (in moderation) and mono-unsaturated fat properties of
olive oil may also have cancer protective properties, especially in relation to breast
cancer. More recently there has been considerable interest in a substance called
lycopene found in tomatoes and some other red fruits. Lycopene is one of the
beta-carotene *anti-oxidants* and is responsible for the red colour of tomatoes. Laboratory studies suggest it may have protective properties against a number of cancers
including cancers of the prostate, breast, lung, stomach, pancreas and bowel.

2.9   Stomach Cancer

Early in the twentieth century, cancer of the stomach was much more common
than it is today. The reason for the decreasing incidence is not completely understood but it has been suggested that it may be associated with the increased use
of refrigeration and less use of artificial chemical preservatives such as pickling
and salt curing of meats and vegetables.

Stomach cancer is seven times more common in Japan and Korea than in the
US, Canada, Britain, Australia or New Zealand. This may be genetic or due to
the high consumption of smoked fish or chemical preservatives or other food
additives or both in Japan and Korea.

An interesting comparison is the high incidence of stomach cancer in northern
Iceland where crude *smoked* salmon is part of the staple diet, compared to a lower
incidence in southern Iceland where the residents prepare their fish differently.

In other studies, a higher incidence of stomach cancer has been found in people who have a highly refined starch diet and high animal fat diet as opposed to

Early in the
twentieth century,
cancer of the
stomach was much
more common
than it is today.

2

a lower incidence in people who eat a diet with a high content of nuts, grains, fruit and vegetables.

2.10   Bowel Cancer: Cancers of the Colon and Rectum

In contrast to stomach cancer, for reasons already stated, large bowel cancer is more common in Europe, the US, Britain, Canada, Australia and New Zealand than in Asian and African countries. It has been called one of the "Western cancers" and is associated with a Western type diet. In Australia and New Zealand, after skin cancer, cancers of the colon and rectum are now the most common cancers in both sexes. As discussed above people who eat little animal fat or refined foods and have a high intake of plant food, crude fibre and roughage with increased phytoestrogens, have a lower incidence.

2.11   Other Cancers

Several reports have suggested a relationship between high consumption of animal fat with increased risk of several cancers not only bowel, breast and prostate cancers but, possibly also pancreas cancers.

2.12   Vegetarian Diets

Members of the Seventh Day Adventist Church have a lower than average incidence of most cancers, including cancers of the oesophagus, stomach, pancreas, prostate, colon and rectum. However, as well as being vegetarians with a high-fibre and low meat and animal fat consumption, these people are usually non-smokers and non-consumers of alcohol which may well be more significant. One study in male members of the Seventh Day Adventist Church found that those church members whose diet included eggs, cheese and milk had a greater incidence of prostate cancer than did those who refrained from all animal products.

2.13   Special Dietary Ingredients: Phytoestrogens and Lycopene

All plant foods contain phytoestrogens. Studies now suggest that these, especially the isoflavone phytoestrogens of legumes, have protective properties against breast and prostate cancers, as well as colon and possibly pancreas cancer.

In tissue culture and animal models, prostate and breast cancer cells appear to be especially inhibited by lycopene, the anti-oxidant red-colouring matter of tomatoes and some other plant products. Laboratory studies also suggest that increased and synergistic cancer-cell inhibitory properties are achieved if lycopene is used in conjunction with beta-carotenes or vitamin D. Whether lycopene and isoflavone phytoestrogens might also have anti-cancer synergistic activity is also under study. Possible clinical or cancer preventive use of these agents used synergistically is awaited with interest.

2.14 Vitamins, Anti Oxidants and Trace Elements

Direct anti-cancer protective qualities of additional vitamins, anti-oxidants, and trace elements, are the subject of many claims, counter-claims and special studies.

Some claims of protection and cure with vitamins are undoubtedly exaggerated, but there is some evidence that the anti-oxidant vitamins A and C and possibly E as well as selenium may offer some protection. More clearly however there is general agreement that a deficiency of any of these dietary ingredients will make people more susceptible to health problems including a greater risk of cancer.

There is a direct relationship between the level of economic development in a country, its diet and the incidence of cancers, especially large bowel cancer. In developed Western countries with more dairy products, meat and animal-fat, and less fibre, large bowel cancer is common in men and women whilst in many developing countries with more predominantly vegetarian diets, large-bowel cancer is rarely seen.

However the association of diet with cancers in parts of the digestive system other than stomach and large bowel is less clear because other factors appear to be of major significance, especially alcohol and tobacco. For example cancer of the oesophagus, pancreas and head and neck, as well as the stomach, are all more common in smokers but the risk is greater if they are also heavy drinkers of alcohol. In Western countries primary liver cancer is most often seen in alcoholics with cirrhosis of the liver although in Asian countries it is usually associated with a history of hepatitis infection.

2.15 Race

Some cancers are more prevalent in people of some races than in other races. Whether the significant factor is genetic or racial or whether it is more likely due to environmental factors, diet, social habits like smoking, or other influences such as the general health and age of the people, is often uncertain.

There are many examples of increased incidence of certain cancers in some races and some parts of the world. These include a high incidence of stomach cancer in Japan, Korea, and to a lesser extent in Scandinavia, Holland and Czechoslovakia, and the high incidence of cancer of the post-nasal space in

Chinese. There is also a high incidence of cancer of the oesophagus in certain African tribes including the Bantu in South Africa but not in the white population. There is a high incidence of primary liver cancer in Malaysians, East Asians and Africans. Europeans and people of European decent have a high incidence of breast, prostate and large bowel cancer so much so that these are sometimes known as "The Western Cancers".

The high incidence of melanoma and other skin cancers in northern Europeans and especially people of northern European descent, who live in tropical and sub-tropical climates, is due to genetic factors associated with fair skin that does not tan readily plus the environmental factor of sunshine.

In Israel, a country with one of the highest incidences of thyroid cancer, the disease is more common amongst Jews born in Europe than in those born in Asia. In South Africa, Bantus have a distinctly higher incidence of thyroid cancer than do blacks from other regions.

Whilst there are genetic influences that predispose people of different races to develop different cancers, it is hard to know with any particular cancer whether the most significant factors are genetic or environmental.

2.16   Geographic Associations

The incidence of a particular type of cancer varies from country to country and even varies within countries according to geographic conditions but it is often difficult to know whether geography is the predominant cause of this difference.

The association of skin cancer and melanoma with fair-skinned people living in a sunny climate is obvious. The incidence is highest in fair-skinned people living in sunny climates in Australia and in the sunny southern parts of the United States. In Australia, not only is there the world's highest incidence of skin cancer and melanoma but the incidence varies from state to state. It increases proportionately with the proximity of the state to the equator. For the more common forms of skin cancer (squamous and basal cell carcinoma) the incidence is directly related to areas of skin most often exposed to the sun. These skin cancers thus occur most frequently on the face, neck and on the backs of the hands and arms. On the other hand, as noted above, the distribution of melanoma is not closely related to the areas of skin most constantly exposed they are most common on the trunk in men and on the thighs and lower limbs in women. For melanoma the association is not especially the amount of direct exposure of skin to sunlight but the intensity of episodes of acute sunburn, especially if episodes of sunburn occurred in childhood.

Primary cancer of the liver (hepatoma or hepato-carcinoma) is common in South-East Asia and East African countries but whether there is a racial predisposition or a dietary or some other environmental factor is not known. However it is clear that longstanding infection with hepatitis B or C are significant. It is uncertain whether the high incidence of stomach cancer in Japan and Korea is mainly genetic or dietary.

2.17 Environment

2.17.1 Sunshine

See Sect. 2.7.1.

2.17.2 Air Pollution

In Western societies, city dwellers living in a more highly polluted atmosphere have a slightly higher incidence of lung cancer than their country cousins. This factor, however, is not nearly as significant as the smoking habits of the people concerned. Atmospheric pollution with asbestos in some workplaces in mining and building industries was, in the past, responsible not only for increased lung cancer but also for development of an aggressive cancer of pleura or peritoneum called *mesothelioma*. This is further discussed below under Sect. 2.18.

Paradoxically, atmospheric pollution may produce a reduction in *skin* cancer rates by reducing the amounts of ultraviolet radiation reaching the surface of the earth.

2.17.3 Ionising Irradiation

The increased incidence of leukaemia and some other cancers (including breast, thyroid and skin cancers) in the survivors of Hiroshima and Nagasaki atom bomb explosions and the Chernobyl atomic energy plant disaster, confirms the environmental effect of ionising irradiation as a cause of some cancers.

2.17.4 Goitre Belts

Cancer of the thyroid is more common in communities where goitre (thyroid gland enlargement) is common. Goitres are most common in places where there is a deficiency of iodine in local food and water supplies. Such areas are known as goitre belts and are usually found in mountainous regions where iodine has been washed out of the soil over millions of years. Goitre belts are found particularly in the Swiss Alps, the Rocky Mountains, the Andes, the Himalayas and the mountainous regions of New Guinea. The Great Lakes district in the United States is also a goitre belt. It is believed that the iodine has been washed out of the soil in the region into the Great Lakes and lost through the rivers into the sea. It is also likely that in some areas, after many years of cultivation of crops, iodine has been leached out of natural soils. Eventually it is transferred into the sea where fish is a good source of iodine in food.

2.18   Occupation

Present-day industrial laws should protect workers against most industrial dangers, including the risks of exposure to carcinogens. A number of cancers were previously linked to working conditions (as discussed), but these have now been largely eliminated.

Industrial laws compelling stringent improvements in working conditions now protect asbestos workers from their otherwise high incidence of lung cancer and *mesothelioma*.

Another less obvious risk is the increased incidence of cancer in the air passages under and around the nose (the para-nasal sinuses) in wood workers, leather workers, metal workers, and especially nickel workers. This is probably due to constantly breathing small particles of these materials. There was also said to have been an increased risk of cancer of the larynx in people who misused their voices, such as old time bookmakers who would shout a great deal in calling the odds, and in clergymen who would spend hours using a high-pitched chant. However, if they truly existed, these risks would be very small in comparison to the risk of cigarette smokers developing the same sort of cancer.

2.19   Habits and Lifestyle

2.19.1   Smoking

Lung cancer in cigarette smokers is increased ten times compared to non-smokers.

Certainly the most striking carcinogen in present day society is tobacco. As well as causing a lot of other health problems the habit of smoking outweighs all other known influences as a cause of serious cancer in present day men and women. Lung cancer in cigarette smokers is increased ten times compared to non-smokers and the risk is directly related to the amount of tobacco smoked and inhaled.

Similarly, cancers in the mouth and throat are closely associated with smoking.

Similarly, cancers in the mouth and throat are closely associated with smoking. It has been estimated that heavy smokers have about six times the risk of developing cancer in the mouth and throat than non-smokers. The risk is increased to 15 times if the smokers are also heavy drinkers.

In the case of lung cancer, the risk appears to be greater in cigarette smokers than in pipe or cigar smokers, whereas with mouth cancers there is no apparent difference whether the smokers use cigarettes, pipes or cigars. Cigarette smokers are more likely inhale smoke into their lungs but there is a similar risk of tobacco products entering the mouth with all forms of smoking.

Apart from tissues in direct contact with tobacco smoke, a number of other cancers also have increased incidence in smokers. These include cancer of the oesophagus, stomach, pancreas, kidney, bladder, cervix and even breast cancer.

2.19.2 Alcohol

Heavy alcohol drinkers have an increased incidence of cancer of the mouth and throat, oesophagus, stomach, liver and pancreas and breast but the risk is greater in those heavy drinkers who are also smokers. Alcohol is sometimes considered to be a co-carcinogen as it does seem to potentiate carcinogenic effects of other products especially tobacco.

Alcohol does seem to potentiate carcinogenic effects of other products especially tobacco.

2.19.3 Sun-Exposure

See Sect. 2.7.1.

2.19.4 Betel Nut

The habit of some Asian and Oriental people of chewing betel nut or tobacco leaf or especially both together, sometimes with lime, is associated with an increased incidence of cancer in the buccal mucosal lining of the cheek.

2.19.5 Pregnancies and Breast Cancer

The incidence of breast cancer is lowest in women who have given birth to babies at an early age and have had multiple pregnancies. In communities where the custom is for women to marry early and have their first babies whilst still in their teens, the incidence of breast cancer is low, whilst in Westernised societies where first babies are commonly born to women over the age of 30 years, the incidence of breast cancer is higher. There may also be some protection against breast cancer by prolonged breast feeding as is common in most developing countries, although the evidence for this is less clear. Women who have never had a child, such as nuns, have the highest incidence of breast cancer.

2.19.6 Cultural and Social Customs

Cultural and social customs may also have a relationship with development of cancer.

Cancer of the penis is extremely rare in Jewish males who are circumcised at birth but is occasionally seen in Muslim males who are not circumcised until about the age of 10 years. Although not a common cancer, the incidence is greatest in uncircumcised males.

Nuns, who practice chastity, have a low incidence of cancer of the cervix of the uterus but an increased incidence of breast cancer. On the other hand, cancer of the cervix is more common in women who commenced intercourse at an early age and who have had multiple male partners. Prostitutes are especially at risk of cervical cancer. The single most significant factor, especially in prostitutes, is the incidence of the sexually transmitted human papilloma virus.

Women who have taken the contraceptive pill for some years appear to have a somewhat reduced incidence of developing both cancer of the ovary and cancer of the uterus. On the other hand, prolonged use of contraceptive pills, and especially the high-dose oestrogen contraceptive pill formerly used, has been associated with a slightly higher risk of developing breast cancer. The low-dose contraceptive pill presently in general use has not been shown to have any significant association with breast cancer, some studies suggest that it may even have some protective value.

Lifestyle in strict vegetarian, teetotal and non-smoking communities and in different geographic, economic and racial communities has been discussed.

2.20   Psychological Factors: The Possible Role of Stress or Emotion in Cancer Development

Among the more unusual theories for causes of cancer has been a suggestion that like emotional and some mental (psychosomatic) illnesses, cancer may be triggered by an unnatural suppression of the "fight or flight" response to anxiety or stress. It has been suggested that if a stressful situation persists over a long period and the person concerned feels that whatever action he or she takes will be wrong, a subconscious decision to escape through death by cancer may result. There is no substantial evidence to support such a theory although some retrospective studies have indicated that a high proportion of cancer patients have experienced some form of severe stress in the period 6 months to 2 years before the onset of their illness.

Most psychologists would not claim that stress is a direct cause of cancer but some consider that it may play a part.

Most psychologists would not claim that stress is a direct cause of cancer but some consider that it may play a part alongside known chemical, genetic, dietary, geographic, viral or radiation causes. People become psychologically disturbed on hearing a diagnosis of cancer and many need additional psychological support by psychiatrists, clinical psychologists, specially trained and experienced nurses, social workers and other trained medical or paramedical health workers.

The belief of many "alternative" health practitioners that stress may stimulate cancer is given as a reason by a variety of such practitioners to support practices in faith healing, meditation or other alternative treatments.

2.21 Cancer Registries

The value of having accurate cancer records in registries kept on a national or state basis must be stressed. Most countries try to keep registries of cancer incidence categorised by age, gender, race, income, geography, environment, culture and/or other relevant group, (see Appendix). They do so with different levels of detail and different levels of success and accuracy. However it is through these registries that information is gathered that can often lead to valuable indications of causes of specific cancers, knowledge of people at high risk and introduction of appropriate public health measures to either prevent such cancers or facilitate their early diagnosis and treatment. One example is knowledge of the relatively high incidence of breast cancer in women in Western countries that has lead to knowledge of lifestyle associations of this cancer and establishment of an awareness among women, especially of the value of mammography screening clinics and specialised breast-cancer detection and treatment centres. This has resulted not only in better treatment outcomes but also a greater interest in supporting research in breast cancer causes, preventive measures and treatment.

The value of having accurate cancer records in registries kept on a national or state basis must be stressed.

EXERCISE

List the factors that are known to contribute to an increased cancer risk.

Summary of Practical Measures to Prevent Cancer

3

Is this chapter you will learn about:

> *Smoking*
> *Viral and bacterial protection*
> *Genetic protection*
> *Skin cancers*
> *Diets – cancers of stomach, bowel, breast, prostate and thyroid cancer*
> *Breast cancer – other potential preventive measures*
> *Industrial cancers*
> *Ionising irradiation*
> *Early detection and treatment of pre-malignant or potentially pre-malignant conditions*

Prevention is so much better than cure. There are many cancer preventive measures that should become lifestyle habits but one of the most important is for people to seek medical advice if they have any suspicion of anything going wrong (Fig. 3.1).

3.1 Smoking

The most obvious preventive measure in reducing the risk of serious cancer is to avoid smoking. By not smoking, the risk of developing many cancers is greatly reduced. Even spending frequent long periods in a smoky atmosphere (passive smoking) is associated with increased cancer risk and should therefore be avoided.

The most obvious preventive measure in reducing the risk of serious cancer is to avoid smoking.

3.2 Viral and Bacterial Protection

Condoms have been the most practical way of providing an immediate practical protection against the human papilloma virus (HPP). However Professor Ian Frazer working in Brisbane, Australia, has shown in recent trials that a vaccine

F. O. Stephens and K. R. Aigner, *Basics of Oncology,*
DOI: 10.1007/978-3-540-92925-3_3, © Springer-Verlag Berlin Heidelberg 2009

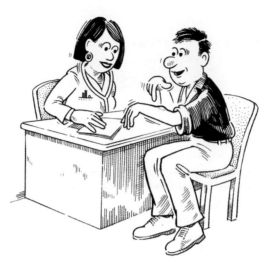

Fig. 3.1. People should be encouraged to seek early advice about any suspicious lesion

against the human papilloma virus has given a 100% effectiveness in immunity to the virus that is responsible for most cancers of the cervix and some skin cancers. Hence in the future people at risk, especially girls and young women who are sexually active or approaching sexual maturity, will be advised to have immunization against the human papilloma virus.

Vaccination against Hepatitis B is also a cancer-protective measure. Widespread vaccination programs are currently being conducted in several countries.

3.3   Genetic Protection

Expert advice is now realistically worthwhile for avoiding or reducing the risk of inheriting or passing on a genetic risk (Chap. 2).

3.4   Skin Cancers

The risk of the common skin cancers – basal cell carcinoma (BCC) and squamous cell carcinoma (SCC) – can be greatly reduced by avoiding unnecessary direct exposure to sunshine or other forms of ultra-violet light such as in solariums. Nature's protection is pigment in the skin in coloured races. For fair-skinned people, the use of wide-brimmed hats, long-sleeved shirts and other appropriate clothing plus ultra-violet filtering skin lotions or creams offers considerable protection. The same measures may help to avoid melanoma to some extent but, intermittent and severe episodes of sunburn should especially be avoided by young people. Sunburn causes permanent damage to the immune defence cells in skin called *Langerhan's cells.*

3.5   Diets: Stomach and Bowel Cancer, Breast Cancer

3.5.1   Prostate Cancer

As previously discussed important factors of diet are the proportions of natural fibre and animal fat and the presence of chemical preservatives or other chemicals in food. Diets that are high in fibre (including cereals, nuts, grains, fresh fruit and vegetables) and low in meat, animal fat, highly refined foods and chemically preserved foods, offer some protection against development of stomach, bowel and possibly pancreatic cancers as well as breast and prostate cancers. Apparently protective factors may include the dietary amounts of phytoestrogens, lycopenes, anti-oxidants, certain vitamins and trace elements. These and some other ingredients are under study but as yet no firm conclusions can be made.

The amount of fat in the diet, especially saturated animal fat, ideally should be lower than in most present Western diets. Omega-3 oils present in oily fish (e.g. salmon, sardines, mackerel, tuna) and soya beans and kidney beans, may have some protective effect against the development of cancer and also against the latter stages of some cancers where there is dramatic loss of weight.

3.5.2   Thyroid Cancer

The addition of iodine to the diet (usually as iodised salt) in iodine-deficient "goitre belt" areas reduces the incidence of goitre and to some degree the risk of thyroid cancer.

3.5.3   Dioxins

Plastic containers of foods and fluids, especially fatty foods, have been under study as having possible carcinogenic potential. There have been recent recommendations to avoid heating fatty foods in plastic containers in microwave ovens. It has been recommended that plastic containers are better avoided for long-term storage of fatty foods; glass or ceramic containers are recommended.

3.5.4   Breast Cancer

Encouragement of breast-feeding may be of some help in reducing the incidence of breast cancer, so too is regular exercise, avoiding obesity, not smoking and attention to diet. Especially breast-screening is widely encouraged as an anti-breast-cancer measure. Whilst regular self-examination is encouraged and may reveal an otherwise unnoticed breast lump women should be advised that it must not be regarded as an alternative to regular mammography in screening for early cancer; that is women and doctors too, should not assume that cancer cannot be present because they have not felt a breast lump (Fig. 3.2).

HRT can slightly increase the risk of subsequent development of breast cancer.

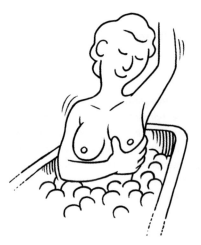

Fig. 3.2. Palpation of breasts in the bath or shower with wet soapy fingers is a good method of self-examination

BREAST SELF EXAMINATION

In the past it was common practice to help relieve post-menopausal symptoms with small doses of hormone replacement therapy (HRT). It is now known that if used over 5 years or more HRT can slightly increase the risk of subsequent development of breast cancer so that if such treatment is now prescribed at all, it is only to treat postmenopausal women with symptoms that cannot be relieved in some other way. Even then it is given for a limited period of time only.

3.6   Industrial Cancers

Industrial laws that protect workers from a number of known industrial carcino-genic agents, such as asbestos and certain chemicals especially in the petroleum and pest control industries, play a significant role in cancer prevention.

3.7   Ionising Irradiation

The lessons of irradiation from atomic bomb explosions and the Chernobyl atomic plant disaster in causing cancers have been well documented, as has the need to avoid excessive irradiation from X-ray plants or nuclear energy plants. There has also been much discussion and study about risks of living near high voltage wires, microwave irradiation and of mobile telephones (cell phones) but as yet the studies are inconclusive.

3.8   Treatment of Pre-Malignant and Potentially Malignant Lesions

3.8.1   Pre-Malignant Conditions

Treatment of any long-standing ulcers or chronically inflamed or irritated lesions may prevent development of cancer. This may involve such different lesions as long-standing varicose ulcers and ulcers in the mouth from a jagged tooth. Good care should also be given for gastric ulcers, persistent gastric reflux, ulcerative colitis of the colon or rectum, long-standing gallstones, kidney or bladder stones or chronically discharging sinuses such as from osteomyelitis. Certain skin lesions may also need attention including a pigmented skin lesion that is chronically irritated by virtue of its position under a belt or bra strap or a pigmented lesion under a fingernail or on the sole of the foot.

All people affected by familial polyposis coli will eventually develop colon cancer.

Another preventive measure is to remove or otherwise properly treat known pre-malignant conditions such as polyps, papillomas, hyperkeratotic skin lesions, leukoplakia in the mouth or moles that show any sign of irritation or change, especially in irregular dysplastic lesions.

Benign tumours that show any evidence of enlarging or that are known to have a risk of malignant change, should be removed to reduce the risk of cancer developing. Such tumours might include dysplastic naevi on the skin, adenomas in the parotid or thyroid glands, papillomas or adenomas in the breast, cysts in the ovary, papillomas or polyps in the stomach, colon, rectum or uterus, papillomas in the bladder, or enlarging soft-tissue tumours of fat (lipomas), nerve tissue (neuromas), muscle (myomas), tumours of blood or lymph vessels (hemangiomas or lymphangiomas) and occasionally of cartilage (chondromas) or bone (osteomas).

Total removal of the colon and rectum before cancer has developed will prevent cancer in those people affected by familial polyposis coli.

Part II
General Features of Cancer-Presentation and Management

Symptoms of Cancer: Local and General

4

In this chapter you will learn about:

> *Lump, ulcer, pain, bleeding, interference with tissue or organ function, unexpected weight loss*
> *Symptoms of metastatic spread: lymph-nodes, liver, lungs, bones, fat and muscles, bowel, the brain, the "unknown primary" syndrome*

A symptom is something that is reported or felt by a patient. A sign is something that can be observed, felt, measured or otherwise demonstrated by another person. Symptoms may result from two effects of a cancer—first the local effects of the cancer itself, and second, the more general effects of the cancer as it affects the person's body as a whole.

Usually *local* effects are noticed first. The main local effects include one or more of the following—a lump; an ulcer that does not heal; a persistent cough possibly with blood stained sputum; persistent local pain; abnormal bleeding from the stomach, bowel, bladder, vagina or elsewhere; or interference with function of the organ or tissue involved. Such functional interference may be seen in obstruction of the bowel in the case of bowel cancer, persistent cough or interference with breathing in the case of lung cancer, difficulty with swallowing with oesophageal cancer or difficulty with passing urine in the case of prostate cancers. These symptoms of local trouble will thus depend upon the site of the cancer; the organ or tissue in which it started; the type of cancer cells that have developed; the size of the tumour; and the possible involvement of other organs or tissues near to the cancer.

The main *general* effects that may be noticed by a person with cancer are lassitude, malaise, fatigue and loss of energy, anorexia and weight loss. General symptoms are usually related to advanced cancers and may result from damage to, or interference with, function of any organ or tissue involved, as well as the body's reaction to the presence of cancer.

F. O. Stephens and K. R. Aigner, *Basics of Oncology,*
DOI: 10.1007/978-3-540-92925-3_4, © Springer-Verlag Berlin Heidelberg 2009

4

In Part 3 each of the above features will be mentioned in more detail in relation to various cancers, but some general features are outlined below.

4.1   Lump

A lump, swelling or tumour of some sort is present in virtually every cancer but the lump may or may not be noticed by the patient or be able to be felt by the doctor. The lump may be obvious if it is in the skin, head and neck (e.g. mouth or tongue), breast, lymph nodes or fat, muscles or bone (especially in an arm or leg). On the other hand, most lumps are non-malignant, but if a new lump is found anywhere in the body it is important to determine what it is. The most common symptom of breast cancer, for example, is finding a lump in the breast. The lump is often felt whilst the patient is in the bath or shower, because most breast lumps are more easily felt with wet soapy fingers.

4.2   Ulcer

If there is any doubt about the origin of an ulcer arrangements should be made to perform a biopsy.

An ulcer in the skin that does not heal readily may be a cancer and should be examined carefully. Skin ulcers are usually noticed easily but ulcers in the mouth or throat may be less obvious, especially if they are painless. Any such ulcer may be of potential concern if it has been present for more than 2 or 3 weeks with no evidence of healing. However, it should be remembered that most long-standing ulcers are not malignant. Chronic ulcers may be caused by such conditions as varicose veins or poor arteries giving poor blood supply to the lower legs or by repeated trauma such as a jagged tooth, ill-fitting dentures or infections in the mouth. If there is any doubt about the origin of an ulcer arrangements should be made to perform a biopsy. This involves taking a small piece of tissue, usually from the edge of the ulcer, and examining it microscopically to be sure exactly what cells are present and what sort of ulcer it is and what has caused it.

4.3   Pain

In general, a small painless lump is more likely to be a cancer than a small painful lump.

Most cancers are painless in their early stages. Pain may develop after a tumour has become big enough to invade or to press upon and damage surrounding tissues or nerves. In general, a small painless lump is more likely to be a cancer than a small painful lump and people should not wait for pain to develop before seeking medical advice.

4.4   Bleeding

Intermittent bleeding can be a feature of many cancers of surface tissues. For some internal cancers such as the stomach, bowel, kidney, bladder, uterus or lung, bleeding is often the earliest or one of the earliest features. Any evidence of abnormal bleeding should be investigated. For example, bleeding from the bowel may be fresh blood that is bright red or it might be altered blood that is dark red or black. Other sites of bleeding may be in the urine, from the vagina (especially between periods or after the menopause), in the sputum (either from the mouth or throat or from the lung after coughing), from a mole in the skin, or from a nipple. While bleeding may be an indication of cancer, it does not necessarily mean cancer; there are many other causes of bleeding. Bleeding or bruising at several sites or small haemorrhagic spots in the skin (*petechial spots*) may be an indication of a blood disorder including those caused by leukaemias or lymphomas.

4.5   Weight Loss

Approximately two-thirds of all cancer patients will experience weight loss, and in many cases this is the first symptom that prompts them to visit their doctor. An involuntary weight loss of greater than 5% in 6 months is often a prognostic indicator for cancer.

The weight loss is often associated with anorexia (premature satiety or lack of interest in food), but this is not the cause, as the weight loss is much more dramatic than the actual reduction in calorific intake. The weight loss is due to a condition known as cancer cachexia, and the patients look gaunt and malnourished. Cancer cachexia is caused by a tumour becoming metabolically adapted to the anaerobic utilisation of glucose (glycolysis), such that it consumes a lot of glucose and produces a lot of lactic acid (as muscles normally do under intense activity). The lactic acid is taken away by the blood and is used in the liver to newly synthesize glucose (by gluconeogenesis) and requires three times as much energy as that yielded by glucose consumed anaerobically. In effect glucose becomes part of a futile and expensive cycle (the Cori cycle) in addition to anaerobic utilisation representing only ~6% of the energy yielded from glucose in aerobic conditions. With generally a reduced energy intake and an increased energy expenditure (to recycle the glucose) the body needs energy and it obtains it via breaking down fat reserves in adipose tissue and proteins in skeletal muscle. Patients can lose up to 30% of their pre-illness weight, and up to 75% of skeletal muscle protein. It is the loss of skeletal muscle that leads to asthenia (muscle weakness), which can affect breathing and heart function, and is often the cause of death. The weight

Weight loss is due to abnormal and inefficient metabolism of glucose.

Weight loss is pre-dominantly from adipose tissue and skeletal muscle, but it is the loss of muscle mass that causes death.

4

loss is not related to the size of tumour because it is directly related to cytokines (small proteins that act like hormone) produced by either the tumour and/ or the host immune system. Cancer cachexia is most commonly seen in children and the elderly, and cancers such as gastric, pancreas, lung and prostate cancers, but is rare in breast cancer and sarcomas. This involuntary weight loss is associated with poor prognosis and a poor response to chemo- and radio-therapy.

4.6   Interference with Tissue or Organ Function

These symptoms vary a great deal depending upon the site of a cancer. For example a cancer in the mouth or throat may make speaking or swallowing difficult. A cancer of the larynx will usually cause hoarseness or change in voice. A cancer of the oesophagus is usually first noticed because of difficulty with swallowing, initially of solid food and later of liquids. A cancer of the stomach may cause difficulty with eating or a change in appetite or vomiting, and a cancer of the bowel may cause a change in bowel habits (diarrhoea or constipation or alternatively intermittent diarrhoea and constipation) or may partially or fully obstruct the bowel causing colic, in the first instance and possibly bowel perforation in the second.

Cancer of the prostate may interfere with the passage of urine, and cancer of the bladder may also cause difficulty or frequency of passing urine.

Cancer of the lung may cause a persistent cough, local obstruction of air passages or localised pneumonia.

Cancers of the liver, bile ducts or pancreas may block the flow of bile from the liver, causing jaundice.

Obviously, there are many other causes of these symptoms but if any of them is noticed for the first time in someone who was otherwise well, especially if the symptoms persist, they should be investigated promptly and thoroughly.

4.7   Symptoms of Metastatic Spread

These symptoms will depend upon the tissues or organs into which the cancer has metastasised.

Enlargement of lymph nodes may sometimes be the first feature of the presence of a cancer nearby.

4.7.1   Lymph Nodes

A common site of spread is to nearby draining lymph nodes in the neck, axillae, groins or elsewhere depending on the site of the primary cancer. Enlargement of lymph nodes may sometimes be the first feature of the presence of a cancer nearby (see Fig. 22.1).

4.7.2 Liver

Spread of cancer to the liver may cause jaundice or pain as well as swelling in the upper abdomen under the ribs on the right side. It may also lead to malnutrition with wasting and weight loss, or to fluid (*ascites*) collecting in and possibly filling the abdominal cavity.

4.7.3 Lungs

Cancer that spreads to the lungs may cause a cough, difficulty with breathing, fever, pneumonia or chest pain.

4.7.4 Bones

Spread of cancer to bones may cause bone pain or a fracture. Metastases in spinal vertebrae risk spinal cord compression and paralysis. Bone metastases sometimes cause anaemia due to destruction of the blood-forming bone marrow tissues and *hypercalcaemia* may result from release of calcium from damaged bones.

4.7.5 Fat and Muscles

Metastases to soft tissues may cause swelling or lumps that may be felt under the skin.

4.7.6 Bowel

Spread to bowel or elsewhere in the abdominal cavity may cause bowel obstruction with colic or swelling and fluid in the abdominal cavity (*ascites*).

4.7.7 The Brain

Cancer that spreads to the brain may cause severe headaches, vomiting, blurred vision, confusion, fits or unconsciousness, convulsions or coma.

4.7.8 The Unknown Primary Syndrome

A patient will sometimes notice symptoms associated with a cancer metastasis without being aware of trouble at the site of a primary cancer. For example a woman may first complain of a lump in her axilla. A biopsy has shown this not to be a primary lymph node tumour, but a lymph node containing metastatic breast cancer, although she was not aware of any breast problem, and no lump can be felt in the breast. A patient may complain of a lump in the neck that is found to be caused by metastatic involvement of nodes from a cancer in the

4

mouth or throat or post-nasal space that has not caused symptoms. Similarly an enlarged liver with or without jaundice or bone pain may be caused by metastatic cancer and can cause the patient to seek attention when the primary cancer was elsewhere but not causing any symptoms. Sometimes a secondary cancer mass may be noticed by a patient or found by a doctor without any evidence of the site of the primary cancer – referred to as the "unknown primary" syndrome.

EXERCISE

List patient symptoms that are commonly associated with cancer.

EXERCISE

Why are breast lumps often first noticed when women take a bath or shower?

Signs of Cancer: Local and General

5

In this chapter you will learn about:

› *Lump, ulcer, bleeding and evidence of blood loss, lymph node enlargement*
› *Other swellings*
› *Findings of general examination including examination of mouth, throat, abdomen, rectum and anus*
› *Rare and seemingly unrelated indications of cancer*

Physical signs of cancer include *local* lumps or other abnormal swellings, ulcers, tender or painful areas, evidence of blood loss from bowel, urine, uterus, etc. and *general* effects on the patient such as weight loss, pallor, and general unwell appearance. There may also be evidence of cancer spread to other organs or tissues (metastases). Different cancers tend to spread in a usually predictable way to different organs or tissues but no matter what signs are present the only proof of cancer depends on a biopsy demonstrating the presence of malignant cells.

5.1   Lump

It is important to recognise features of lumps that are most likely to be associated with cancer in general and particular forms of cancer. For example, cancer lumps are usually harder than lumps from other causes. Cancer lumps usually are not cystic (although on occasions they may be) and they are usually not tender unless quite advanced. As they enlarge, cancer lumps adhere to and invade nearby structures and therefore become less mobile.

Cancer lumps are usually not tender unless quite advanced.

F. O. Stephens and K. R. Aigner, *Basics of Oncology,*
DOI: 10.1007/978-3-540-92925-3_5, © Springer-Verlag Berlin Heidelberg 2009

5

5.2   Ulcer

Malignant ulcers often have raised or heaped up edges. They tend to grow into nearby tissues on which they lie and there is usually surrounding swelling and induration. They may bleed easily but usually not profusely. They may or may not be tender. Ulcers due to skin cancer are usually not tender, whereas malignant ulcers in the mouth and throat, usually become quite tender in the later stages.

5.3   Bleeding and Evidence of Blood Loss

There may be obvious blood loss or hidden (*occult*) blood loss with evidence of anaemia due to chronic blood loss. Blood in the faeces may be detected chemically even when it is not obvious to the naked eye and this may be an early feature of cancer of the stomach or bowel. In fact occult blood loss is often used as a screening test for people with a high risk of developing gastric or bowel cancer even though they may have no symptoms.

Blood in the urine may sometimes be found on microscopic examination of the urine even when it is not obvious to the naked eye. This can be a feature of cancer of the kidney or bladder although there are also other more common causes of blood in the urine.

5.4   Lymph Node Enlargement

Evidence of metastatic spread of cancer may be revealed by examination of the draining lymph-node areas.

Evidence of metastatic spread of cancer may be revealed by examination of the draining lymph-node areas. For example, if a head and neck cancer is suspected the submandibular, submental and cervical (neck) nodes must be examined (Fig. 5.1a, b). If breast cancer or cancer of the skin of the arm or chest wall is suspected, the axillary lymph nodes must be examined. If cancer in the lower limb or of the skin of the abdomen or lower back, scrotum, anus or vulva, is suspected the inguinal lymph nodes must be examined.

Abdominal lymph nodes may be involved from cancers of the stomach, bowel, pancreas, testes, uterus, ovaries or elsewhere in the abdominal cavity but these are usually not palpable unless very large. Nowadays they are often first seen in CT studies. Sometimes lymphatic channels allow a tumour to spread from the abdominal organs to supraclavicular lymph nodes in the neck (usually the left side), so these too need to be examined; they are easily felt if enlarged. The name given to a palpable metastatic lymph node in the lower neck from a primary cancer in the abdomen or pelvis is Virchow's node. Finding this node to be present is called Trousseau's sign.

Lymph nodes in the chest may be involved from cancers of the lung or oesophagus or sometimes the breast. Although these cannot be felt with the hands,

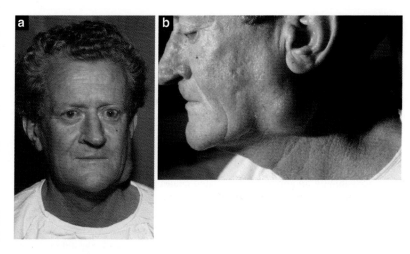

Fig. 5.1. (**a**, **b**) Enlarged cervical (neck) lymph nodes that became obvious 3 years after apparently successful treatment of a squamous cell cancer of upper lip

evidence of mediastinal node enlargement can sometimes be seen in a chest X-ray or in CT studies.

Lymph nodes may also be enlarged in the lymphomas or leukaemias. If enlarged, these lymph nodes are usually somewhat rubbery, and less hard than nodes involved with cancer. They are also likely to be smoother in outline, less likely to become fixed to other structures and often lymph nodes on both sides of the neck or lymph nodes in other places may also be involved. The spleen also behaves like a large lymph node, and although a normal spleen cannot be felt, it may become enlarged and palpable in patients with a lymphoma or leukaemia.

5.5   Other Swellings

There can sometimes be evidence of lumps or swellings due to metastases in other parts of the body, especially a subcutaneous lump or a lump in the abdomen, the liver or any other tissue or organ. Metastases in such sites can arise from virtually any cancer.

5.6   Findings of a General Examination Including Mouth, Throat, Abdomen, Rectum and Anus

Part of the examination of the alimentary tract should be an examination of the mouth, tongue and throat, and most importantly, an examination inside the anus with a gloved finger. Most cancers of the rectum can be felt with a gloved finger in the rectum and many other conditions such as an enlarged or lumpy prostate, an enlarged uterus or tumour in the pelvis can be felt by this simple examination or by a bi-manual examination: a finger in the rectum (or vagina) and the other hand palpating the lower abdomen. Also by examining the glove used, the colour and nature of the faeces and presence of blood that can be seen and an abnormal finding might give a clue about the possibility of a cancer being present.

5.7   Rare and Seemingly Unrelated Indications of Cancer

Very occasionally an apparently unrelated health problem may be the first evidence of an occult cancer. An unexplained anaemia is the most common, but a neuropathy or other neurological disorder or the onset of herpes zoster in an elderly person may indicate a weakened immune response possibly associated with an undetected malignancy. An unexplained deep vein thrombosis with no obvious initiating factors may occasionally be the first clinical feature of a cancer (Fig. 5.2).

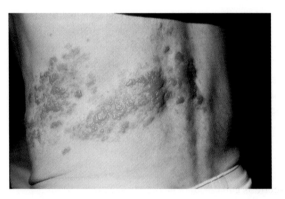

Fig. 5.2. A typical outbreak of herpes zoster (shingles) that was the first evidence of this 72-year-old man's cancer of pancreas

EXERCISE

List patient signs that are commonly associated with cancers.

Clinico-Pathology of Cancers

6

In this chapter you will learn about:

> *Typing, grading and staging of cancer*
> *Clinical decisions based on pathology information*

The ultimate diagnosis of any benign or malignant tumour will depend upon a pathologist's examination of a specimen of tissue. This can be a surface scraping of tissue, a small sample of cells taken by aspiration with a syringe, a small core of tissue taken with a small core cutting instrument, a small sample of representative tissue (incision biopsy) taken by a surgeon using a scalpel or other cutting instrument or even the whole tumour mass (excision biopsy) taken by a surgeon. The ultimate diagnosis is sometimes not confirmed until after death of the patient with specimens taken at autopsy.

No matter how the tissue sample is taken, the pathologist will, if possible, report on the macroscopic as well as the microscopic features of the tissue and its cells. Before the pathologist can report on the microscopic features of the tissue and cells in it, the tissue must be prepared in a solid block, usually a wax block, so that fine sections can be cut. The prepared tissue will be stained with appropriate stains to best display special features. Unless immediate cell smears or frozen section specimens (described later in this chapter) are prepared, most tissue preparations and staining procedures require at least 24 h and usually 2–3 days.

The pathologist will be able to report not only on the type of tissue but whether it is normal or abnormal tissue and if abnormal, whether it shows features of a tumour–benign or malignant.

If it is found to be a malignant growth the pathologist will report on the range of relative normality and maturity of cells in it (i.e. the degree of anaplasia), and other more abnormal and aggressive features. If possible, a sample of surrounding tissue should be taken with the biopsy specimen so the pathologist can also report on the degree of invasion or infiltration of cancer cells into surrounding or underlining tissues.

F. O. Stephens and K. R. Aigner, *Basics of Oncology,*
DOI: 10.1007/978-3-540-92925-3_6, © Springer-Verlag Berlin Heidelberg 2009

6

6.1   Typing, Grading and Staging of Cancer

Best management of cancer will depend on many factors including patient factors (age, state of health, family, social and emotional considerations), hospitals or other treatment facilities with or without specialised nursing care and allied health professionals, as well as particular factors of the cancer itself.

The cancer factors include three special pathology considerations: the type, grading and staging of the cancer. These will be made with information provided by both the pathologist and the cancer treatment team.

6.2   Cancer Typing

The treatment team depends on the pathologist for confirmation of the presence of cancer, the cancer type and other features of the cancer. The most common malignancies are carcinomas from cells of epithelial surface or glandular type and usually retaining some of the features of these types of cells.

Other malignances include those of connective-tissue cell origin (sarcomas), germ-cell origin (testicular cancers and some ovarian cancers) and blood-forming cell origin (leukaemias and lymphomas). Malignancies that do not readily fit into any of the preceding group types include gliomas of brain and myeloma, an uncommon tumour that develops in bone but is not of bone cells. Myeloma or multiple myeloma is a malignancy of plasmacytes in bone.

The pathologist will recognise features of these various types of cells. Often they are obvious to the expert and closely resemble their tissue of origin but sometimes there is so much anaplastic change it can be very difficult or impossible to recognise the original cell type. Special facilities such as use of special stains, electron-microscopy or immunochemistry can be helpful in making a more accurate tissue typing determination.

In cases where the site or history of an original primary cancer is uncertain the pathologist might also be of special help in deciding whether malignant tissue in a biopsy is from a primary cancer or has features indicating that it is more likely to be metastatic tissue.

6.3   Cancer Grading

Cancer grading gives an indication of the likely aggressiveness of the cancer. In general, highly differentiated tumour cells that closely resemble their cells of origin may be either benign or may be very low-grade cancers with little tendency to grow rapidly or to metastasise early. Whereas poorly differentiated, anaplastic cancer cells that have often lost all special features of their tissue of origin are much more likely to behave in an aggressive fashion and invade nearby tissues as well as to metastasise to other sites.

In general, cancers that remain localised, or invade surrounding tissues by pushing into them and infiltrating only as a continuous growth, are less aggressive than cancers with cells that break free from the original tissue of origin and invade more deeply into surrounding tissues.

Nuclear pleomorphism is the degree to which cell nuclei vary in size, shape and in staining patterns. The more pleomorphic the cell nuclei, the more aggressive the likely behaviour of the cancer.

Along with the number of pleomorphic cells, the number of mitotic figures (indicating dividing cells) gives an additional indication of the aggressive potential of the cancer.

Sometimes the cancer growth is surrounded to a greater or lesser degree of infiltration by lymphocytes. Such lymphocytic infiltration may give an indication of natural body immunological defence against the cancer and therefore a potentially lower grade of cancer than one with no evidence of a protective reaction.

With these features all considered: well differentiated or poorly differentiated cancer cells, presence or absence of cancer cells separating from the primary cancer site and infiltrating into surrounding tissues, the degree of nuclear pleomorphism, the number of mitotic figures and the amount of lymphocytic reaction, the pathologist will be able to give an indication as to the potential for aggressive behaviour of the cancer. That is the grade of the cancer from low grade and less aggressive to high grade and a potentially more aggressive cancer. This all depends on a truly representative biopsy sample being made available to the pathologist. The grade of the cancer may be different in different samples of tissue. In general the cancer growth pattern is likely to follow the highest grade of tissue sample rather than the lowest so that the grade report given by the pathologist will depend on the highest grade of cancer tissue seen.

6.4 Clinico-Pathological Staging of Cancer

Cancer type and cancer grading will depend on findings of the pathologist. The third important pathology information is the staging of the cancer and this will depend on combined information of pathologist and surgeon or clinical team.

Cancer staging expresses how much the cancer has grown and has spread from its site of origin. The important elements of the most commonly used clinical staging indices are:

1. Local primary growth: The size of the tumour and the extent of its spread into local tissues is indicated by the letter "T" and the scale of 1–4; T1 being a small localised cancer; T4 being an advanced cancer that is destroying surrounding tissues and unlikely to be curable.

Cancer staging expresses how much the cancer has grown and has spread from its site of origin.

2. Lymph-node involvement: The extent of spread into the nearest local lymph nodes or more distant lymph nodes in the region is indicated by the letter "N" and the scale 0–3. NO indicates no lymph node involvement; N1 indicates involvement of adjacent lymph nodes only; N2 indicates that a further set of lymph nodes is involved; and N3 indicates distant involvement of lymph nodes.
3. Metastatic growth: Evidence of metastatic spread (usually by bloodstream) into distant organs or tissues is indicated by the letter M and the scale 0–1. MO indicates no evidence of metastatic growth in distant tissues and M1 indicates metastatic spread into one or more distant sites.

The best prognosis cancers are T1, N0, M0 and the worst prognosis cancers are T4, N3, M1.

The symbol X is used to indicate an uncertainty of classification. When there is insufficient information to classify one or more of the clinico-pathological stages the symbol X is used. TX suggests that there was not sufficient information to make a staging of the primary tumour; NX indicates that node staging was not known; and similarly MX suggests that evidence for or against the presence or absence of metastases was not known.

Tumour staging can be based on clinical assessment compiled after all clinical information is known. This is *clinical staging.* Alternatively staging may be based on the pathologist's examination of tissue biopsies. This is *pathological staging.* Clinical staging is more readily available to the examining doctor but ultimate decisions are better based on pathological staging which should be more accurate.

6.5 Clinical Decisions Based on Pathology Information

All of these pieces of pathology and clinical pathology information together with knowledge of the habits of cancers of different tumour types will allow the medical team responsible for the patient's care, to make an assessment of the prognosis for the patient as well as the most appropriate treatment schedule and likely response to treatment. However in each case advice must be modified by the knowledge that not every tumour will respond in a predictable way. With few exceptions, advice about likely response should be guarded and given in general terms only. Usually statistical likelihood is the most appropriate method of making clinical decisions and in giving clinical or prognostic advice.

Sometimes special tests on biopsy tissue will indicate appropriate treatment choices. For example tests of breast biopsy tissue for hormone receptor activity, oestrogen receptor ER or Progesterone receptor PR can indicate a likely response to hormonal management if positive. ER +ve and PR +ve cancers are more likely to respond to hormone management than ER −ve and PR −ve breast cancers. Another more recent test, an immuno-histochemistry test for HER2 growth receptors, is for likely response of breast cancers to Herceptin. If there is an over-expression of extracellular growth receptors on the cell surface then Herceptin is recommended for treatment, as it targets the cancer cells for destruction.

What pathology features help in determining curability or prognosis cancers?

. . . .

. . . .

. . . .

. . . .

. . . .

Investigations That May be Useful in Detecting Cancer

7

In this chapter you will learn about:

› *Screening tests*
› *Organ imaging*
  − *X-rays, isotopes, CT, ultrasound*
  − *MRI (magnetic resonance imaging)*
› *PET (positron emission tomography)*
› *Indirect evidence of cancer blood and serum tests*
› *Direct evidence of cancer biopsy*

A large range of tests is now available to help detect cancer. Some of the most useful of these became available only during the last decade or two of the twentieth century. These range from screening tests, that may help detect the possibility of cancer in people who are at risk but without any symptoms, to organ-imaging tests when symptoms are being investigated. Helpful tests include X-rays, CT scans, ultrasound scans, isotope scans, MRI scans and PET scans. Each of these may reveal the presence, the site and likely dimensions of a deep-seated tumour. Endoscopic tests that use flexible mirrored endoscopic tubes allow the operator to look at, photograph and even biopsy lesions in the alimentary tract, thorax, peritoneal cavity or in other body cavities. A number of blood and serum tests may reveal evidence of reactions to a tumour somewhere in the body. The ultimate investigation, however, is a biopsy because microscopic examination of biopsied material can very often tell the type of malignant cells and the organ or tissue from which they originally developed, as well as the degree of anaplasia or potential aggressiveness of the cancer.

F. O. Stephens and K. R. Aigner, *Basics of Oncology,*
DOI: 10.1007/978-3-540-92925-3_7, © Springer-Verlag Berlin Heidelberg 2009

7.1　Screening Programs

Screening programs are simple, non-invasive and relatively inexpensive methods of detecting early cancers in people in high-risk categories. Early detection before symptoms or signs of cancer have become evident results in significantly better prospects of cure. When certain cancers are known to have a high incidence in a community, governments and health authorities have established on-going screening programs in many countries.

7.2　Screening Tests

7.2.1　The Cervical Smear or "Pap" (Papanicolaou) Test

One of the first, and still one of the most useful, specific screening tests is the Papanicolaou (cervical smear) test for detecting early cancer of the cervix of the uterus. Cancer of the cervix is the most common cancer of the uterus. Women over the age of 40 and especially those who have had several sex partners or several pregnancies are at increased risk for this type of cancer, and many such women now have a cervical smear test every year. Women who have been exposed to infection with the human papilloma virus, especially sex workers who have had multiple male partners, have the greatest risk and should be tested more frequently. This test has the advantage of being simple, painless, cheap, and in most cases, highly reliable. In this test a swab or scraping is taken from the uterine cervix through the vagina. Fluid from the swab or scraping is smeared over a glass slide and examined for cells. If malignant cells are found, cancer may be detected early and treated with good results. Other abnormal cells may suggest pre-malignant changes that could become cancer if not treated, so simple treatment at that stage can often prevent a cancer developing.

7.2.2　Occult Blood Tests

A number of chemical and other tests have been used to detect small amounts of blood in the faeces. As stated earlier, blood in the faeces that is not obvious to the naked eye, is called "occult blood". Its presence indicates some abnormality in the stomach or bowel that might be a cancer or possibly a pre-cancerous condition such as a polyp. Occult blood tests are not always reliable and sometimes produce false-negative and false-positive results. Positive tests can be caused by a number of inflammatory or other benign conditions. However occult blood tests can be useful screening tests to help detect people who are most at risk of cancer and help determine those in need of further investigation. For people with a high risk of bowel cancer regular screening of the colon and rectum by colonoscopy is advisable.

7.2.3   Gastro-Oesophageal Screening

For people in countries where oesophageal cancer is common, gastro-oesophageal screening by regular endoscopy is advisable. In recent years in Western
countries Barret's ulcer of the lower oesophagus has become more common. A
Barret's ulcer is an ulcer in the lower oesophagus associated with long-standing
gastro-oesophageal reflux. An unhealed Barret's ulcer is now regarded as a pre-
malignant condition requiring regular endoscopic observation for early detection
of a malignant change.

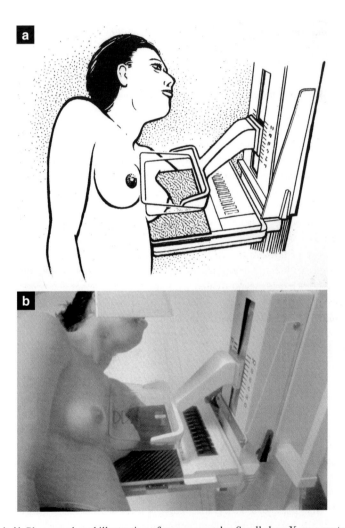

Fig. 7.1 (a, b). Photograph and illustration of mammography. Small-dose X-rays are taken
with the breast held firmly between two plates

7

7.2.4   Breast Screenings: Mammography

Although there is no
single screening test
that is totally reliable,
a number of tests
can be combined
to help detect early
breast cancer.

Other than skin cancer, breast cancer is the most common cancer in women
in most Western countries. Although there is no single screening test that is
totally reliable, a number of tests can be combined to help detect early breast
cancer. These include the teaching of self-examination and examination for
lumps in screening clinics by a doctor or specially trained nurse. Mammography, ultrasound studies and biopsy using a fine needle or similar instrument
to aspirate or otherwise remove a sample of fluid or cells from any suspicious
lump for microscopic examination, are important screening tests. These are
often performed in special clinics supported by government-funded screening
programs. Most large cities in developed societies now have breast-screening
clinics in a city hospital or elsewhere in conveniently located central positions
(Figs. 7.1 and 7.2).

7.2.5   Skin Cancer Screening: Especially the "Mole Check"

In countries where skin cancer is common, annual "mole checks" are often
arranged for members of clubs or particular workforces. This is now commonly
practised in many Australian surf clubs. Although called "mole checks", with
particular interest in detecting early melanoma, many "non-mole" pre-malignant

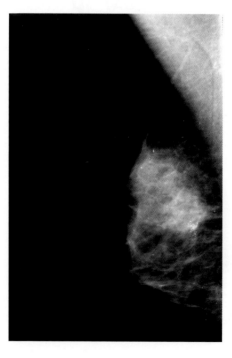

Fig. 7.2. Mammogram showing a
rather dense area of breast with a
cluster of spicules of calcification
suggestive of breast cancer

or early malignant lesions of skin are detected, especially hyperkeratoses, basal cell carcinomas and squamous cell carcinomas.

7.2.6   PSA Screening Test

Other than skin cancer, prostate cancer is the most common cancer affecting men in Western societies. It is not common before the age of 50 but thereafter becomes increasingly common in older men. Previously, digital rectal examination (DRE) with a gloved finger to detect evidence of a hard or lumpy prostate was the only useful screening test but the prostate specific antigens (PSA) blood test is now commonly used. The PSA is a simple test in which a raised level is suggestive of a prostate disorder that might be cancer. PSA tends to increase naturally with increasing age in all men. At age 50, the upper level should not be above 3 ng/mL; at 60 it should not be above 4 ng/mL. Higher levels indicate an abnormality of the prostate, most commonly benign prostatic hyperplasia, but progressively increasing levels (up to 6, 8 or 10) or greatly increased levels above about 12 are more suggestive of cancer. Prostate biopsy might be indicated when there is a progressively rising PSA or when the initial PSA is significantly elevated, even if no lump or other abnormality can be detected by DRE.

7.2.7   Genetic Testing

The genetic basis for a familial incidence of some types of cancer such as some cases of breast, prostate, ovary, and large bowel cancers is becoming better understood. In most cases, cancers associated with inheritance of abnormal tumour suppressors and oncogenes tend to appear at an earlier age than those not found to have an hereditary association.

Genetic testing is time-consuming and, as yet, has not become available for general cancer screening but there is potential for early detection and cancer prevention in individuals with a strong family history of a particular cancer. People found to be at special risk should be referred to special counselling and risk-management clinics.

7.3   Organ Imaging

7.3.1   X-Rays

Radiological studies or X-rays are a relatively old but still useful method of medical examination for cancer. Techniques are constantly being improved and the doses of X-rays needed are becoming smaller. X-ray films are only able to detect spots or lesions that have different permeability for X-rays than that of normal tissue in the region. This difference is seen as a relatively light or relatively dark shadow on a film. For example, X-rays pass easily through air in the lungs or gas in large bowel and this is shown as a dark shadow on a film. If a tumour is present in a chest X-ray, the X-rays will penetrate the tumour tissue less well than the air-filled lungs so that the tumour will show as relatively lighter or whiter part in the area normally showing as dark shadow from the air-filled lungs. On the other hand, X-rays are blocked by dense bone that shows as a white area on film. If a tumour is present in bone, the bone destruction may show as relatively dark or grey areas in the bone that is otherwise white due to lack of penetration of normal bone by X-rays. Other tissues such as muscle and fat are intermediate between the dark shadow of air or the white shadow of bone in their penetration by X-rays. These tissues are of similar consistency and have similar penetration to X-rays as do tumours so that it is not so easy to detect tumour shadows in soft tissues by simple X-rays, and more sophisticated investigations may be required.

7.3.2   Barium (Baryum) and Iodine Contrast X-Rays

Barium (baryum) or iodine compounds and some other materials (often called "dyes" or "contrast" material) are impervious to X-rays and these are often used in the body to outline cavities that are otherwise not easily seen in a plain X-ray film. A barium meal is a barium sulphate mixture swallowed into the stomach. This outlines the shape of the stomach. If a cancer is present it may show as an abnormality in the shape or in the outline of the stomach. Similarly, a barium enema in the lower bowel may allow X-rays to help detect a cancer in the colon or rectum (Figs. 7.3 and 7.4).

Iodine compounds are also used as "contrast" material as they are excreted in the urine after injection into a peripheral vein. These may be used to show the position, shape, size and outline of the kidneys or bladder. This is called an *intravenous pyelogram* (IVP) or excretory urogram. Iodine compounds can also be injected into the bladder or the kidneys from below, through the urethra and/ or the ureters, and X-rays taken. Such X-ray studies of the kidneys are called *retrograde pyelograms* or *retrograde urograms*. Iodine compounds have in the past been injected into other body cavities such as the fluid-filled space around the spinal cord, and an X-ray called a myelogram may show some abnormality of the filling if a tumour is present. Nowadays myelograms have been replaced by CT or MRI studies.

Some iodine compounds are also excreted in bile into the gall bladder and bile ducts. X-rays can then be used to outline the shape and contents of the gall bladder (cholecystogram) and bile ducts (cholangiogram) that again may show abnormalities if tumours or other defects, such as gallstones, are present. Injection of contrast backwards up the biliary tree into the pancreatic duct is

Fig. 7.3. A barium (baryum) meal X-ray showing a "filling defect" of the greater curvature of the stomach due to a gastric cancer

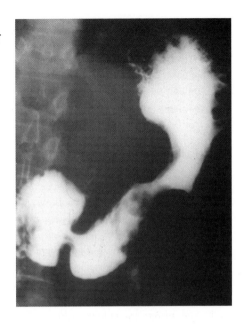

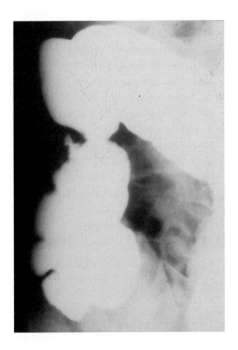

Fig. 7.4. A barium (baryum) meal X-ray showing a "filling defect" of the greater curvature of the stomach due to a gastric cancer

7

possible if a fine tube is passed into the Ampulla of Vater in the duodenum (through which bile and pancreatic juice normally pass). This test is known as *endoscopic retrograde cholangio-pancreatogram* (ERCP). It is endoscopic because passage of an endoscope through the mouth and down the oesophagus and stomach into the duodenum is necessary to insert the fine tube into the duodenal papilla.

7.3.3   Radiographic Screening

Whereas in years past all X-rays were recorded on a film as still photographs, nowadays techniques are used to allow the radiologist to study on a television screen the movement of a radio-opaque material (dye or contrast) such as barium or iodine in a body cavity. After a barium meal or barium enema the patient is taken into a dark screening room where the radiologist can change the position of the patient to allow the radio-opaque material to flow into different parts of the organ being examined. This manoeuvring helps to visualise more accurately on the television screen the size, shape, position and outline of the organ under study, and allows the radiologist to see, for example, if a lump in the bowel is faeces that can be moved, or tumour attached to the bowel wall.

Air can be used to replace fluid in certain cavities and shows up as a dark shadow in X-rays. Air is sometimes used in the large bowel together with barium so that the barium coats onto the bowel wall and the air fills the bowel cavity. This allows X-rays to show more precisely the shape of the wall of the bowel and any lump projecting into the cavity of the bowel. This is called an air *contrast barium enema* and can be a very useful examination to detect tumours or polyps attached to the bowel wall. Air can also be used to replace some of the fluid in the cavities (ventricles) of the brain. This allows X-ray films to detect evidence of some brain lesions by the contrasting penetration of X-rays passing through air as compared to a tumour that might be distorting the shape of the brain ventricles. This study is known as an *air encephalogram*. This test was used much more often before CT and MRI scanning facilities became widely available.

In most cases, the X-ray density of a cancer is similar to the X-ray density of surrounding tissues and X-ray films alone are unlikely to show evidence of a deep-seated cancer. For cancers that are not so deep-seated, however, such as breast cancer, X-ray (mammograms) can be used to detect any small differences in penetration of the tissues that may indicate the presence of a cancer.

A negative mammogram in a woman with a breast lump does not in itself negate the necessity of having other tests.

7.3.4   Mammography

A mammogram is a special X-ray of the breast that may show the presence of cysts, dense fibrous tissue, or a cancer in the less-dense fatty tissue of the breast. Small amounts of X-rays only are needed so this examination is safe if not used excessively. Although mammograms produce some false negatives and some false positives they are nevertheless very useful, safe and inexpensive in screening for breast cancer. However even the small doses of X-rays needed for mammography are better avoided in women who may be pregnant or wish to have further pregnancies as even this exposure to irradiation can cause genetic mutation of foetal cells or of actively functioning ovarian tissue. This usually means that mammography is not routinely recommended in women younger than 40.

It is important to appreciate that, like any other test, a mammogram is not infallible. A negative mammogram in a woman with a breast lump does not in itself negate the necessity of having other tests such as ultrasound and, more importantly, a fine needle biopsy.

7.3.5 Chest X-Ray

Chest X-rays are most useful investigations for detecting abnormalities in the lungs, including tumours, which may show as white opacities within the dark air-filled lungs (see Figs 11.1a, b, Figs. 11.2a, b). Sometimes the size and shape of the lungs, or the tissues between the lungs (the mediastinum), may be altered. Lymph nodes in the chest are grouped around the midline between the lungs. If lymph nodes are enlarged as in the lymphomas, the normal mediastinum or central area of white density in a chest X-ray may be widened.

7.3.6 Skeletal X-Rays

These will show the outline of bones and give an indication of their density. Primary cancer of bone (i.e. cancer starting in the bone, called osteosarcoma) may sometimes be seen as an abnormal shape and abnormal density of one part of the bone, usually towards one or other end of a long bone. Sometimes a primary bone cancer may give a "sunray-like" appearance in an X-ray. Secondary (metastatic) cancers in bone usually show as rounded less-dense areas in the bone due to local destruction of bone tissue. They may sometimes show as fractures in damaged bone (a form of pathological fracture). Some metastatic cancers containing calcium may even show as rounded areas of increased density in the bone. However, X-rays are not infallible and will not always detect malignant lesions in bone, especially if the lesions are small.

7.3.7 Angiography

Radio-opaque materials (dyes) may be injected into arteries, veins and even lymph vessels for films to be taken or for immediate viewing on a television screen. The radiologist can then determine whether the vessels are in their normal position or whether they may have been pushed aside by a lump of some

Fig. 7.5. An angiogram taken during injection of an iodine compound into the upper end of the femoral artery. A mass in the lower thigh is seen to flush with blood due to a vascular sarcoma seen to be distorting the normally straight femoral artery. Such vascularity in a tumour is known as a "tumour blush"

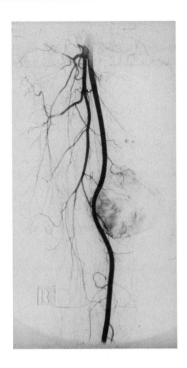

sort, which may be a cancer. Some cancers also develop a distinctive blood supply showing, with this technique, as a cluster of small blood vessels called a "tumour blush" (Fig. 7.5).

Modern angiography has allowed arteries in virtually every part of the body to be outlined by radiographic (X-ray) techniques and may be helpful in detecting and treating deep-seated tumours.

Lymphangiography, by injecting radio-opaque "dyes" into lymph vessels, will also allow X-rays of the lymph nodes to be taken to determine whether they are enlarged or partly replaced by abnormal tissue that may be cancer.

7.3.8   Isotope Scans (Nuclear Scintigraphy)

Isotope scans have some similarity to X-rays in that the shadows of a radioactive source are recorded on a film plate. In this case the radioactive material is injected into a peripheral vein and is distributed in the bloodstream. The radioactive dose used is very small. The radioactive material is made of, or combined with, various agents depending on which organ or tissue is to be examined. Radioactive iodine, for example, is concentrated in the thyroid gland and the amount of uptake, size, shape, position, and consistency of tissue in the thyroid gland can be determined from such a test. Another such material, called technetium, is concentrated in bone, particularly in areas of the bone with cellular activity or growth. Thus a bone scan

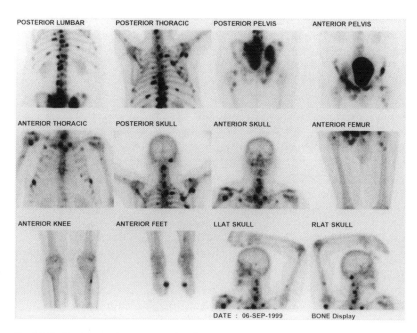

POSTERIOR LUMBAR   POSTERIOR THORACIC   POSTERIOR PELVIS   ANTERIOR PELVIS

ANTERIOR THORACIC   POSTERIOR SKULL   ANTERIOR SKULL   ANTERIOR FEMUR

ANTERIOR KNEE   ANTERIOR FEET   LLAT SKULL   RLAT SKULL

DATE : 06-SEP-1999   BONE Display

Fig. 7.6. Radio-isotope bone scans showing many metastatic cancer deposits in bones (*dark spots*). The patient had advanced metastatic prostate cancer

will not only outline the position, size and shape of bone but will also show areas of abnormal cellular activity that may be due to cancer (Fig. 7.6).

Similar scans are used to outline the size, shape and any abnormal activity in the liver and spleen. In these organs, cancer may show up as one or more areas of decreased activity.

Similar radioisotope scan tests are now available for a number of other organs or tissues including the brain, lungs and lymph nodes. An isotope of gallium can be used to help delineate between normal and abnormal patterns of lymph nodes. Scanning is carried out with the patient lying on a special table. Apart from a needle prick to inject the material into a vein, it is quite painless.

7.3.9 CT Scan or CAT Scan (Computerised Axial Tomography)

In the early 1970s British workers developed a technique in which small doses of X-rays were used to construct a picture of tissues in a cross-section of the trunk, head and neck, or limbs. Many cross-sectional pictures of the abdomen for example, are taken, thus allowing a three-dimensional image concept to be developed. The position, size and shape of all the organs, major blood vessels, bones and muscles in the abdomen can be seen and the position, size and density of any abnormal tumour can often be assessed with considerable accuracy. CT scanning requires highly specialised equipment and skilled personnel and is

7

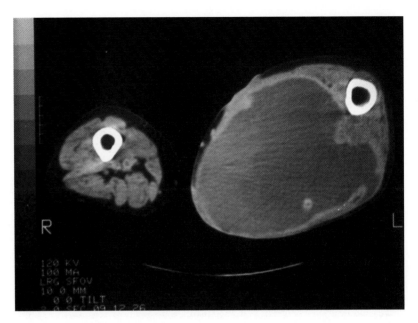

Fig. 7.7. CT scan showing a cross-section of both thighs with a large sarcoma in one thigh

therefore relatively expensive in comparison to standard X-rays. CT scans have proven to be of great value in investigating cancers and tumours in otherwise inaccessible areas of the head, abdomen, chest and limbs.

CT scanning is carried out with the patient lying on a table and, like other types of X-rays, it presents no discomfort to the patient except for the need to lie still for several minutes on a thin foam mattress in a relatively confined space (Fig. 7.7).

EXERCISE

What advantages do CT scans have over plain X-rays, and what disadvantages

7.3.10   Ultrasound Scans

X-rays, nuclear scans and CT scans all depend on penetrating X-rays and gamma rays. Although the small doses now required are safe if used with proper care, there are occasions when even these are probably better avoided. One of these situations is during pregnancy because the developing foetus is highly sensitive to irradiation. The ovaries and testes of people of reproductive age are also better not irradiated even with small doses of radiation.

In more recent years, use of ultrasound waves has been developed to give a somewhat similar cross-sectional picture of body tissues and organs as does the CT scan. The ultrasound waves are quite harmless and can be safely used in the region of a pregnant uterus or active ovaries. The principle depends upon sound waves being reflected or bounced back in different degrees by body tissues of different densities somewhat like a radar or a depth sounder.

The degree to which sound waves bounce back depends on the nature or qualities of the underlying tissues. The principle is similar to that used by fishing crews to detect schools of fish or oceanographers to measure the depth of the ocean floor. It is certainly not a new or original physical adaptation of sound waves. Dolphins use a similar system to locate schools of fish. The same principle is used by bats flying in the dark.

Ultrasound scans in general do not give as much information as CT scans but for some lesions, for example cysts, they are more accurate in showing the position and type of lesion. This is especially true in examining breasts of young women because the ultrasound shows more information in the more dense breast tissue of younger women. It is also completely safe in studies during pregnancy or ovulation. Hence they may be used as an alternative to CT scans in some situations or in conjunction with CT scans in other situations.

Like taking X-rays and CT scans, ultrasound examinations are carried out with the patient lying on a table with a small handpiece moving over the patient. The procedure is harmless, painless and causes no discomfort.

EXERCISE

Under what circumstances would ultrasound be preferable to mammography in breast examination?

7.3.11   MRI (Magnetic Resonance Imaging)

A MRI scan shows tissues on cross sectional images similar in appearance to those of a CT scan although based on quite different principles of physics. The images are based on computer analysis of absorption and penetration of high frequency radio waves by water molecules in a strong magnetic field. There is no exposure to X-rays or other damaging forms of irradiation. In some parts of the body and in some body tissues such as in bone, muscles and in the brain and spinal cord an MRI scan may show more detail and provide more information than a CT scan but in other situations a CT is preferred. Whereas a CT scan only shows pictures horizontally, with MRI pictures can be taken from almost any angle. MRI scanning is now recognised as the preferred method of imaging of musculo-skeletal structures and of intra-cranial and spinal cord investigation. In some situations both CT and MRI studies are used. They may complement each other by giving different information about the size, shape and other character-istics of a tumour and its possible extent of spread into surrounding tissues.

The scan is usually performed as an outpatient procedure. The patient must lie still. It is painless and no anaesthetic is required, except possibly in children to keep them perfectly still. Since the procedure is conducted in a powerful mag-netic field it is important for the patient not to wear jewellery or metal objects.

7.3.12   PET (Positron Emission Tomography) Scan

The PET scan is the most recent of presently used non-invasive studies – that is studies that do not require an instrument to be put inside the body or for a piece of biopsy tissue to be removed or a surgical operation. At the time of writ-ing this innovative but very costly equipment is available only in a relatively small number of centres where intense research studies are being carried out to determine exactly how it can help in the diagnosis and treatment of cancers and other serious medical conditions.

PET scans are quite different to X-rays, CT or MRI studies. X-rays are used to produce films that are shown as black/white shadows with shades of grey. These are inexpensive and readily available but do not give nearly as much information as CT or MRI scans. Both CT and MRI scans give more three dimensional information about the position, size, shape and consistency of tumours or lumps deep to the surface and their position in relation to other tissues like arteries, nerves, muscles, bone and important organs. They are also produced in black and white pictures with shades of grey. They are based on laws of physics using penetration of X-rays and radio waves under different conditions including a change in magnetic fields in the case of MRI.

Although PET scans produce three-dimensional pictures that may be in black and white or in colour, they are based not so much on laws of physics but on different chemical activity in different types of tissues and different cells. The basic principle is that cancer cells use more glucose than normal cells. They demonstrate areas of activated uptake of glucose which is a feature of cancer cells. PET scanning therefore represents functional as opposed to anatomical imaging. PET scans are often able to show something of the activity of the cancer such as its rate of growth and any changes made to the cancer by treatment given. For some cancers, such as lung cancers, they are better able to show whether the cancer has spread (metastasised) to other places. For lymphomas they are better able to show the extent of the disease. They may also indicate whether a cancer has totally responded to treatment or whether it might be starting to recur after treatment.

PET scanning is a very safe study but it is expensive. The equipment costs the equivalent of several million dollars. Because it is not yet known what help it can give that cannot be given by less expensive methods, many more studies must be made and costs contained before PET scanning can be made more widely available. However in the United States PET scanning it is now recognised as a unique tool in cancer investigation and is supported financially by health authorities.

More recently combined imaging of PET and CT or PET and MRI have been used to more precisely demonstrate both anatomical and functional activity of cancer deposits.

7.4   Endoscopic Examinations: Rigid and Flexible Scopes

7.4.1   Rigid Scopes

Most people are familiar with a dentist using a mirror to examine the back of the teeth and the stereotypical image of a doctor using a head mirror to reflect light waves into the mouth to examine the throat, larynx, or back of the nose. The principle of using mirrors and lenses with a light source to examine the inside of body cavities has been extended and refined to remarkable degrees of precision, that were inconceivable a few decades ago. Previously, non-operative examination of the inside of body cavities was limited to the larynx, trachea and air passages (bronchi), oesophagus, stomach, rectum and lower large bowel, bladder and vagina, through rigid or semi-rigid tubes. These are still useful methods of examination as they allow ready visualisation of these organs. They are reasonably simple to use, cheap to buy and are readily available both in doctors' surgeries and hospitals.

> Some internal organs such as the oesophagus or prostate may be well examined for presence of cancer by the use of an ultrasound probe passed through a scope.

7.4.2   Sigmoidoscopy

Although largely replaced by more flexible colonoscopes, old-fashioned readily available rigid metal sigmoidoscopes are still used in isolated country practices and developing countries. Examination of the rectum and lower bowel by a sigmoidoscope can still be a valuable examination for large bowel cancer. More than half of all large bowel cancers are within reach of a rigid sigmoidoscope. Sigmoidoscopy can be performed in a doctor's surgery without anaesthesia and a biopsy of any suspicious tissue can be taken at the time of examination. Some precautions are first taken to empty the bowel of faeces. During the examination the patient usually lies on one side and the sigmoidoscope is passed through the anus. The instrument is fitted with a small light and air is blown into the bowel to inflate it and so open up the lumen or bowel cavity. This air and the passage of the instrument are uncomfortable but not unbearable.

7.4.3　Proctoscopy

Examination of the anus and lower rectum can be carried out quite simply in a doctor's surgery with a small metal tube-like instrument called a proctoscope or anal speculum. Although it does not penetrate far into the rectum, it is fitted with a small light and can be useful for detecting or treating lesions in or near the anus such as haemorrhoids or cancer of the anus, which is rather rare.

7.4.4　Vaginal Speculum

A vaginal speculum is a metal instrument that allows a doctor to examine the walls of the vagina or cervix of the uterus in the surgery without significant discomfort to the patient.

7.4.5　Laryngoscopy and Bronchoscopy

The larynx can be examined indirectly with a mirror in the doctor's surgery but a more direct examination of the sensitive larynx or main air passages is usually carried out with a rigid laryngoscope or bronchoscope in hospital under general anaesthesia.

7.4.6　Oesophagoscopy

Similarly, in the past, examinations of the oesophagus were usually carried out in hospital under general anaesthesia using a rigid oesophagoscope.

7.4.7　Cystoscopy

The bladder too may be examined with a rigid cystoscope usually in hospital under general anaesthesia

7.4.8   Echo-Endoscopy

Some internal organs such as the oesophagus or prostate can be examined for presence of cancer by the use of an ultrasound probe passed through a scope. The combined use of scope and ultrasound probe is referred to as echo-endoscopy.

7.4.9   Flexible Scopes

In recent years advances have seen great progress made in fitting a series of lenses and mirrors and a light source to flexible fibre-optic endoscopes and colonoscopes as well as a great variety of flexible scopes to replace many of the rigid metal scopes previously used.

7.4.10   Gastroscopy or Endoscopy

Skilled gastroenterologists can pass the modern gastroscopes or endoscopes without general anaesthesia. Provided the patient is suitably sedated these instruments are passed with little discomfort. They allow examination, not only of the oesophagus and stomach, but also of the first part of the duodenum. Through the duodenum and at the ampulla of Vater they also allow examination of the opening of the bile duct from the liver and gall bladder and the pancreatic duct. Radio-opaque material (dye) can be injected into these ducts allowing ERCP X-rays to be taken for more detailed examination.

7.4.11   Colonoscopy

The colonoscope is similarly a flexible instrument that can be passed through the anus and around the whole length of large bowel to allow examination of all the length of the large bowel. The instrument can be used to remove pre-malignant polyps or to take biopsies of a suspected cancer. Special preparation is required to empty the bowel clear of faeces before the colonoscope is used. This instrument may be passed without undue discomfort if the patient is well sedated, although for some patients general anaesthesia may be preferred.

A less invasive bowel examination is by *virtual colonoscopy* in which the bowel is prepared as for a colonoscopy, an enema mixture is given and the colon is scanned by CT. Anaesthesia is not required and accuracy of detection of colorectal lesions is probably comparable but if a lesion is detected and biopsy or removal of a polyp is required a true colonoscopy is still required.

7.4.12 Laparoscopy (Peritoneoscopy) and Thoracoscopy

The body cavities – the peritoneal cavity and the pleural cavities can also be examined by passing an instrument called a laparoscope (or peritoneoscope) or a thoracoscope through a small incision into the cavity. This is carried out under general anaesthesia in the operating theatre. Through these instruments the surgeon can examine the contents of the body cavities. First a harmless gas (CO_2) is used to fill the peritoneal cavity to separate movable organs and allow manipulation of the instrument between loops of bowel and other tissues and viscera. The examiner may be able to take biopsies if suspicious lesions are seen. Special equipment is now available to carry out some surgical operations using similar scopes with surgical instruments passed through a second or third small opening in the abdominal or chest wall. Some cancer operations can be carried out in this way.

7.4.13 Culdoscopy

Culdoscopy is a similar examination of the pelvis. The instrument is passed into the pelvic cavity through a small incision made in the top of the back wall of the vagina.

7.5   Indirect Evidence of Cancer

Blood tests may show either direct or indirect evidence of cancer.

7.5.1   Blood and Serum Tests

Haemoglobin and red cell count (RCC)
    Most cancers eventually cause some degree of anaemia, which manifests as decreased haemoglobin and red blood cell counts but some tumours might be quite advanced before this becomes apparent.

7.5.2   White Cell Count (WCC)

The total white cell count might also show a reaction to some types of cancer but most significantly the number and type of white cells might be the first direct indication of leukaemia.

7.5.3   Erythrocyte Sedimentation Rate (ESR)

The ESR is an index of blood sedimentation and increases with elevation of certain proteins in the blood due to ill-health. Many organic disease processes, including cancer, are associated with a raised ESR, but apart from giving an indication of the severity of disease, the test can be useful in giving an indication of response to treatment given. If a raised ESR falls after cancer treatment it suggests that the treatment has been effective although it cannot be regarded as a guarantee of complete cure.

7.5.4   Serum Biochemistry

Some types of cancer are likely to change biochemical components in the blood. For example cancer of the prostate gland may cause an elevation of the enzyme *serum acid phosphatase,* advanced breast cancer may cause elevation of serum calcium and a particular type of large bowel cancer, papillary adenocarcinoma, may cause loss of potassium from the bowel resulting in fall in serum potassium. Cancers in the liver may cause a degree of liver failure which may also be detected in changes in serum biochemistry after checking that the patient is not suffering from cirrhosis.

7.5.5   Tumour Markers

The potential for using biological tumour markers to help detect early cancer or recurrent cancer is constantly under study. Many tumour markers are now useful in determining the presence of cancer. Some are already in regular clinical use with varying degrees of reliability. The most regularly used are the PSA for prostate cancer (as previously discussed); the carcino-embryonic antigen (CEA) test for cancers of the alimentary tract, especially large bowel cancers; and the alpha-foeto-protein (AFP), a test for primary liver cancer and germ-cell cancers and the CA125 test for ovarian cancer. Useful markers in detection of germ-cell cancers are AFP, human chorionic gonadotropin (HCG) and lactate dehydrogenase (LDH). No doubt further tumour markers will be found to be clinically valuable in detecting early cancers as well as in determining response to treatment or tumour recurrence.

> Valuable and reliable tumour marker tests, indicating the presence or absence of specific cancers will be available for more specific clinical use in the not too distant future

Tumour markers are also used to estimate the success or otherwise of treatment of the cancer. A fall will indicate a good initial result of therapy but a subsequent rise might indicate the presence of recurrent or residual cancer either at the original tumour site or elsewhere.

7

7.5.6   The Future

As yet, no tumour marker test is totally reliable on its own, but a great deal of work is being carried out in this field. The major issue is one of specificity and sensitivity being inversely related – the more specific the criteria (higher concentrations) for a tumour marker the less cancers are identified, and these pre-dominantly are more advanced, conversely the less specific criteria identify more cancers but there will be more false positves.

It seems certain that valuable and reliable tumour marker tests, indicating the presence or absence of specific cancers, will be available for more specific clinical use in the not too distant future.

7.6   Direct Evidence of Cancer

7.6.1   Biopsy

The ultimate test for cancer is in the tissue biopsy in which a piece of tissue is taken from a suspected cancer and examined microscopically. Provided a truly representative sample of tissue is taken, examination of the cells in the biopsy specimen will usually allow the pathologist to determine not only whether a cancer is present, but also the type of cancer, the tissue of origin of the cancer and even the degree of malignancy. In some cancers the biopsy may also give a good indication of the most appropriate treatment and likelihood of a cure being possible.

Ideally a biopsy is taken before any treatment, including surgical treatment, is started. This helps the clinical team to decide upon most appropriate treatment. Often biopsies are also taken by a surgeon during an operation. Usually the surgeon will take a small representative sample of a suspected cancer (incision biopsy) or if the tumour is small the surgeon may remove the whole tumour for examination (excision biopsy). Sometimes the surgeon will biopsy tissues or an organ nearest to the cancer to be sure that it does not have cancer cells spread into it, that is to be sure of a "clear margin" of tissue free of cancer (Fig. 7.8). A number of techniques have been developed to help make a diagnosis by biopsy.

EXERCISE

List features of microscopic appearance that suggest a biopsy shows a highly malignant tumour.

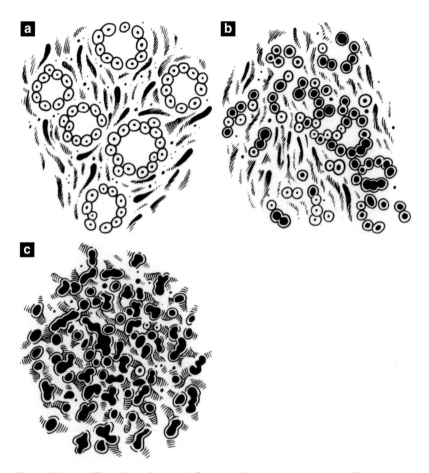

Fig. 7.8. Diagrams illustrating microscopic features of **(a)** normal prostate gland, **(b)** changes of early "in-situ" or "latent" prostate cancer and **(c)** more advanced, invasive prostate cancer.

7.6.2   Needle Aspiration or "Punch Out" Biopsy

For some tumours – as for example, some lumps in the breast, a special needle can be inserted into the lump to aspirate or suck out sufficient cells or tissue for biopsy examination. There is also a special needle called "Trucut" with a "punch out" mechanism that allows a small core of tissue to be "punched out". This might be done under local anaesthesia without admission to hospital or sometimes a general anaesthetic may be required. Provided a representative specimen is taken and an expert team is readily available to examine the specimen, a diagnosis might be made rapidly with little disturbance to the patient.

Needle aspiration or "punch out" biopsy may now be used for a number of different types of tumours in a variety of other tissues such as the prostate gland, the liver, the thyroid gland, or deep-seated tumours in the limbs or in the chest.

7.6.3 Aspiration Cytology

This is similar to aspiration biopsy except that it applies to the examination for cells in cysts or other fluid. A cyst in the breast or elsewhere may be aspirated and by special preparation the contents are examined for the presence of malignant cells. If malignant cells are found, a positive diagnosis of cancer can be made. If, however, no malignant cells are found there may still be some doubt as to whether cancer is present and a further biopsy may be necessary. It is still possible that cancer cells could be in the cyst or adjacent lump but not in the sample of fluid taken.

7.6.4 Bone Marrow Biopsy

A similar aspiration technique is used to obtain specimens of bone marrow, which is especially important in determining the presence and type of any suspected leukaemia. Bone marrow biopsies can also be valuable in confirming the presence of metastatic cancer in bones.

7.6.5 Standard Paraffin Section Biopsy and Frozen Section Biopsy

Preparation and staining of a biopsy specimen for microscopic examination usually takes several days. The tissue is prepared embedding it in a wax block and staining it to reveal special features of the cells. In some circumstances it may be important for the surgeon to know the diagnosis immediately, so that any necessary cancer operation can be completed without delay. An experienced pathologist can often make a diagnosis without delay by using the technique of *frozen section*. In a frozen section examination the biopsy specimen is prepared by immediately being frozen solid so that it can then be finely sliced. Fine slices are then stained with a simple stain and examined microscopically. The pathologist may then be able to give the surgeon an accurate diagnosis within a few minutes. If the patient is anaesthetised and prepared for operation, the surgeon may then be able to completely remove any cancer at the same operation. Frozen-section techniques are now highly accurate for most cancers if used by skilled pathologists, but for some cancers it may not be possible to determine an accurate diagnosis until special pathology sections embedded in wax have been prepared some days later. Sometimes a variety of special stains or even other tests, such as immunohistochemistry tests, using antibodies against tumour markers, are needed.

EXERCISE

List the most useful investigations that help in establishing a diagnosis of cancer.

Treating Cancer

8

In this chapter you will learn about:

> *Can cancer be cured? An outline of prognostic factors*
> *Methods of treatment*
> *Surgery*
> *Radiotherapy, including brachytherapy*
> *Chemotherapy – anti-cancer drugs*
> *Hormone therapy*
> *Immunotherapy*
> *Cell mediated anti-cancer activity*
> *Other treatments under study*
> *General care*
> *Supportive care and supportive care teams*
> *Psychological and spiritual help*
> *Follow up care*
> *The specialty of palliative care*
> *"Alternative medicine"*

8.1   Can Cancer Be Cured? An Outline of Prognosis

Although cancer is a frightening word, it is a fact that in modern developed societies most cancers are cured. The possibility of cure of a cancer depends upon a number of factors, especially the tissue from which it has grown and the type of cancer cells in it, the size and position of the tumour in the body, the degree of abnormality of the individual cancer cells, the structures into which the cancer may have grown and the presence and site of any metastatic spread. The age and general health of the patient are also significant. The patient's natural defence reactions may be highly significant although, as yet, not clearly understood and not yet able to be measured with any confidence.

Many of the most significant factors will depend upon how quickly the cancer is detected and treated. A small cancer detected early and before it has spread or involved other tissues may be eminently curable whereas the same cancer

F. O. Stephens and K. R. Aigner, *Basics of Oncology,*
DOI: 10.1007/978-3-540-92925-3_8, © Springer-Verlag Berlin Heidelberg 2009

8

neglected, perhaps for some months, until it has enlarged and spread to other sites, may be quite incurable.

Many years ago a great American pathologist, Arthur Purdy Stout, said:

"The best chance of curing cancer lies in the hands of the therapist who makes the first attempt".

Nowadays this should be paraphrased as:

"The best chance of curing many advanced and aggressive cancers lies in the hands of the team of therapists that makes the first attempt".

That is, a cancer that has recurred after a failed attempt at treatment is more difficult to cure than it would have been at the first attempt. The quality of treatment given to the patient, especially in the initial treatment, is a most important factor in determining whether or not a cure is likely. For difficult cancers, this is often now best achieved with integrated treatment and a team approach.

8.2   In Western Societies More Cancers are Cured than Not Cured

This is certainly true because the most common cancers are basal cell cancers of skin and squamous cell cancers of skin. Not only do these cancers grow relatively slowly and spread relatively late, if at all, they are usually obvious to the patient and doctor when they are quite small, and if properly treated at that stage they are eminently curable. Even the more aggressive and dangerous pigmented skin cancer, the melanoma, is usually eminently curable in its early stages. With people becoming more aware of the danger of any change in a pigmented mole, or other dark spot on the skin, most melanomas are now detected before they have spread. If properly treated at this stage they are effectively cured.

All this is good news but, even better, is the fact that even excluding skin cancers, more cancers can now be cured than not cured.

The common cancers of the breast and bowel and cancers of the uterus are usually curable now that methods of early detection are widely practised. It is most important that these cancers should be detected early as the outlook is so much better if treatment is initiated when these cancers are small. For this reason, a great deal of effort has been spent in establishing cancer screening clinics to detect potentially curable cancers before they reach an incurable stage. This is now likely to need a diagnostic and therapeutic team effort.

Cure can now be expected for most cancers in the head and neck region, including the lips, mouth and throat, larynx, salivary glands and thyroid gland.

Until fairly recently, cancers that develop in cells scattered widely throughout the body tissues, such as the lymphomas and leukaemias, were considered incurable but with modern treatment methods, increasing numbers of patients with these malignancies are being cured including the majority of children who develop leukaemias.

The most common internal cancer in men, prostate cancer, can now usually be diagnosed at a curable stage. However because most of these cancers are slowly growing and not necessarily life threatening during the patient's otherwise expected lifespan, there may be uncertainty as to whether radical treatment to establish a cure is justified. Sometimes the outlook without curative treatment does not justify the severe side effects of curative treatment, especially in elderly men with other health problems.

The outlook for germ-cell cancers of the testis underwent dramatic change over the last two to three decades of the twentieth century. From being cancers with a poor prognosis except when treated at a very early stage, most are now cured when treated with combined and integrated therapy programs using modern chemotherapy, radiation therapy and surgery.

Integrated treatment methods have also improved the curability of a number of other cancers including more advanced head and neck cancers, sarcomas, especially in limbs, and previously high-risk stomach and breast cancers.

Cancers with the worst prognosis (least likely to be cured) are often those that develop in deep body tissues and are usually not obvious until they have spread to lymph nodes or other tissues. These include cancers of the oesophagus, pancreas and lung. Hence the search for methods of earlier detection of these cancers. Other cancers with poor prognosis include those in organs that cannot be easily dispensed with such as the liver or a major part of the brain.

With modern endoscopic techniques, stomach cancer can now also be detected at a curable stage. In Japan, where this cancer is common and screening tests are becoming a routine, most are now diagnosed at an early stage and are cured.

8.3 Methods of Treatment

The three mainstays of cancer treatment are surgery (meaning operative surgery), radiotherapy and chemotherapy.

8.3.1 Principles of Treatment of Potentially Curable Regional Cancers

The main principle of treatment of any new and potentially curable cancer is to treat one step beyond the apparent limits of the cancer.

With an inflammatory condition, such as an acutely inflamed appendix, only the appendix needs to be removed to cure the condition. Similarly in treatment of benign lesions such as benign cysts, adenomas or polyps, only the lesion needs to be removed. Best treatment of cancer however, requires surgical removal of more than just the apparent cancer. Tissues adjacent to the cancer into which cancer cells might have spread are also removed. Similarly if treatment involves radiotherapy, it is given to tissues beyond the apparent edge of the cancer, that is tissues into which microscopic cancer cells might have spread. Chemotherapy is often given in addition to surgery and/or radiotherapy if the cancer being treated is one that has significant risk of having already spread beyond the local primary

The main principle of treatment of any new and potentially curable cancer is to treat one step beyond the apparent limits of the cancer.

8

site or region being treated even though there may be no evidence of more distant spread.

8.3.2   Surgery

The discipline of surgery is that part of medicine and medical practice that is likely to involve need of a surgical operation. The word surgery is also often used to mean operative surgery and it is in this context that the word surgery is used in the following paragraphs.

Before the discovery of general anaesthesia and the first use of ether as a general anaesthetic by Dr Crawford Long in America in 1842, operative surgery was very primitive but nevertheless it was the only available effective cancer treatment.

Early use of general anaesthesia for operative surgery was followed by rampant cross infection with a high mortality rate. The situation changed after the discovery of micro-organisms in infected wounds by great world scientists Pasteur in France, Koch in Germany, Semmeilweiss in Hungary and Lister in England (Fig. 8.1).

These changes in operating under general anaesthesia with aseptic conditions allowed operative surgery to develop and progress to what it is today. Thus operative surgery became the first widely used effective and generally applicable anti-cancer treatment.

Surgery was thus the first effective form of cancer treatment. It is now used to establish a diagnosis, to effect a cure or in some advanced or incurable cases, to give good palliation and relief of symptoms. When possible the surgeon's primary objective is to excise the cancer in its entirety, together with all adjacent tissues into which cancer cells may have spread. For many cancers, especially for early skin cancers and small cancers on lips or in the mouth, surgery offers a relatively simple, straightforward, quick and effective method of eradicating cancers. A complete cure can be expected without any residual problem. For more advanced cancers that have spread to or are likely to have spread into draining lymph nodes, the surgeon removes not only the primary cancer but all the draining lymph nodes likely to be involved. The primary cancer and lymph nodes are best removed in continuity in one block of tissue where this is feasible. This is called a "*block dissection*" and a high incidence of long-term cure can also be expected. If a great deal of tissue has to be removed, the surgical team may need to do some form of plastic or reconstructive surgical procedure to leave as little defect or deformity as possible. The surgical removal of a tumour is also the most effective cure for the cancer associated weight loss (cancer cachexia), as the cellular source of the abnormal metabolism driving the weight loss is removed.

Used alone successful surgery depends upon establishing diagnosis and treatment early in the disease and before the cancer has spread into tissues that cannot be resected with the primary cancer.

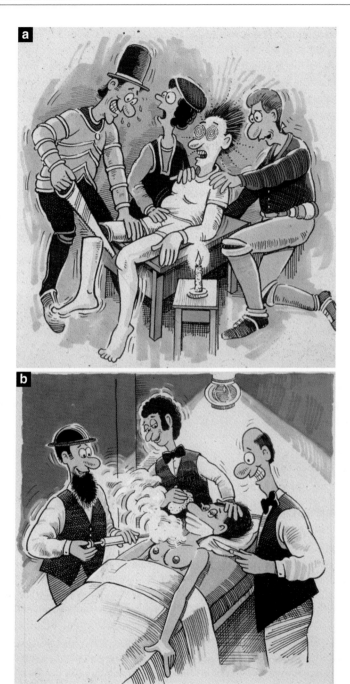

Fig. 8.1. (**a**) Operative surgery before 1842. (**b**) Lister using lysol spray to help create asepsis in an operating theatre

8

For breast cancer that is confined to the breast with possible early involvement of lymph nodes in the axilla, the most common surgical treatment over the past 100 years has been total removal of the affected breast and lymph nodes from the axilla as one block of tissue. This operation, called a *radical mastectomy*, has cured many women with breast cancer over the years but nowadays less radical operations have been equally successful.

For deep-seated cancers the whole or part of the involved organ is usually excised together with nearby draining lymph nodes. Such has been standard treatment for cancer of the stomach, colon, rectum, uterus, ovary, oesophagus, lung, and sometimes the pancreas. For some the cure rate by surgery alone has been good but for others the cure rates by surgery alone have been dismal.

Sarcomas in limbs tend to recur locally in the limb unless widely excised and sometimes the best chance of cure by surgery, especially for big sarcomas, has been by amputation of the affected limb. Newer techniques of combined treatment (discussed later in this chapter) have reduced the need for amputation in many cases.

EXERCISE

What are the possible objectives of surgical operations in treatment of cancer?

8.3.3   Radiotherapy

Radiotherapy is the second oldest effective form of treatment for cancer but has been clinically available only since about the year 1900 following the work of the Curies in France and Dr Roentgen in Germany. Treatment depends upon the sensitivity of dividing cells being destroyed by X-rays or gamma rays emitted from a radioactive source. Treatment, equipment and computer assisted techniques are constantly being improved with improved results in eradicating cancer cells and causing minimal damage to surrounding tissues and cells (Fig. 8.2).

Radiotherapy has the advantage of avoiding a surgical operation but in many cases treatment over 5–8 weeks is required. Radiotherapy has the disadvantage of causing some damage to normal tissues and cells covering and surrounding the cancer in the area treated (the irradiation field). The radiotherapist must have the patient in a correct position so that the radiation beams will include the whole tumour in the irradiated field with minimal exposure of normal tissue. This will

Fig. 8.2. Photograph of a patient
ready for treatment with super-
voltage external radiotherapy

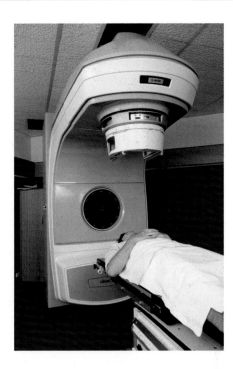

allow greatest destruction of tumour cells with as little as possible damage to
surrounding normal tissues and cells.

Radiotherapy alone is effective treatment for many skin cancers, some head
and neck cancers and for some deep-seated cancers that cannot be totally removed
by surgery. It is also used as a palliative treatment to give relief by reducing the
size of some cancers that cannot be cured by surgery or other means.

The dose of radiotherapy used is critical and must be given by experts. Too
little will not destroy cancer cells but too much will destroy normal tissues and
may result in loss of tissue sometimes with painful ulceration of overlying skin
which may not heal, and other long-term local problems such as damage to an
underlying lung or other tissue. The dose is also cumulative, that is, that once
radiotherapy has been given to a part of the body in a therapeutic dose it cannot
ever be given again to the same site without risk of serious tissue damage.

The actual administration of radiotherapy is quite painless although it may
leave some skin changes, like an erythema resembling sunburn, and may make the
patient feel listless and tired, adding to his or her feeling of depression. Depression is a natural feature of having a cancer. Radiotherapy sometimes adds to the
depression but it usually improves when active treatment has been completed.
Although the red flush of skin change settles a few weeks after radiotherapy,
some minor skin changes with small, visible blood vessels called *telangiectasia*
are often a permanent feature of an area that has in the past been irradiated.

**Radiotherapy is
now often used
in combined,
integrated
treatment
programs,
especially with
surgery and/or
chemotherapy.**

8

8.3.3.1 Brachytherapy

Brachytherapy is a form of radiotherapy in which radio-active needles or "seeds" are inserted into a tumour to give a measured dose of irradiation directly to the cancer. The dose of irradiation given by such needles (withdrawn after the required dose has been administered) or "seeds" (left permanently in place in the cancer) is critical. It is also critical to place the radioactive material in such a position that all of the cancer tissue receives a satisfactory dose of irradiation. Traditional external irradiation can more reliably cover the needed irradiation field but will irradiate surrounding tissues. Brachytherapy will more specifically deliver a dose of irradiation into the cancer but has a greater risk of missing some of the outlying cancer cells. In some clinics, combined use of these two forms of radiotherapy can be used in treating some cancers. In some clinics brachytherapy or combined external irradiation with brachytherapy is becomingly increasingly used in treating prostate cancer when there is a localised limited cancer focus. Results are now believed to be equivalent to radical surgery but with the advantage of fewer side effects.

Radiotherapy is now often used in combined, integrated treatment programs, especially with surgery and/or chemotherapy. For many advanced and aggressive cancers combined and integrated treatment will effect cures that would have been unlikely by using one treatment modality alone. This is why it is becoming increasingly important for patients with aggressive or advanced cancers to be seen by clinicians working in cooperative multidisciplinary teams.

EXERCISE

What are the advantages and disadvantages of treating a cancer by brachytherapy as opposed to external radiotherapy?

8.3.4 Chemotherapy (Cytotoxic Drug Treatment)

Doctors, scientists and others have been searching over the centuries for chemical substances that might cure cancer. The first effective such treatment was reported by Dr George Beatson from the Glasgow Royal Cancer Hospital early in the twentieth century. Dr Beatson reported that oophorectomy (removal of the ovaries) depressed growth of some breast cancers. Hormonal management of breast cancer followed that observation. Next was a report in 1941 by two Americans doctors, Charles Huggins and Clarence Hodges that some prostate cancers responded to treatment with the female hormone stilboestrol. Four years later in 1945 it was first observed that a gas that had been used during World War I, destroyed dividing cells, and so nitrogen mustard was discovered as being a drug that could be used clinically against cancer cells in patients. This was the beginning of modern anti-cancer chemotherapy. Since that time a large number of effective anti-cancer drugs have been developed. These drugs have their greatest effect on dividing cells and because cancer cells are more constantly dividing than normal cells, they are more likely to be affected than normal body cells. The present anti-cancer drugs are grouped or classified according to how they affect dividing cells (Fig. 8.3).

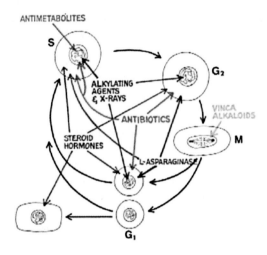

Fig. 8.3. Diagram illustrating the sites of greatest activity on dividing cells of some of the anti-cancer agents

Why are cancer cells more likely to be affected by chemotherapy than normal cells?

8.3.4.1   Anti-Cancer Drugs

Just as details of surgical procedures must be left to trained surgeons and the details of the best use of radiotherapeutic procedures must be left to specialist radiotherapists, so too details of best use of anti-cancer agents are highly complex. The use of complex anti-cancer agents is best guided by experts who are appropriately trained and experienced in their use. However some knowledge of the agents most commonly used should be helpful as a basis for further understanding.

The number of anti-cancer drugs is constantly increasing as newer agents with more selective actions against particular tumour types are discovered. In general they are grouped as:

Antimetabolites. This group of anti-cancer agents predominantly interfere most with synthesis and metabolism of DNA and, to some extent, RNA. They include methotrexate, 5FU (5-fluorouracil), cytarabine, gemcitabine and 6MP (6 mercaptopurine).

DNA damaging agents. These include alkylating agents like cyclophosphamide and ifosfamide and melphalan; antibiotics like adriamycin, actinomycin D and bleomycin; nitrosoureas (such as BCNU and CCNU) and platinum derivatives like cisplatin and carboplatin.

Mitosis inhibitors. This group includes vinca alkaloids (like vincristine and vinblastine) and taxanes (Taxol).

Cancer cell enzyme inactivators. This is a new class of anti-cancer agent recently discovered and undergoing much research. The first, code-named STI 571 (trade name Gleevec or Glivec), is the enzyme *tyrosine-kinase* inhibitor. Tyrosine-kinase is an essential for cancer cell reproduction. STI 571 was first found to counteract the *Philadelphia chromosome* of chronic myeloid leukaemia and, in treating this leukaemia, results have been very encouraging. STI 571 is now being used in trials of treating other cancers, particularly with certain gastrointestinal stromal cancers and renal cancers, with encouraging results. There may be a place for similar management of some breast cancers and prostate cancers.

All effective anti-cancer drugs presently available have side effects. Unfortunately all effective anti-cancer drugs presently available have side effects that affect some people more than others. Some become manifest early as acute toxic side effects. Some are long-term or late side effects and may not be apparent for months or even years. Until all adverse side effects of such agents are well understood experienced specialists should oversee their clinical use.

8.3.4.2   Using Combined Anti-Cancer Agents

In treating cancers, the specialist cancer clinician (oncologist) selects drugs that are known to be effective against the type of cancer being treated with least possible damage to normal body cells. In general, appropriate combinations of effective drugs are more effective than large and increasingly toxic doses of

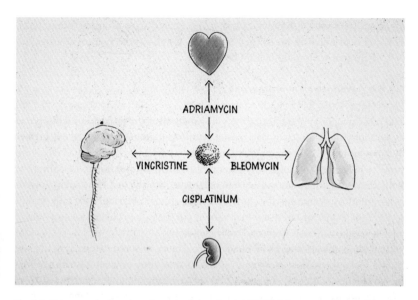

Fig. 8.4. Diagram indicating the principle of use of multiple agents in combination in treating a cancer rather than using larger and more toxic doses of just one agent. As illustrated, provided the drugs are known to be active against the type of cancer being treated, a selection of two or more agents should have increased activity against the target cancer cell. It is like hitting the cancer cell in two or more places at the same time. It is safer to avoid using drugs with the same side effects so that normal cells are less likely to be damaged by multiple agents

one drug only. Much research is constantly being carried out to discover the most effective and safest combinations and dose and timing schedules of drugs against different types of cancer with minimal damage to normal dividing cells (Fig. 8.4).

8.3.4.3 Time and Concentration of Anti-Cancer Cytotoxic Drugs on Different Cancer Cell Types

Another aspect of the use of anti-cancer drugs is the sensitivity of the cancer cells being treated in relation to the length of time of their exposure to the drugs and their relative sensitivity to drug concentration. For example 5FU is generally more effective if given by continuous infusion over several days whereas melphalan seems to have a greater impact given in greater concentration over a shorter period, possibly an hour or so. Similarly cancers of different types respond differently to different periods of exposure and to different concentrations of agents. Gastrointestinal cancers and mouth and throat cancers seem to respond best to continuous prolonged drug exposure over days or weeks whereas melanoma responds best to a more intense concentration of agents that can only be given over a short period. There is still much to be learned about dose, combinations, length of time of exposure and concentration of agents to achieve

There is also much to be learned about when anti-cancer cytotoxic drugs are best integrated with radiotherapy or surgery.

greatest effect on the type of cancer being treated with minimal side effects. There is also much to be learned about when anti-cancer cytotoxic drugs are best integrated with radiotherapy or surgery.

8.3.4.4   Palliative Chemotherapy

The most widely applied use of the anti-cancer drugs is in treating widespread cancers or cancers that for one reason or another cannot be treated effectively by surgery or by radiotherapy. Although some drugs will, on occasions, cure some widespread cancers, in general this form of treatment is palliative. Palliation means that the cancer may be reduced in size and the patient may be given relief of symptoms for some time, but almost invariably the cancer will re-develop sooner or later, at which time it will be more resistant to anti-cancer agents. Eventual death from the cancer is likely.

Palliative chemotherapy, by reducing the cancer, will usually prolong life and should make the patient more comfortable. Sometimes, however, because of the inconvenience and problems associated with treatment and the possible distress of side-effects (see "*side effects*" below) there is doubt as to whether palliative chemotherapy is worthwhile. In each case the medical attendants should discuss the likely benefits and possible problems with the patient and members of the patient's family before a final decision is made about having this form of treatment. Although it is the doctor's responsibility to give informed advice, the final decision as to whether to have palliative chemotherapy should be made by the patient. If doubt exists in the patient's mind about the desirability of having such treatment, a trial course of treatment may be appropriate, that is, that treatment be commenced with the proviso that if the patient finds treatment too distressing, treatment can be modified or stopped at any time.

8.3.4.5   Adjuvant Chemotherapy

Adjuvant chemotherapy is chemotherapy given following surgery or radiotherapy and is used to treat cancers where it is known there is a significant risk that scattered cancer cells may be present somewhere even though they cannot be detected.

The most proven value of adjuvant chemotherapy is in treating women who have had a breast cancer treated by surgery (mastectomy, segmentectomy or lumpectomy) or a combination of surgery and radiotherapy to the breast region. These are patients who have certain prognostic factors that suggest that, although undetectable, there is a significant risk of some cancer cells already having spread beyond the treated region. Adjuvant chemotherapy is also given as part of the treatment for people (usually young people) who have had bone cancer (osteosarcoma) treated by surgery. The surgery may have been amputation of a limb. Post-operative chemotherapy is now standard even with small osteosarcomas because there is a high risk that some cancer cells will have already escaped from the local tissues and formed micro-metastases in the lungs. Treatment of ovarian cancers and some colo-rectal cancers also now often includes administration of adjuvant chemotherapy to get best long-term results.

8.3.4.6 Systemic and Regional (Intra-Arterial) Chemotherapy

(a) Systemic chemotherapy

The most convenient and simplest way of giving a measured dose of chemotherapy is by intravenous delivery, either by bolus injection or by slow infusion into a vein. After intravenous delivery, drugs are distributed by the bloodstream more or less equally to all parts of the body and should affect cancer cells wherever they may be.

Whilst surgery is limited to treating cancers localised in a particular region that can be excised, and radiotherapy is limited to treating cancer cells in a limited radiation field, chemotherapy is generally given systemically, that is, to treat the body as a whole. Some anti-cancer drugs can be given by mouth but most are given by intravenous injection or infusion. This method of chemotherapy is likely to be the most effective as adjuvant therapy when there is a significant risk that there may be widespread cancer cells remaining somewhere after a primary cancer has been eradicated.

(b) Regional (intra-arterial) chemotherapy Fig. 8.5

When cancers appear to be limited to one particular body region and that region is supplied with blood by one particular artery, it is sometimes possible to concentrate anti-cancer drugs to the cancer by injecting or *infusing* the drugs directly into the artery supplying blood to the cancer. This is called regional or intra-arterial chemotherapy. The initial activity of the agents is concentrated in the tissues supplied by the artery infused before most of it flows into the systemic circulation and then functions as systemic chemotherapy. An alternative to this intra-arterial *infusion* chemotherapy is intra-arterial *perfusion* chemotherapy, with regional vascular isloation. With perfusion chemotherapy, carried out under general anaesthesia, a "closed circuit" pump is often used and the part containing the cancer (usually a limb) has its circulation separated or isolated from the general circulation. A high dose of the drugs is thus concentrated in the isolated tissues containing the cancer without flowing into the general circulation where in such high concentration they would cause severe toxicity. This is a form of delivery used in treating some cancers that may be confined to a limb but respond only to a high concentration of an anti-cancer drug, such as some cases of melanoma or some limb sarcomas.

It is sometimes possible to concentrate anti-cancer drugs to the cancer by injecting or *infusing* the drugs directly into the artery supplying blood to the cancer.

8.3.4.7 Other Regional Chemotherapy

Chemotherapy is sometimes used to achieve a greater regional effect by intra-thecal or intra-ventricular injection, or by intrapleural or intraperitoneal injection. Some drugs do not pass the blood/brain barrier so that to be effective

8

Fig. 8.5. Diagram illustrating the principle of intra-arterial chemotherapy. If all active anti-cancer agents are infused into a small artery that supplies the cancer with all its blood (illustrated in the *bottom* of the diagram) the cancer will be exposed to a greater initial concentration than if the agents are infused into the venous circulation. Infused into the venous circulation they will be distributed more or less equally but in lower concentration to all body tissues. The value of this technique depends on the agents used being active in the form in which they are given. Some agents, e.g. cyclophosphamide, need to be activated by passage through the liver so that for them intra-arterial infusion has no advantage. For some other agents exposure over a prolonged period of time may be of greater importance than a more concentrated exposure

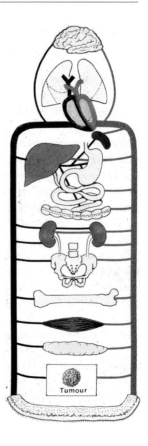

against tumours in the brain they must be given intrathecally (i.e. directly into the cerebro-spinalfluid). Some drugs can be effective in treating skin cancers when incorporated into creams or ointments for local (topical) application.

EXERCISE

Under what circumstances might there be potential advantages in delivering chemotherapy to a cancer by the intra-arterial route?

Intraperitoneal chemotherapy is a form of regional chemotherapy that can be useful in treating some intra-abdominal cancers. The activity of the agents is first concentrated in the peritoneal cavity but some is then absorbed into the general circulation as systemic chemotherapy.

8.3.4.8 Combined Integrated Treatment

For relatively small and uncomplicated localised cancers that can be readily and effectively treated by surgery or radiotherapy, these forms of treatment are best used in a straightforward and usually simple fashion.

For some cancers, however, surgery alone or radiotherapy alone or even surgery and radiotherapy together may not be able to cure most of the patients. Or possibly, a surgical operation required to eradicate the cancer may be so mutilating as to be unacceptable to the patient. In these circumstances, better results can sometimes be achieved by combining surgery and/or radiotherapy and/or chemotherapy.

Present-day treatment of some breast cancers is an example of a widely accepted use of combined treatment. Often nowadays, for women with moderately advanced breast cancer, the breast and axillary lymph nodes are removed surgically and radiotherapy is given to the breast region after surgery. Nearby lymph nodes if not removed at operation may be treated by radiotherapy. However adjuvant chemotherapy is given systematically to control any cancer cells that may have escaped further than draining lymph nodes into the circulation and could be the seeds of future metastatic growths in distant organs or tissues. With such combined and integrated treatment programs survival rates have been improved considerably.

Treating advanced cancer of the cervix is an example where statistics have now shown improved survival rates for women treated by integration of chemotherapy with radiotherapy and surgery rather than by radical surgery alone.

8.3.4.9 Induction Chemotherapy

Induction chemotherapy (sometimes called neoadjuvant, primary, initial, basal, or reducing chemotherapy) is chemotherapy given before any other treatment in order to induce tumour changes. In treating some cancers that appear to remain localised to the site of origin but which are so advanced locally that they are unlikely to be cured by surgery or radiotherapy alone, induction chemotherapy given first can reduce the size and extent of the cancer. This may make it possible to totally remove the reduced tumour either by surgery or using with radiotherapy or using a combination of both.

The primary advantage of administering *induction* chemotherapy is to allow the chemotherapy to flow into the cancer before its vascularity has been compromised. Both surgery and radiotherapy will damage blood vessels and compromise blood

Both surgery and radiotherapy will damage blood vessels and compromise blood flow through tumours.

flow through tumours. If the chemotherapy flows through undamaged arteries supplying the cancer with blood, the cancer should be maximally affected and reduced in size and viability, thus improving the chance of success by subsequent surgery or radiotherapy as well as being immediately effective as systemic pre-operative adjuvant chemotherapy.

If *induction* chemotherapy can be given by regional infusion, directly into the tumour arterial supply, with its greater concentration, it should have an even greater impact on the primary cancer and most of it will still flow off throughout all body tissues and should be effective as immediate systemic "adjuvant" chemotherapy. This means that both the concentrated induction chemotherapy reducing the primary cancer and the immediate pre-operative systemic adjuvant effect on possible micro-metastases are given to best advantage. Hopefully in this way the primary cancer is reduced and small undetected clusters of cancer cells distant from the primary site are completely or partially destroyed before curative surgery or radiotherapy of the primary cancer is carried out. Work investigating this form of combined treatment is showing encouraging results especially in treating some cancers in the head and neck (including the mouth and throat), some stomach cancers, some breast cancers and some cancers and sarcomas in limbs.

In treating locally advanced cancers whether or not induction chemotherapy can be given by regional infusion there should be an advantage in giving at least some chemotherapy before surgery. This should reduce and destroy as much of the cancer as possible whilst its blood supply is still intact, and avoid waiting for a surgical or radiotherapy procedure to be completed before adjuvant chemotherapy is started.

8.3.4.10   Side Effects of Chemotherapy

The risk of using cytotoxic anti-cancer drugs that cells in normal tissues may be damaged. Expert supervision should ensure maximum damage to cancer cells and minimum damage to normal cells and normal body tissues.

Because cancer cells are the most constantly dividing of all cells, they are more susceptible to chemotherapeutic agents than normal cells. However, a number of cells in normal tissues are at risk because they also divide frequently. These include blood-forming cells (in the bone marrow), surface skin and growing hair cells, mucosal cells lining the mouth, throat, stomach and bowel, and cells lining the air passages.

Using chemotherapy and radiotherapy over the same treatment period, has been shown The most serious acute or short-term side effect of most anti-cancer agents is a fall in the white cells or platelets in the blood – this may lead to reduced ability to resist infection or to bleeding problems (granulocyte stimulating factor or G-CSF, stem-cell infusion and bone marrow transfusion are methods of helping to correct this side-effect in more severe cases). Hence regular blood counts are taken and doses of drugs may need to be adjusted. Other common acute side effects are mouth and throat ulcers, nausea and vomiting, hair loss, or bleeding from the bowel. Whilst some side effects are common, provided the patient survives their toxicity, almost all of them are reversible and they abate after drugs have been stopped.

A small number of anti-cancer drugs may affect function of the heart, lungs, kidneys, central nervous system or peripheral nerves, but these effects are not often seen because they are unlikely to occur with normal doses of drugs. Even so, it is still necessary to watch closely and stop treatment at any sign of these problems. With proper supervision by oncologists, the risk of very serious problems is small (Fig. 8.6).

If chemotherapy is infused intra-arterially or otherwise given regionally, the risk of damaging local tissues with local or regional side effects will be greater because the chemotherapy is concentrated in tissues near the cancer that are supplied by the artery that is infused. Such regional infusions should be given only by clinicians experienced in these techniques.

to be more effective than using the two treatment modalities separately. However potential damage to surrounding normal tissues is also greater.

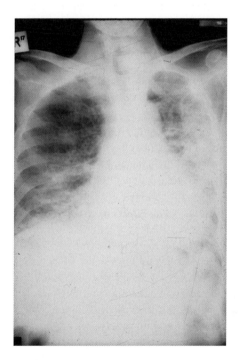

Fig. 8.6. Major side effects of different anti-cancer agents are often different. This chest X-ray shows pulmonary fibrosis that developed as a serious side-effect in a patient being treated with bleomycin

Fertilisation and Pregnancy

Cells in the ovaries of young women and cells in the testes of men are constantly dividing to produce ova or spermatozoa for potential reproduction and development of a new embryo. If chemotherapy is necessary for such people, they are advised to avoid pregnancy during treatment and for at least 12 months afterwards due to the risk of abnormal ova or spermatozoa. There is even a risk of permanent sterility. In the case of young males, keen to become fathers, spermatozoa can be produced and kept in cold storage (in liquid nitrogen) before chemotherapy is started so that it can be used for fertilisation at a later date. Sometimes it may also be possible to take and store ova from young females before commencing chemotherapy. These can be fertilised and implanted into the uterus at a later date if subsequent cancer treatment has been successful.

Late or long-term side effects of chemotherapy have been less apparent than the more acute side effects and in fact not all long-term side effects have been confirmed. Such delayed side effects as impairment of hearing or balance, bone marrow dysplasias and delayed haematological toxicity are becoming well documented although fortunately they are not common. Prolonged use of some anti-cancer drugs can even cause a second cancer. All alkylating agents can be associated with bone marrow dysplasia *(myelodysplastic syndrome)* or rarely acute leukaemia. This small risk is highest with the alkylating agent *melphalan*. A second group of drugs *(the topoisomerase II inhibitors doxorubicin, epirubicin, etoposide, teniposide etc)* can also be associated with a mild increased risk of myelodysplastic syndrome or acute leukaemia. The risk of leukaemia is further increased when chemotherapy is combined with radiotherapy.

8.3.4.11   Concomitant Chemotherapy and Radiotherapy: The So Called "Sandwich Treatment"

Using chemotherapy and radiotherapy over the same treatment period, has been shown to be more effective than using the two treatment modalities separately. Some chemotherapeutic agents e.g. cisplatinum, appear to sensitise cells to radiotherapy. Although responses in the cancer are likely to be significantly greater, it is apparent that the potential damage to surrounding normal tissues is also greater, thus greater regional side effects. Programs for such concomitant treatment schedules are under study but until further clarified they should be used with great care and limited to experts in specialised cancer centres. Some reports of using intra-arterial chemotherapy concomitant with radiotherapy in treating locally advanced primary and secondary melanoma masses have also been encouraging but because there is potential for serious tissue damage such treatment schedules must be restricted to specialised centres.

8.4   Other Important Treatments

8.4.1   Hormone Therapy

8.4.1.1   Breast Cancer

Since 1896 when Dr George Beatson observed regression of breast cancer after removal of the ovaries, it has been shown that in a number of women, especially young (pre-menopausal) women, breast cancer is to a greater or lesser extent dependent upon the female sex hormone oestrogen. Just as removal of the major source of the patient's own circulating oestrogen (by oophorectomy) results in regression of breast cancer in many patients, giving more oestrogen to women with breast cancer can result in the cancer growing more rapidly. Removal of the ovaries is still sometimes used in treating cancer of the breast in pre-menopausal women (i.e. women with active ovaries) if the cancer is widespread or is so advanced that it cannot be cured by surgery or by radiotherapy. Unfortunately, removal of the ovaries or other hormone treatments rarely, if ever, results in complete cure, although it often results in a period of worthwhile regression.

When the cancer enlarges again in younger women whose ovaries have been removed, or in older women whose ovaries are not actively functioning, a further improvement may be gained by giving male hormones, the androgens. An even greater number may respond to one of the more recently developed anti-oestrogen products. The first and still most widely used anti-oestrogen agent is called *Tamoxifen*.

Hormone manipulation has a distinct advantage over other forms of chemo-therapy because hormones are less likely to cause serious side effects. However, the male hormone, androgen, will cause most female patients to develop certain male characteristics such as a deepening of the voice and growth of hair on the face. It may also cause an increase in sexual desire (libido) that can be distress-ing for some patients such as women without a partner. Modified androgens with reduced side effects are an improvement but none is without any side effects.

Another form of hormone therapy used in the past was to remove or other-wise put out of action other glands – the adrenal or pituitary that are responsible for oestrogen production after the ovaries have ceased to function or had been removed. Nowadays their actions can be suppressed by the use of luteinising hormone releasing hormone (LH-RH) agonists and *aromatase inhibitors*. If this is done, other precautions must be taken and medications given to replace other essential functions of these glands.

The original hormonal treatments of breast cancer have now been largely replaced by more modern hormone treatment schedules that should be adminis-tered carefully by specialist oncologists.

Anti-Oestrogens: Tamoxifen

The anti-oestrogen compound, Tamoxifen, has a somewhat similar effect to androgen but has the distinct advantage of being relatively free from side effects. Tamoxifen is also more likely to be effective in a larger number of patients (including older women), than androgens or other agents.

Whilst Tamoxifen is often effective and is the most widely used hormonal agent (actually it acts in competition with oestrogen) it rarely causes any upset to the patient in the short term. When used over several years there is some risk that it may alter the uterine mucosa and can even stimulate a cancer in the uterus. This risk is small but most doctors now limit the use of Tamoxifen to 5 years unless it is clearly essential to use it for longer periods. Studies have now shown that

8

used as adjuvant chemotherapy, after treatment of breast cancer in women with hormone receptor positive cancers, hormone therapy can significantly reduce the risk of both recurrent disease and mortality.

Cortisone

The adrenal gland hormone, cortisone, may also suppress some cancers. It is often used in combination with cytotoxic chemotherapeutic agents in treatment of breast cancer, some cases of leukaemia, the lymphomas, especially Hodgkin disease, (*Chap. 19*), adenocarcinoma of the kidney (*Chap. 17.2.2*), advanced prostate cancer (*Chap. 16.2.4*) and a rare cancer of plasmocytes in bone called multiple myeloma (*Chap. 19.8*).

Hormone Side Effects

Most patients tolerate hormone therapy better than chemotherapy. However hormones may sometimes have some serious long-term side effects after prolonged use. Oestrogens can cause thrombosis and, in males, some feminising effects. Androgens in females can cause hypertension as well as troublesome mascularising effects. Removal of the adrenals or pituitary glands also leaves problems of endocrine balance that must be managed.

Hormone treatment is often more readily accepted by patients and the medical profession as being more "natural", more scientific, and less toxic than cytotoxic chemotherapy. Unfortunately, however, the good responses of hormone treatment of widespread cancer are usually relatively short-lived and eventually most of the cancers re-develop. Each time they re-develop they are less responsive to other forms of hormone management and eventually become unaffected by all forms of hormone management.

Long-Term Hormone Therapy

Small doses of oestrogen were commonly given to menopausal and post-menopausal women to relieve hot flushes, depression, vaginal dryness loss of sexual libido and other menopausal symptoms. This hormone replacement therapy (HRT) given over a prolonged period, was known to be associated with a slightly increased risk of breast cancer as well as a small risk of deep vein thrombosis. Oestrogen therapy was then replaced by medications combining small doses of oestrogen with progesterone. However it has now been shown that there is still a small risk of side effects from oestrogen which are possibly even greater, from the combined medication, including increasing the risk of osteoporosis, thrombosis and cardiac problems. From recent studies there is no apparent increased risk of breast cancer if HRT is given to post menopausal women for no longer than 2 years and very little risk if given for no more than 5 years. However women who have already been treated for breast cancer or women in other high-risk groups are not given such treatment.

New Agents

New more effective agents are constantly being developed and tested. Herceptin is discussed in a later chapter (Sect. 12.7 in Chap. 12). Tests on biopsy specimens indicate likely response to Herceptin if needed.

8.4.1.2 Prostate Cancer

In 1941 Charles Huggins and Clarence Hodges, showed that a large percentage of cancers of the prostate regressed after either the removal of male hormone (by castration) or administration of a female hormone (oestrogen). This was the first study that showed that some hormone dependent cancers can be influenced by giving the patient an antagonistic hormone. Castration is sometimes still used in treatment of prostate cancer, and can be worthwhile, but it gives only temporary control in the majority of patients. Oestrogen is no longer used because there are better hormonal agents now available that don't cause the desire and ability to have sexual activity to be so suppressed and there is less likelihood of other changes in sexual characteristics such as enlargement of the man's breast tissue. Anti-androgen drugs luteinising hormone releasing hormone agonists (LH-RH) have a similar cancer suppressive activity with fewer side effects than with oestrogens (*see Chap. 16*).

8.4.1.3 Other Possible Hormone Sensitive Cancers

Other cancers that respond to hormones include cancer in the male breast, which often responds to castration, although a more acceptable treatment is Tamoxifen to which it will often respond. Cancer of the lining inside the uterus (endometrial cancer) may respond to progesterone. Sometimes cancer of the kidney will respond either to male or female hormones, and some cases of thyroid cancer will be at least temporarily suppressed by the thyroid hormone, thyroxine.

8.4.2 Immunotherapy

The body's natural defence against invasion by organisms and other foreign matter is through its immune defence system. The body also has some immune defences against malignant cells and, possibly, development of cancer may be caused by some fault or breakdown in these protective mechanisms. (Some present concepts of these defence mechanisms are discussed below under *Cell mediated anti-cancer activity.*)

Attempts have been made to develop immunity against cancer but the only real success has been vaccines against viruses that are associated with cancer directly against HPV (the human papilloma virus) and indirectly by immunising against Hepatitis B.

Three groups of immunological substances of particular interest are interferon, the interleukins and tumour necrosis factor (TNF).

A great deal of research is concerned with determining the nature of these immunological defence mechanisms and trying to improve them or assist them in people with cancer. These approaches will one day be of considerable practical value in cancer treatment.

Injections of certain relatively harmless organisms such as the cowpox virus, BCG or (*Corynebacterium parvum*). Both are harmless bacteria and have been used in trials in the treatment of some malignancies to stimulate natural immune defence mechanisms. Some isolated successes have been reported, especially in the treatment of melanoma and lymphomas. Unfortunately as yet for most cancers, little if any clinical benefit has resulted although further worthwhile studies are in progress, especially in vaccine treatment of advanced melanoma. There is still a place for clinical use of BCG in treatment of some bladder cancers and prolonged cancer control is well established in many of these patients.

8.4.2.1 Monoclonal Antibodies

Many attempts have been made to develop antibodies with specific activity against a particular cancer. In animal studies this has been possible in a number of different models, especially with several tumours types in mice. There have been three somewhat different therapeutic objectives:

1. One is to develop "killer antibodies" that specifically act against a particular cancer.
2. Another is to develop "magic bullets" where antibodies are used to carry an anti-cancer chemotherapeutic agent or a radioisotope or other such agent directly to the cancer cells wherever they might be.
3. The third potential use of monoclonal antibodies is to identify the presence of cancer cells by reaction to specific antibodies.

The application of these principles to treatment of clinical cancers in humans has met with some encouraging results, especially in treating metastatic breast cancer.

Recently developed techniques in biotechnology have made it possible to manufacture so called monoclonal antibodies that are aimed at specific vital targets in certain cancers. These include malignant lymphoma, breast and bowel cancers. The use of these antibodies is relatively new, e.g. mabthera for lymphoma, herceptin in breast cancer and erbitux for bowel cancer. In general these antibodies are used in combination with chemotherapy. Despite their great expense they are showing considerable effectivity, although their final role is still being evaluated.

Herceptin (trastuzumad) is a commercially available humanised monoclonal antibody medication that specifically targets cancer cells. In fact it specifically targets a certain protein, human epithelial growth factor (HER2). HER2 is responsible for normal cell growth and cell division but HER positive cancer cells have raised HER receptors on their surface and grow more quickly than normal cells. Herceptin can also activate the immune system to kill HER2 positive cancer cells. This explains why cancer growth is more specifically retarded by Herceptin. In some patients Herceptin is considerably more effective if used in combination with chemotherapy, especially taxones. Herceptin is expensive but is relatively non-toxic in clinical doses.

Three groups of immunological substances of particular interest are interferon, the interleukins and tumour necrosis factor (TNF).

8.4.2.2   Interferon

It was first recognised in the 1930s that infection of animal cells with one virus would for a time "interfere" with infection by other viruses. Thirty years later it was discovered that a protein substance was released from cells infected with a virus and this substance protects other cells against other viral infections. This interfering substance is called "interferon".

Interferon is found to be species specific. That is, interferon produced by chicken cells is protective to other chicken cells against virus infection but is not protective for cells of any other animal species. Similarly, interferon produced from human cells is protective for other human cells but not for cells of other animal species.

Because it is difficult and expensive to prepare large quantities of interferon, trials to study its clinical value in large numbers of patients have been difficult to arrange. There is evidence that it may be protective in some viral infections but is too expensive for general use. A rare form of leukaemia called "hairy cell" leukaemia is one malignancy that often does respond well to interferon treatment (*Chap. 19*).

AIDS (acquired immune deficiency syndrome), is due to a virus infection. This condition is an infection and not a cancer but a particular type of cancer called *Kaposi's sarcoma* was found to develop in some of the first patients with AIDS. Over a longer term some types of lymphoma, cancers of the cervix and some other cancers have been found to develop more commonly in AIDS patients than in the community at large. Early hopes that AIDS might respond well to Interferon or any other immune treatment has so far not been fulfilled.

8.4.2.3   The Interleukins

The interleukins are protein substances, known as cytokines, and are produced from white cells and are found to activate the immunological defence system. The first interleukins were Interleukin 1 which is produced from macrophages (giant white cells) and Interleukin 2 that is produced from lymphocytes (small white cells). They stimulate reproduction and activity of immune cells against a cancer to which the cells have been specifically sensitised. In experimental animals, interleukins have been shown, under certain conditions, to stimulate the animal's natural lymphocyte activity against implanted cancers to such an extent that the cancers have been eradicated. At the time of writing this book neither Interleukin I nor Interleukin 2 nor several more recently discovered Interleukins have made any widespread impact on cancer treatment.

However some cancers, including melanoma and kidney cancers, sometimes appear to have increased response when certain interleukins are used in conjunction with other treatments.

8.4.2.4 Tumour Necrosis Factor (TNF)

TNF is a more recent cytokine protein product of immunological research. TNF does cause cancer cell destruction in some experimental models but is too toxic for direct use in human patients. However recent work has shown that TNF enhances the anti-cancer effect of certain other chemotherapeutic agents and can be used safely and effectively when given exclusively to a limited part of the body. At the time of writing this book it can be given with safety only in a closed circuit by regional perfusion or regional infusion to treat malignancies such as melanoma and sarcoma when confined to a limb (as discussed under *"Regional Chemotherapy"*) but it can not be used systemically with safety.

TNF in combination with Interleukins 1 and 6 has been implicated in promoting cancer cachexia. Indeed, TNF was originally called cachetin, as the agent that caused cachexia. Drugs that suppress the production of TNF, e.g. corticosteroids and thalidomide, have shown promise as agents that suppress cachexia and tumour growth, respectively. The omega-3 oils are thought to work by suppressing Interleukin 6, which promotes breakdown of adipose tissue and skeletal muscle.

Small Molecule Target Inhibitors

Basic cancer research has identified a number of key signalling pathways that co-ordinate cancer cell growth. Growth signalling cytokines circulate in the blood and bind to cancer cells via special receptor molecules. Receptors become activated by the binding cytokine, and send a complex series of chemical signals to the cell nucleus stimulating cell growth and division The principle oncogene proteins responsible have been identified and successfully targeted for direct inhibition by small molecules (low molecular mass compounds) that specifically inhibit the enzyme activity that stimulates growth. Examples are: Imatinib mesylate (Gleevec), inhibit the tyrosine kinases, c-ABL + PDGF and c-KIT, that are activated in chronic leukaemia and gastrointestinal stromal tumours respectively. Small molecules can also inhibit other protein functions or block regulatory protein–protein interactions.

8.4.2.5 Cell-Mediated Anti-Cancer Activity

Cell-mediated anti-cancer activity starts with a *dendritic cell*, a specialised type of white blood cell produced in bone marrow and lymph nodes. Dendritic cells are responsible for initiating and coordinating the body's defence and immune system. They stimulate macrophage activity. Macrophages have scavenger (phagocytic) activity and are present in connective tissues and many organs including bone marrow, lymph nodes, spleen, liver and the central nervous system. Macrophages are also called *antigen-presenting cells (APC)*. They process antigens for presentation to "T" (tissue) lymphocytes.

Helper "T" cells recognise foreign antigen on the surface of foreign cells and stimulate the production of cytotoxic "T" lymphocytes or *killer cells*. The killer cells destroy cancer cells and virus-infected cells by targeting foreign antigen that has been presented by macrophages.

This is all like a rather interdependent cycle of immune-cell activity and many of the immune therapy factors described in this chapter are derived from different cells involved in this intriguing cycle. Each is aimed at boosting natural defences against cancer cells.

8.5   Some Further Treatments Under Study

8.5.1   Heat Therapy

Because cancer cells are more sensitive to heat than normal cells heat-therapy is now used in conjunction with chemotherapy in treating some tumours confined to a limb, for example melanoma. When chemotherapy and heat can be confined to the limb circulation there is a greater anti-tumour impact than with the use of chemotherapy alone. However the safe and effective level of temperature elevation must be kept in a narrow range and even then there is an increased risk of damage to normal muscles, skin and other tissues in the limb.

Investigations continue into methods of applying localised heat selectively to internal organs or tissues containing cancer in a manner that will safely destroy the cancer cells without damaging the normal body tissues. This approach could be particularly valuable for treating cancer cells in a vital organ that cannot be safely removed (such as in the liver). Several types of microwave emitting machines have been designed for this purpose. A number of problems have yet to be solved, particularly in maintaining the heat at a critical level for a significant period without overheating the patient or causing damage to normal tissues and cells. Studies are continuing but after several years the most that can be said is that some interesting and hopeful results continue to be reported.

8.5.1.1   Cryosurgery

This is another technique of destroying tumour tissue by using an extremely cold temperature application to freeze-thaw and so destroy the tissue. It has been used topically for years to treat small skin pre-malignant lesions (CO_2 snow, or liquid nitrogen) but more recently an internal probe has been developed to destroy metastatic deposits of cancer cells, especially in the liver. Good results have been reported from cancer centres specialising in this treatment.

8.5.1.2   Laser Surgery

In general the somewhat romantic objective of developing a laser gun that could be specifically aimed at cancer cells and initiate their destruction sadly still remains largely in the realm of science fiction. However some studies using laser in treating some early cases of prostate cancer are encouraging, otherwise to date the closest application of this principle is with photodynamic surgery as discussed below.

In its more general application, laser surgery is simply development of surgical technique in cancer treatment in which laser light is used to cut tissues in some ways similar to diathermy. However studies of the use of laser light in combination with other agents such as in photodynamic therapy continue and their future expanded clinical application is almost certain. These techniques have already be used in some clinical areas such as vascular surgery in which endoscopic tubes are used to reach pathological lesions or tumours in organs or tissues of otherwise difficult access.

8.5.1.3   Photodynamic Therapy

This is a type of light sensitive treatment being further investigated for some cancers.

The small new capillary blood vessels that develop with a cancer to supply it with blood are poorly formed and fragile. They easily break down if damaged and also allow some chemicals to leak out into the cancer tissues. In photodynamic therapy patients are injected with certain photo-sensitising chemical substances, that leak out of the fragile blood vessels in the cancer. The cancer is then subjected to laser light of certain wavelengths. The reaction of the substances to laser light destroys the cancer cells. As laser light does not penetrate any distance into tissues this treatment has so far only been used to treat certain surface cancers, such as skin cancers and cancers in the mucous membrane lining the mouth. Studies to date are being carried out only in specialised clinics as precautions must be taken to avoid side effects, especially general sunlight hypersensitivity from photosensitising agents.

Any advantages of this treatment over other more standard treatments are as yet uncertain but in the future there may be potential for developing similar techniques to treat other less accessible cancers, for example bladder cancers.

Dermatologists have now developed an effective photodynamic therapy for skin cancers using a local application of a photosensitive cream and a strong light wave, not necessarily laser light. Many superficial skin cancers are now treated very effectively by this relatively simple technique.

8.5.2   Gene Therapy

Among the more exciting areas of progress of both understanding cancer and treating cancer is the study of genes and their activity and genetic abnormalities. In the near future genotypic tumour changes will be relevant in deciding treatment.

Gene therapy is in its infancy, but the Chinese Government has licensed in 2005 a recombinant adenovirus that produces a functional p53 protein when the virus is injected into head and neck squamous-cell carcinoma (HNSCC), and it has shown to be effective in combination with radiotherapy (to induce apoptosis and tumour regression).

8.5.2.1 Matching Treatment to Cancer-Associated Genes and Molecular Characterisation of Cancers

As well as traditional matching of treatment to histological features of cancer cells, progress is now being made in matching treatment to cancer-associated genes and molecular typing. Progress is especially being made in using the tyrosine-kinase inhibitor STI 571 or imatinib (Gleevec) with successful treatment of chronic myeloid (or myelocytic or granulocytic) leukaemia and gastrointestinal stromal tumours *as mentioned in Chap. 19.4.3.*

More of this progress is outlined in Chap. 24.19 under the heading "Molecular Characterisation in Future Cancer Treatment".

8.5.2.2 Anti-Angiogenesis

Following the principles mentioned in photodynamic therapy, agents are now being developed specifically aimed at damaging or preventing development of the small blood vessels (capillaries) that supply the cancers with blood. Without a blood supply the tumours can't grow or survive. At this stage successful experiments have been conducted against tumours in mice and other animals. One such product is called "angiostatin" but it is likely that a number of new agents, aimed specifically at tumour blood vessels, will be developed in the near future.

People who remember the deformed limbs of some babies born about in the early 1960s to some mothers who took the anti-nausea drug thalidomide, may be interested to know that thalidomide caused the defects in the growing foetus precisely as a result of interfering with the important blood vessels growing in the developing foetus limbs in at a crucial time of foetal development. Thalidomide and similar products are now being investigated to destroy the small blood vessels in some growing cancers.

8.6 General Care

8.6.1 Care of General Health

The presence of cancer in the body sooner or later will have a profound effect on the sufferer's general state of health. Anorexia (loss of appetite), weight loss, anaemia, lassitude, and general malaise and debility are common general features and specific problems will develop according to the site of the cancer and the tissues or organs involved. The ability of the body's natural defence mechanisms to control cancer is affected by the patient's general state of health, as will the patient's mental and emotional state and ability to tolerate the various forms of treatment.

The ability of the body's natural defence mechanisms to control cancer is affected by the patient's general state of health.

8

For these reasons, it is important that special attention should be paid to the patient's general health and well-being. The diet should be nutritious yet tempting and interesting. Adequate vitamins must be provided either in the food or in vitamin supplements and omega oils should be part of the treatment of cachexia. Any anaemia should be appropriately treated and there should be provision for adequate rest and gentle healthy exercise. There must be adequate provision for pain relief. Emotional support from family, friends and the treatment team including friendly concern and support of a good family doctor make a big difference in the prospects of the patient living comfortably and making achievable progress.

8.6.2   Treatment of Complications

Special problems associated with particular forms of cancer will need appropriate attention. These include nutrition for patients with obstructive cancer of oesophagus or stomach. Surgical measures can give relief of obstruction for patients with obstructive bowel cancer or patients with pancreatic cancer obstructing the bile duct and causing jaundice. Surgical relief can also be given for urinary obstruction of patients with obstructive cancer of the prostate gland. Local treatment and dressing is essential for cancers fungating through the skin. Diuretics and some other measures sometimes give partial relief from pressure on the lungs with breathlessness caused by fluid accumulated around the lungs in the pleural cavity (pleural effusion). However removal of pleural fluid or ascites fluid accumulated in the chest or abdominal cavity may be needed to achieve temporary relief from pressure in the abdomen and chest.

Raised intra-cranial pressure may cause headaches, vomiting, papilledema (with blurred vision) convulsions or coma. This may be caused by tumours with surrounding swelling in the brain and the patient can often be relieved by radiotherapy or the use of certain drugs, especially steroid drugs, that reduce the swelling.

Complicating infections due to cancer, such as pneumonia associated with cancer obstructing the air passages or infections associated with weakened leukocyte defences of leukaemias, will also require appropriate attention.

Bleeding, bruising or thrombosis also commonly associated with blood disorders of leukaemias will also require special attention.

Anaemia is also a common association with many cancers including the leukaemias; cancers of stomach, bowel or uterus with abnormal bleeding; or primary or secondary cancers destroying or replacing bone marrow. Anaemia secondary to chemotherapy can be improved with judicious use of the bone marrow protective agent *erythropoietin*. Haemoglobin should be maintained at or above 12 g/L. This reduces the need for blood transfusion and improves the patient's quality of life.

Bones involved with cancer may not only be painful but may fracture spontaneously – known as *pathological fracture*. The use of *bisphosphonates* has been
shown to decrease the risk of complications (fractures, hypercalcaemia, spinal
cord compression etc) as well as relieving bone pain. Bisphosphonates become
incorporated in the weakened area of bone, restoring some strength to the bone
and helping it to resist further destruction. Bisphosphonate treatment requires the
patient to attend the hospital or oncology unit for a couple of hours. A slow drip of
fluid containing the drug is infused into a vein. The patient simply sits comfortably during the procedure, possibly reading a book or watching television. The
treatment should not worry the patient or cause side effects and can be repeated
at about monthly intervals if necessary. Bisphosphonates are used to advantage
in managing metastases from breast, prostate and lung cancers.

Pathological fractures need to be treated on their merits but healing is often
helped by local radiotherapy. Metastatic cancers not only in bones but also in
liver, lungs, brain, bowel and other situations may also need special treatment.

8.6.3 Supportive Care and Supportive Care Teams

Because of the complexity of cancer treatments, their inevitable side-effects,
and the need for both acute and long-term specialised care, professional "supportive care" teams have been established in some clinics. These teams consist
of doctors, nurses, allied health professionals, social, psychological and spiritual
helpers. These teams have particular skills and interest in care of cancer patients
who have developed complications of treatment and patients who have residual
complications but an otherwise good, long term prognosis. The skills of these
teams range from administration of haemopoetic growth-factors and blood transfusions to restore depressed bone marrow activity, management of infections or
nutritional problems as well as longer term restoration of physical activity, long-
term pain relief and restoration of social and income producing activity.

This is an area of care that has been historically shared between the cancer
treatment team and the palliative care team.

In most clinics "supportive care" is still provided either by the cancer treatment team or the palliative care team but in some clinics, especially where the
clinical workload is increasing, specialised supportive care teams have become
a valuable asset in cancer care.

8.6.4 Pain Relief

Nothing is more wearing, debilitating and distressing for people than to suffer
constant and unrelieved pain. Whilst most cancers causing severe pain are usually
advanced and some are incurable, at least patients suffering severe pain can be
given relief. For curable cancers, the best pain relief is achieved by eradicating
the cancers, but for incurable cancers many pain-relieving measures are available.

8

Radiotherapy will often give pain relief by reducing the size of the tumours and surrounding swelling and pressure. This is especially so for metastatic cancers in bones and the brain. Operations to relieve obstruction of bowel, bladder or other organs will give pain relief. Hormones or anti-cancer drugs that reduce the size of tumours, thus reducing any associated pressure, may also be used on occasions to effect pain relief.

Nerves that transmit pain may also be put out of action by injecting them with local anaesthetic or with alcohol or possibly by cutting them surgically. Occasionally the nerve pathway in the spinal cord that conducts pain sensation to the brain can be cut to give permanent loss of pain sensation from a region of the body.

Meditation, hypnotherapy or even acupuncture is used at times for pain relief. Whilst they are undoubtedly helpful for some patients, for others, their greatest value may be in providing emotional support rather than physical relief of severe or constant pain.

The most common and quickest method of pain relief is with simple pain-relieving drugs (analgesics) or the stronger and addictive pain relieving drugs (narcotics). Simple analgesics such as aspirin and aspirin-like products, paracetamol and the like, are usually used first. If not effective, agents containing small amounts of the least dangerous narcotic agent, codeine, are often used. The stronger narcotic agents, Pethidine (meperidine), methadone, and the opium derivative, morphine, may be given for immediate relief of severe pain usually as a temporary measure until other treatment has given more permanent pain relief. They may also be given on a permanent basis for pain-relief in people, who have a limited life expectancy, from an incurable cancer.

One of the most frequent treatment errors in oncology is under-treatment of pain, especially chronic pain in a palliative setting. Combination analgesic therapy, with narcotic and non-narcotic drugs, as well as tricyclic drugs for stress relief is an important aspect of management for people with advanced incurable cancer. In some countries heroin is also used very effectively in these circumstances but only when life expectancy is strictly limited.

8.6.5 Psychological and Spiritual Help

As mentioned in Chap. 2.20, some psychologists, alternative medicine practitioners and well-qualified psychiatrists postulated that sometimes cancer may be a result of anxiety, emotional trauma or depressive states. This may or may not be so but at least it must be acknowledged that such emotional states are detrimental to the patient's well-being and often do have an adverse effect on the progress of the disease and response to treatment. Perhaps more importantly, people who rightly or wrongly believe that they have a cancer become anxious and emotionally disturbed even if they were not previously. This is a natural and understandable reaction to what they often regard as a death sentence at worst, or a very serious illness requiring radical or prolonged treatment, and possibly with disfigurement at best.

Such emotional distress will often cause patients to seek alternative medications or fringe medicine therapists, unconventional "faith healers" or tragically unqualified "quacks", especially if they have been told that traditional medicine has nothing to offer.

Every doctor who cares for cancer patients should anticipate these natural reactions and readily support the emotional needs of the patient and the patient's family in all situations. Sometimes this can be given effectively by the responsible clinical specialists with the cooperation and help of the family doctor experienced nurses and other qualified helpers including social workers or psychologists. For most people, support of a member of the clergy can be a great comfort. Sometimes the help of an understanding psychiatrist experienced in this field is mandatory and certainly it is extremely valuable for a cancer treatment team to have the services of an interested and experienced psychiatrist and/or clinical psychologist and a social worker readily available.

Some psychiatrists and paramedical workers have claimed that some patients who have learned techniques of relaxation and meditation or hypnotherapy have shown not only emotional and physical benefit but even regression of the size of the cancer. In some patients such benefits may be real but they are difficult to prove. A strong wish for improvement may cloud any measurable judgment, and very occasional cases of spontaneous cancer regression have been reported in response to no particular therapy. However, an invaluable benefit of an experienced psychiatrist or clinical psychologist and social worker is to help the cancer sufferer and members of his or her family adjust to the new situation with all the emotional, social and other problems associated. An experienced social worker is of great help in advising of financial and other supportive agencies that may be available to help a patient's readjustment and other needs. For many people, especially those with advanced or incurable cancer, member of the clergy or other spiritual adviser will be of great value in helping in this re-adjustment process in which the patient has to come to terms with a changed and possibly fatal situation.

8.6.6 Follow-Up Care

No matter what treatment is used in cancer management it is important that all patients should undergo regular medical follow-up examinations. This is mainly to detect and treat, at an early stage, any problem that might arise but also gives most patients confidence that they are not being neglected and that any new problem will be detected and treated early. It is also important for doctors to keep accurate and continuing records of the long-term success or otherwise of treatment given so that improved treatments can be recorded and further developed.

For some cancers if 2 years has passed since treatment with no evidence of cancer, it can be very hopeful that the cancer has been cured. Indeed for most cancers a period of 5 years free of cancer indicates that cure of that cancer is very likely. Two of the more common cancers however require a longer period of regular

No matter what treatment is used in cancer management it is important that all patients should undergo regular medical follow-up examinations.

follow up as evidence of disease can show up years later. These are melanoma and breast cancer. It seems that for these two cancers in particular, the body's natural "immune" defences can keep the cancer under control for many years until something causes it to show up again, sometimes as a lump under the skin or in a lymph node, or somewhere else. These recurrent or residual cancers are often slowly growing and may be curable provided they have been detected whilst still small and localised. Hence the special need for regular and long-term follow-up of cancer patients.

8.6.7   The Specialty of Palliative Care

In recent years palliative care has developed into a specialty service in its own right. It is especially relevant to the field of oncology.

When cure is beyond all probability and remaining life is, or is likely to become, increasingly miserable, doctors, nurses and other associated experts who develop special expertise in relieving distressing symptoms and making remaining life more comfortable and tolerable make up the palliative care team. Rather than leave the family doctor, or specialist surgeon, physician, radiation oncologist or other specialist oncologist either individually or collectively to do their best to relieve distress, the experts in palliative care form a team dedicated to studying and administering methods to best make life more comfortable for suffering patients. These teams specialise in relieving acute or chronic pain, bladder or bowel incontinence, feeding, respiratory, speech and mobility problems and sleeping difficulties. They are aware of and help avoid problems of prolonged ill health or confinement to bed such as pressure sores, pulmonary congestion or deep-vein thrombosis.

These caring specialists have now become most valuable associates for cancer treatment teams attending to special needs of the patient not only medical and physical but also needs of a social, emotional and spiritual nature. They help families and friends adjust to different circumstances and different needs – specially when there is no prospect of curing the cancer.

Palliative-care specialists initially began their work in hospitals and nursing homes but now many are able to offer services in other institutions or in family homes. In some countries, separate institutions have been established for specialised services in palliative care.

8.6.8   Alternative Medicine

8.6.8.1   *Ranging from Unproven Naturopathic and Herbal Medicine Remedies To Unscrupulous "Quack" Practises*

There are almost limitless numbers of "cancer cures" promoted by a variety of people ranging from thoughtful, well-intentioned and knowledgeable alternative medicine practitioners on the one hand to misguided "quacks" and unscrupulous

Most unconventional "cures" have been investigated one way or another and found to be lacking when analysed scientifically.

charlatans on the other. These "cures" range from large doses of vitamins (especially vitamin C), to pure or blended mixtures of herbs and a variety of plant extracts. One of the most publicised plant extracts is an extract of apricot kernels called Laetrile. Diets (especially low-protein diets) are commonly advocated. Other common recommendations are meditation, acupuncture, hypnotherapy and faith healing.

There are also some contemptible, deceitful unqualified practitioners who use sleight-of-hand manoeuvres in which they pretend to extract cancers painlessly from sufferers and produce a handful of bloodstained tissue as evidence of this.

Some of these alternative remedies are undoubtedly based on incidental observations. Some are based on reasonable observations or hypotheses, as may be so for vitamin C therapy and the other anti-oxidant vitamins A and E. Others however are devoid of any logical or scientific basis. Some of these are based on a figment of imagination or a "one-off" incidental observation in an isolated cancer sufferer who happened to undergo a spontaneous remission.

Unfortunately sometimes a "cancer cure" promotion is purely based on a desire to get rich on the part of the practitioner, at the expense of the cancer sufferer and his or her family. Sometimes cancer cures have been claimed in patients in whom a diagnosis of cancer was never established.

Most unconventional "cures" have been investigated one way or another and found to be lacking when analysed scientifically. None has been more thoroughly studied than Laetrile and, although no medicinal value has been found, it is entirely understandable that people who find themselves unable to face the reality of having an incurable condition or of requiring radical surgery or other radical treatments, will search for a more acceptable alternative. This must be appreciated by cancer treatment teams who need to be prepared to spend time in advising and helping cancer sufferers in their mental and emotional as well as physical distress.

At the same time, medical practitioners should not close their minds to the possibility that one day an idea might be proposed or an observation made by a non-traditional practitioner that could be of value in cancer treatment.

Many valuable medications, including some anti-cancer agents, have been found in plants. Undoubtedly more will be found in the future. The medical profession and research scientists are aware of these possibilities, so that most proposed new or alternative but unproven "cancer cures" undergo some form of examination by appropriate authorities.

For some patients alternative or unorthodox therapy can be comforting and supportive even though specific cancer healing properties are either non-existent, not known or not understood. Provided such therapy is helping or comforting for the patient, is not harmful either physically or financially, and does not conflict with necessary treatment, it should not be dismissed for this patient by the cancer treatment team.

For some patients alternative or un-orthodox therapy can be comforting and supportive even though specific cancer healing properties are either non-existent, not known or not understood.

8

EXERCISE

What are interferon, interleukins and TNF?

Relationship Between Patients, Their Doctors and the Healthcare Team

9

In this chapter you will learn about:

> The importance of selecting appropriate specialists for patient care
> The importance of developing an honest and compassionate relationship between doctor and patient
> Skills in delivering worrying news to patients and their families
> Differences that often exist between men and women in dealing with health issues.

Nowhere in the field of medical practice is it more important for the patient to have good personal relationships, trust and understanding, than between each patient with cancer, or suspected cancer, and his or her medical advisers. Breast cancer and prostate cancer stand out as having special need for good relationships. In the case of breast cancer different possible courses of action are likely to achieve similar long-term results and the patient's preferred treatment option should be discussed. In the case of prostate cancer there may be a question of advisability of any attempt at cure so that the patient's personal life priorities must be considered.

The occasion of breaking bad news to any patient with cancer must be handled with gentleness, compassion and understanding. It must not be hurried and preferably the patient's wife or husband or a particular friend or family member should be present. Questions must be answered truthfully and carefully but without unnecessarily stressing pessimistic aspects.

There is no simple answer and each patient's special needs and priorities and his or her family and social relationships and circumstances are all important in the decision making.

By the time women reach the age of having need for advice about a cancer problem most will know a family doctor in whom they have trust and confidence.

Men are usually less ready than women to seek medical advice and often need to be persuaded by a wife or a friend.

The occasion of breaking bad news to any patient with cancer must be handled with gentleness, compassion and understanding.

F. O. Stephens and K. R. Aigner, *Basics of Oncology*,
DOI: 10.1007/978-3-540-92925-3_9, © Springer-Verlag Berlin Heidelberg 2009

9

After a comfortable, unhurried and mutually thoughtful and honest discussion about the problem with the family doctor, and, at least on one occasion with the patient accompanied by his or her wife, husband, partner or other close family member or friend, arrangements will usually be made for consultation with a specialist.

The specialist is unlikely to be an old family friend, as the family doctor may well be. However it is equally important for the family doctor to arrange referral of the patient to a skilled but compassionate, supportive and understanding specialist who is prepared to listen to the patient's anxieties and take time to answer many asked or unasked questions. The specialist should be chosen because he or she has special skills, facilities and expertise and is also readily able to communicate comfortably with an anxious, worried and often confused patient and his or her family. This is not the occasion for the family doctor to arrange consultation with a specialist predominantly because he or she was an old school mate or one who has just come back from overseas with good training and needs support. The relationship between specialist and patient will probably be prolonged over several months or years. In fact there should be a close three-way relationship with good understanding and communication between specialist or treatment team, family doctor and patient.

Certainly the specialist must have the appropriate skills and facilities and must be up to date with latest information. But over and above this, it is most important for the specialist, and members of the treatment team, to be able to communicate, explain and be ready to answer questions freely and in an unhurried atmosphere and be readily accessible, possibly by telephone, if or when problems or questions arise. Discussions about the most appropriate treatment should not sound like an edict from above but be mutually considered and arranged, having taken into account many factors unique to the individual patient. The specialist must also appreciate that no matter how clearly he or she has explained everything to the patient it is unlikely that the patient will be able to "take it all in" in one visit. One or more further visits are almost essential for probably every patient, if not to the specialist, then at least to the well-informed family doctor.

Part III
Most Common Cancers

Skin Cancers

10

In this chapter you will learn about:

> *Skin cancer prevention*
> *BCC (basal cell carcinoma)*
> *SCC (squamous cell carcinoma)*
> *Melanoma*

Cancer of the skin is the most common cancer affecting people of European descent. It is especially common in fair-skinned people who live in sunny climates. Australians and New Zealanders have the world's highest incidence of skin cancer, followed by the white populations of the southern regions of the United States. In fact more than half of the white-skinned people living in these climates can expect to get one or more of the common skin cancers during their lifetime.

There are three common types of skin cancer – basal cell carcinoma (BCC), squamous cell carcinoma (SCC) and melanoma. BCC is by far the most common and fortunately, the least dangerous. SCC is the next most common but is more aggressive than BCC. Melanoma is fortunately the least common of the three but is the most dangerous.

10.1   Skin Cancer Prevention

As for any health problem, the best treatment for skin cancer is prevention. BCCs and SCCs of skin can be largely prevented by avoiding too much ultraviolet irradiation from strong sunlight or artificial light in solariums. It is particularly important for fair-skinned people, and especially fair and red-headed people, who live in sunny tropical or subtropical climates, to take preventative measures in their everyday lives. If exposed to strong sunlight they are advised to wear protective clothing, broad brimmed-hats, long-sleeved shirts, and long skirts or trousers, and apply sun-screening lotions on exposed skin if any time is

F. O. Stephens and K. R. Aigner, *Basics of Oncology,*
DOI: 10.1007/978-3-540-92925-3_10, © Springer-Verlag Berlin Heidelberg 2009

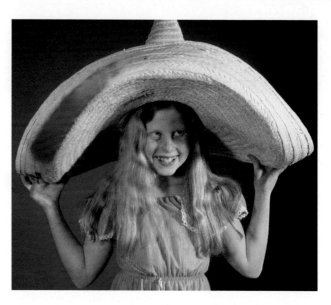

Fig. 10.1. The best preventative measure against skin cancers is to protect the skin, especially fair sensitive skin, against sunshine and other forms of ultraviolet irradiation. A large shady hat, protective skin creams, ointments or lotions and other forms of protective clothing all give protection. The very fair skinned girl pictured is wearing a large shady hat but would have been even better protected if she had worn a long-sleeved dress

spent in strong sunlight. They are advised to confine outdoor swimming or beach activities to early mornings or late afternoons. They are especially advised to protect nose, lips and face in general and the backs of their forearms and hands, because of the risk of long periods of exposure. By taking such measures, the risk of developing BCCs and SCCs can be greatly reduced.

Protective measures against risk of melanoma are similar with special emphasis on the need to avoid getting sunburnt. This applies especially to children and young people who may like to remove clothing from chest, backs and limbs thus exposing relatively white skin when days are sunny and beaches are available. The skin of young people is especially vulnerable to changes that reduce protective cells in skin (*Langerhans cells*), leading to an increased risk of melanoma later in life (Fig. 10.1).

10.2   Basal Cell Carcinoma (BCC)

A BCC is usually first noticed as a small, crusty patch or pearly grey nodule or an ulcer on the skin surface. These cancers occur most commonly in skin that has been constantly exposed to sunshine over many years. Hence they are not common before the age of 40 and become increasingly common with increasing age. More than 70% occur on the face because the skin of the face is most constantly exposed to the sun. The next most common sites are on the skin of the neck, the backs of the hands or forearms, lower legs, chest, shoulders and back.

BCCs are painless, usually slowly growing and may have been noticed for months or even a year or more before medical attention is sought. If neglected, they usually develop as slowly enlarging ulcers, sometimes called rodent ulcers because of the appearance that may look as though a rat had gnawed out a piece of skin. Although, fortunately, they almost never metastasise to lymph nodes or other distant tissues, they do tend to erode locally into tissues around them. Thus if neglected for a long time they may become incurable or even fatal by causing destruction to such tissues as underlying cartilage of the nose or ear, underlying bone of the skull, or large blood vessels in the neck. They can sometimes invade the orbit and paranasal sinuses and may even erode into the brain (Figs. 10.2 and 10.3).

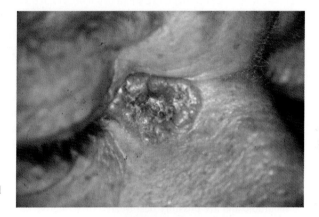

Fig. 10.2. A typical BCC on the face

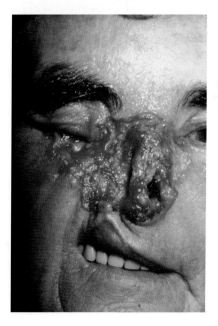

Fig. 10.3. This photograph shows a woman with a tragically neglected advanced BCC on her face. Such neglect before seeking medical attention is extremely rare. When seen it is usually in someone who has been living in isolation. This case does demonstrate that even slowly growing BCCs can become mutilating if improperly treated or neglected for some years

10.2.1   Treatment

Very small superficial BCCs are often treated by cryotherapy, usually with a liquid nitrogen spray. If larger or extending deeper, they are better treated by simple surgical excision, usually under local anaesthesia. The tissue excised is examined by a pathologist to confirm that it was a BCC and that it was completely excised with an adequate margin of normal tissue. Radiotherapy can also be an effective method of treating BCCs but preferably after a small biopsy has been taken to confirm the diagnosis. Radiotherapy has the advantage of avoiding a surgical operation and of being a painless procedure. Radiotherapy has the disadvantage of requiring expensive specialised equipment and personnel, requiring several treatment attendances (often 20 or more) and leaving some permanent radiation damage to a small patch of skin. It also has the disadvantage that if no tissue is removed, there may be some doubt about the exact diagnosis of the lesion and whether it was completely eradicated. Nevertheless, for many small lesions, especially in elderly patients and in difficult places such as over a lacrimal duct, it may be the most appropriate form of treatment. Sometimes small BCCs are removed by dermatologists using cauterisation or a small curette. These techniques should be left to experienced specialists because a mistake in diagnosis or incomplete removal can lead to a greater problem.

BCCs that have recurred after previous attempts at treatment or BCCs that occur close to vital structures such as a lacrimal duct or in an eyelid, present special problems and require expert attention.

Large BCCs invading bone or other tissues may require extensive surgical procedures including reconstructive surgery. Very occasionally they may even be incurable and are possibly best treated by palliative radiotherapy. (Palliative treatment will give a patient relief by reducing the tumour or lessening its symptoms without being likely to cure). Although such advanced lesions are not common, they are disastrous when they do occur and can easily be prevented by correct treatment of BCCs in their early stages. Hence it is important for people with small lesions to seek medical help early, at which time BCCs are easily and completely curable.

10.3   Squamous Cell Carcinoma (SCC)

SCCs are also most common on the skin of the face, especially the lower part of the face and lower lip. However they also commonly occur on the neck, the backs of the hands or forearms, or skin of other frequently exposed areas such as the lower legs, back or chest.

They often develop in skin lesions called hyperkeratoses that are small, crusty or flaky thickened areas of skin, resulting from previous repeated sun-damage over a long period.

An SCC is usually first noticed as a small painless, often crusty, lump growing on the surface of the skin or as an ulcer in the skin. Intra-epithelial hyperplasia

(Bowen's disease) is a very early non-penetrating SCC confined to the most superficial skin layer. It is a carcinoma "in-situ" and often presents as a small red patch of skin, possibly superficially ulcerated.

SCCs usually grow more rapidly than BCCs and, unlike BCCs, after a time they do tend to metastasise to nearby draining lymph nodes. Later, they may spread further to more distant lymph nodes or to other distant tissues or organs such as the lung. They also grow locally and are likely to invade surrounding tissues causing ulceration, bleeding and pain.

Fortunately, however, most SCCs of skin have not metastasised when first diagnosed and treatment of draining lymph nodes is usually not required. However, draining lymph nodes must be kept under close observation and if they enlarge they should be treated without delay – usually by surgical excision (Figs. 10.4–10.7).

10.3.1 Treatment

As for all cancers, the earlier SCCs are diagnosed and treated, the less radical treatment they need and the greater the likelihood of cure.

For any lesion suspected of being an SCC, it is important for a biopsy to be taken. In the case of a small lesion, this may be best achieved by surgical excision of the whole lesion – an excision biopsy. For a large lesion it is usually more appropriate for a small piece of tissue to be taken from its edge for microscopic examination – this is called an incision biopsy. A frozen section examination of a biopsy specimen, (as described in Chap. 7.6.5), is sometimes appropriate to allow immediate complete treatment to be carried out without delay.

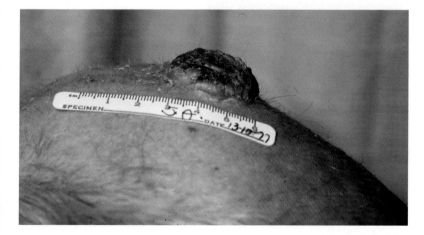

Fig. 10.4. A typical SCC (squamous cell cancer) on the scalp of a bald-headed elderly man who had worked out of doors all his life as a gardener

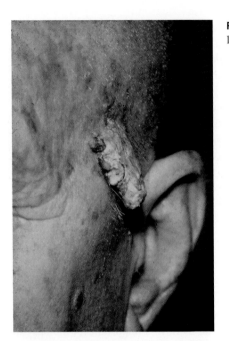

Fig. 10.5. A cutaneous horn that is likely to develop SCC in its base

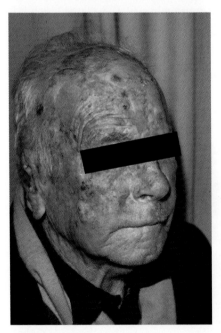

Fig. 10.6. Multiple BCCts and SCCs can develop in fair-skinned people after many years of unprotected sun exposure. This man has almost "wall to wall" cancers

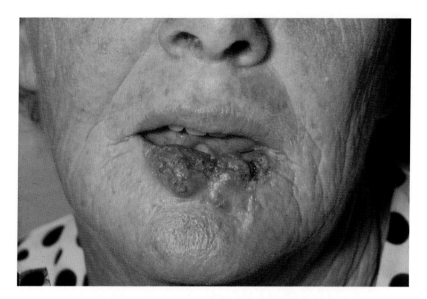

Fig. 10.7. An advanced SCC of the lower lip

Very superficial SCCs (Bowen's disease) can now be treated effectively by photodynamic therapy. The lesion is painted with a photosensitising cream and subsequently exposed to a strong light beam. Cryotherapy is also effective.

Once the diagnosis of an invasive or potentially invasive SCC in skin is established, treatment is usually by surgical excision or sometimes by radiotherapy. Surgical excision is usually the most effective and appropriate treatment. The lesion is widely excised and examined microscopically to confirm that a margin of normal tissue surrounding the cancer has also been excised to be sure that total removal of all the primary cancer has been achieved. If draining lymph nodes are enlarged without evidence that this is due to infection, then the lymph nodes too should be removed in one block of tissue and examined histologically. Depending on the site and how much tissue has to be excised, cosmetic surgery such as a skin graft may be needed to repair the tissue and close the defect.

As in the case of BCCs, radiotherapy is sometimes used to treat some SCCs of skin, especially in elderly patients or in other patients in whom an operation might be risky, or occasionally as palliative treatment when cure by surgery is considered to be impossible.

People occasionally are seen with large SCCs of skin that appear not likely to be curable by radiotherapy or surgery (or only curable by mutilating surgery such as amputation of a limb). These can sometimes be reduced in size and extent by first administering chemotherapy, especially when given regionally by intra-arterial infusion or perfusion (as described under Sect. 8.3.4.6 and 8.3.4.9 in Chap. 8). After the use of chemotherapy, the tumours are usually so reduced in size, extent and viability that they can then be cured by radiotherapy and/ or local surgical excision and usually with surgical excision of any involved regional lymph nodes.

Occasionally when a SCC of skin is very advanced, possibly invading local vital organs or tissues, or if there is metastatic spread into distant organs or tissues, it may be incurable. However, it may still be appropriate to use anti-cancer drugs and radiotherapy as part of a palliative-care program to reduce the extent and size of the cancer and to relieve symptoms.

CASE REPORT

Skin Cancer

Eric is a 64 year-old man of Northern European origin who has lived in Southern California since he was 2 years of age and has spent most of his life in out-door activities.

Between his 40th and 60th birthdays he had many hyperkeratotic skin lesions on his face, neck and backs of hands treated by cryotherapy (liquid nitrogen), four BCCs excised surgically and one SCC on his lower left cheek excised surgically. At the age of 60 when he had many more crusty lesions and a newly-developed reddish lesion, called Bowen's disease (superficial squamous carcinoma in-situ) on his lower right face, he was referred to a specialist dermatologist. The dermatologist suggested that the present lesions, including the patch of Bowen's disease, be treated with a chemotherapy cream called Efudix (Efudix is a skin cream containing the chemotherapeutic agent fluorouracil). The dermatologist advised that the cream should be applied to the lesions twice daily for three weeks during which time Eric should avoid direct sun-exposure as his skin would have increased photo-sensitivity. He explained that the lesions should flake off leaving a clearer complexion.

When Eric returned in one month for follow-up consultation both he and the dermatologist were pleased with the result. The lesions had disappeared and his face had a clear, fresh appearance.

Two years later three further crusty lesions had developed. These too were treated with Efudix cream with a similar result. Now, four years after first using the cream, two more lesions have developed and are to be treated similarly. Eric is otherwise well and is pleased with the result.

10.4   Melanoma

Melanoma is the most dangerous form of skin cancer. A melanoma is a malignant growth of pigment-forming cells in the skin or in an eye. Occasionally it may occur in mucous membranes such as the lining of the mouth or anus.

Whilst melanoma is a highly malignant tumour, present-day general awareness, early detection and better management methods have greatly improved the outlook. From being a lesion with a more than 50% mortality until the mid-twentieth century, the outlook nowadays has so improved that 85–90% of people with melanoma can now be cured.

The outlook nowadays has so improved that 85–90% of people with melanoma can now be cured.

10.4.1   Pathology

There are three main pathological types of melanoma called "lentigo maligna", "superficial spreading melanoma" and "nodular melanoma".

Lentigo maligna melanoma in situ develops in a freckle-type pigmented lesion in which the pigment cells (melanocytes) are in the basal layer of skin as opposed to common freckles which contain pigment in the superficial layers of skin. Lentigo maligna occurs most often in the skin of the face in older age group people after years of sun exposure, when they are known as *Hutchinson's melanotic freckles*. These are superficial, non-invasive melanomas and are less aggressive than invasive melanomas arising in the skin of the trunk and limbs.

Melanomas on invesive sites, especially on the trunk for men and the lower limbs for women, are usually either *superficial spreading melanoma* (and not penetrating deeply early in the disease) or *nodular melanoma* with somewhat thickened or lumpy features and usually penetrating more deeply into underlying skin layers. The deeper the penetration of melanoma the worse the likely prognosis and the more radical the treatment needed to achieve a cure.

10.4.2   Causes and Incidence

Melanoma is most common in fair-skinned people living in sunny tropical or sub-tropical climates but as opposed to BCCs and SCCs, melanoma does not commonly occur on areas of the body most constantly exposed to sunshine. The most usual sites of the more common and more often aggressive melanomas are on the back, particularly in men, or on the thigh or leg, particularly in women, as opposed to the face that is the most common site of other cancers caused by sunshine. However, like other skin cancers, the world's highest incidence is in the white populations of Australia and New Zealand, especially those living closest to the equator and nearest to the seaside. In Australia about 10% of all registered

Melanoma rarely affects children before puberty. After puberty it affects people of all ages including teenagers and young adults.

cases of the more serious cancers are melanomas. The white population of the sunny southern parts of the United States also have a high incidence of melanoma. In Europe the fair-skinned people of Scandinavia and Northern Europe also have a relatively high incidence. Even though they do not live in a tropical or subtropical climate they do tend to take their holidays in sunny climates and often become sunburnt. People of dark-skinned races do occasionally develop a melanoma but in these people it is much more common for the melanoma to be at sites of less pigmentation such as the sole of the foot, under fingernails or toenails or in the mucosa lining the mouth or anus.

Melanoma rarely affects children before puberty. After puberty it affects people of all ages including teenagers and young adults but the incidence rises with increasing age, especially in males. Whilst it affects males and females almost equally in younger years, it becomes more common in males with increasing age. Also the outlook for females is rather better than that for males. In Australia and in Scandinavia it has been found to be more common in upper socio-economic groups, possibly because these families can afford to spend more holiday time in the sun or at the beach. It is also more common in native-born Australians than in immigrants from the UK, Ireland or elsewhere, possibly because they were less likely to have had sunburn in their childhood years in their countries of origin.

A strong family history is a significantly increased risk factor for melanoma and the stronger the family history the greater the risk factor for other members of the family. A previous history of other skin cancers is also an increased risk factor for melanoma. There is also an increased risk in patients who are immunosupply following organ transplants and in AIDS patients.

The danger of melanoma lies in the fact that it tends to metastasise early to draining lymph nodes and to distant organs like liver, lungs, bowel and brain. The outlook has improved in recent years mainly because people in general, and doctors in particular, are becoming more aware of the early indications of melanoma and the need to treat it as early as possible. Most melanomas develop in pre-existing moles in the skin but almost as many develop in areas of skin without any pre-existing mole.

Melanoma sometimes develops in a long-standing, slowly-growing freckle of older age people called a Hutchinson's melanotic freckle.

In 5–10% of cases a melanoma will develop without pigment. This is known as an *amelanotic melanoma* and can be diagnosed with confidence only by microscopic examination. Amelanotic melanomas behave in a similar way to pigmented melanomas and require similar treatment.

10.4.3   Early Features of Melanoma

Any evidence of increasing pigmentation in a spot in the skin, especially on increase in size or pigmentation of a mole, must be regarded with suspicion. Other early features may be itching or crusting of a mole. Bleeding and ulceration are usually late features. Any of these features occurring either in a pre-existing mole or in a newly developed pigmented spot, require immediate attention and if there is any doubt, a biopsy should be taken. In most cases the most appropriate biopsy procedure is for a surgeon to excise the whole lesion as an *excision biopsy*. If an infiltrating melanoma is confirmed by pathology, a wider excision with or without lymphnode surgery should be scheduled. For large lesions, preliminary incision biopsy is sometimes done. If the biopsy is positive, the surgeon can then proceed with appropriate surgical treatment (Fig. 10.8).

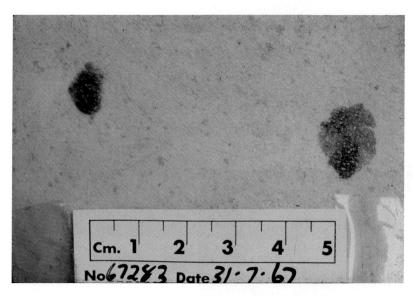

Fig. 10.8. Photograph of two pigmented lesions in skin of a woman's thigh. The larger lesion proved to be a benign dysplastic junctional naevus but the smaller lesion was a melanoma. This illustrates the need to obtain histological confirmation of suspicious lesions

EXERCISE

What features of a mole might indicate malignant change? (Sects. 10.8–10.11)

10

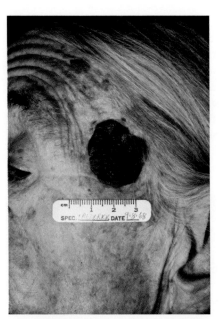

Fig. 10.9. This deeply pigmented lesion in skin of a woman's temple was not a melanoma but a seborrhoeic keratosis (a benign pigmented or "senile" wart). These are most common in elderly people. After the first such wart develops sooner or later others usually start to appear

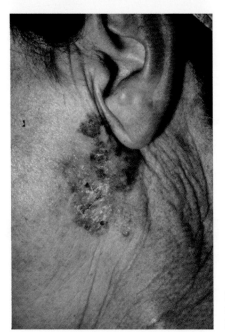

Fig. 10.10. This Hutchinson's melanotic freckle was proven by biopsy to have become malignant (melanoma)

Fig. 10.11. A typical nodular melanoma

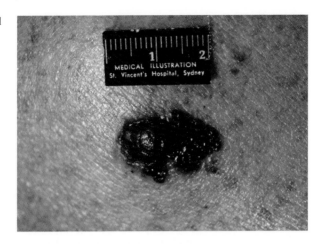

10.4.4 Treatments of Melanoma

10.4.4.1 Surgical Treatment

Surgical excision of early lesions offers the best prospect of cure. The melanoma must be excised with a wide margin of normal tissue surrounding the melanoma (at least 1 cm and at least 2 cm for thicker, more deeply invasive tumorus) because melanoma cells are sometimes present in tissues or even in lymphatic vessels surrounding the tumour. To determine whether there is involvement of drawing lymph nodes, "Sentical" lymph node biopsy may be recommended. If there is evidence of meta melanoma a sentivel lymph node or if metastatic disease ininvasive lymph node is clinically apparent, a complete surgical densure of the lymph node field is the standard treatment.

10.4.5 Investigations to Guide Surgical Treatment

10.4.5.1 Skin Penetration

The likelihood of spread of melanoma is directly related to the thickness and skin penetration or infiltration of the tumour. Thin melanomas, i.e. less than 1 mm in thickness, are unlikely to have spread to lymph nodes, whereas half of all melanomas greater than 4.0 mm in thickness, may have metastasised, especially to lymph nodes. Penetration of skin by a melanoma is also recorded by the level of skin involvement measured as Clark's levels 1–5: Level 1 being a surface lesion only with good prognosis and Level 5 being a melanoma that has completely penetrated all skin layers and has a very guarded prognosis as metastasis is likely.

Ultrasound studies of enlarged lymph nodes are becoming highly reliable in determining whether the node enlargement is caused by metastases.

10.4.5.2   Sentinel Node Biopsy

Surgical excision of early lesions offers the best prospect of cure. The melanoma must be excised with a wide margin of normal tissue surrounding the melanoma

More recently, a test called "sentinel node biopsy" is used in specialised melanoma units. In cases where lymph nodes are normal size despite a distinct possibility of melanoma having spread to them rather than excising all local lymph nodes "just in case they are involved", *lymphatic mapping by lymphoscintigraphy* may be carried out. This helps to detect localised nodes that are first in line for lymph-node drainage from the site of the melanoma. These are called the *sentinel nodes*. In this test a radioactive isotope is injected adjacent to the melanoma and nuclear scanning over the regional nodes will show which node or nodes are first in line for drainage from the melanoma site. Marks are then made immediately over the sentinel node or nodes so that the surgeon can remove these one or two nodes for pathological examination. If melanoma cells are not found in sentinel nodes, no further nodes are removed. If malignant cells are found in sentinel nodes then block dissection of all that group of nodes is carried out because of the risk that adjacent nodes might also be involved.

As well as lymphatic mapping using a radioactive isotope, a "blue dye test", may be used. The test is similar in that a blue dye (Patent blue or isosulphan blue) is injected adjacent to the melanoma just or before operation. At operation the surgeon can then identify the blue-stained lymph nodes that drain the melanoma site and these nodes are removed for microscopic examination for melanoma cells.

Usually the blue dye test and the radioactive isotope test are done together to be more certain of identifying the appropriate node or nodes for biopsy.

10.4.6   Other Treatments

In general, melanomas are not particularly sensitive to radiotherapy although radiotherapy may be helpful in achieving worthwhile palliation in some situations such as for a metastasis in the brain and sometimes for other metastatic deposits. An exception is in treating the rather uncommon uveal melanomas in the eye. Responses have been good using application of a radioactive plaque (containing a radioactive isotope such as iodine 125) for 5–7 days. More recently in some centres a special form of external radiotherapy, proton-beam irradiation, is also being used with good effect in treating a primary melanoma in an eye. When oculor melanoma metastasises it most commonly spreads to the liver. Occasionally metastatic melanoma in the liver can be excised depending on the number and sites of the metastatic deposits.

Chemotherapy has in general been disappointing in treating melanoma. Occasional beneficial responses have been observed but they are infrequent. When advanced melanoma appears to be confined to one limb, treatment by more concentrated regional chemotherapy using a special technique of closed-circuit perfusion of the limb with high dose chemotherapy, usually achieves worthwhile tumour regression, (see Sect. 8.3.4 in Chap. 8). A newer technique of "closed circuit infusion" without needing a perfusion pump may be as effective as closed-circuit perfusion and is more easily carried out. In this technique a tourniquet is applied to separate the circulation in a limb from the general circulation, the anti-cancer drugs are mixed with blood drawn from a vein in the limb and reinjected into the main artery in the limb. This process is repeated several times for upto 30 min or so, thus avoiding the need for a continuous infusion pump.

Regional chemotherapy treatment is more effective if heat is used with the chemotherapy and appears to be even more effective if the immunotherapy agent tumour necrosis factor (TNF) is used with chemotherapy.

Reports of effective use of concomitant radiotherapy and chemotherapy, so-called "sandwich treatment" (see Sect. 8.3.4.11), have encouraged further studies of this approach.

Immunotherapy is also sometimes used to treat advanced or widespread melanoma. Although occasional responses have been observed with general (systemic) immunotherapy, results have been inconsistent and early hopes of a possible new cure have not yet been fulfilled. Some encouraging results have been reported in using Interleukin 2 in combination with other chemotherapy.

Work with chemotherapy and immunotherapy is continuing in large melanoma clinics in the hope of improving treatment techniques so that more reliable treatment methods may be available for patients with advanced melanoma in the future.

10.4.7 Vaccine Studies

There are also studies being conducted with the objective of finding an effective protective anti-melanoma vaccine but as yet there is no preparation for safe, reliable or effective clinical use.

CASE REPORT

1. Thin Melanoma
Mr TD is a 46-year-old teacher. His grandparents had migrated from Scotland to Australia. As a child, he had played outdoor sport and loved the beach.

His wife noticed a new mole on his back about a year ago. Over the last few months she noted that it was darker and had changed shape.

Mr TD went to his general practitioner (GP) who examined the mole and found that it was 1 cm in diameter, was irregular in pigmentation and had irregular borders. No axillary, groin or cervical lymphadenopathy was present.

(continued)

(continued)

The GP performed an excision biopsy of the whole lesion. The pathology showed a melonoma 0.4 mm in thickness, Clark level 2, without ulceration and with only occasional mitotic figures (one mitosis per square millimetre) indicating a comparatively low grade melanoma. A definitive wider excision was performed taking a 1 cm margin down to muscle fascia.

It is now 5 years since operation. Mr TD remains well and returns yearly to his GP for follow-up of his melanoma and for a full skin check.

2. Intermediate Thickness Melanoma

Mr LB is a 58-year-old solicitor who had lived all his life in Southern California. He went to his GP for an annual health check. He was on anti-hypertensive medication but is otherwise well. His GP noticed a pigmented nodule on the right upper chest which was 8 mm in diameter and irregular in shape. An excision biopsy was performed and pathology showed a melonoma 2.5 mm in thickness, Clark level 4, with ulceration present and four mitoses per square millimetre. Mr LB was referred to a specialist surgical unit.

The surgeon recommended a wider excision of the primary melanoma site (taking a 2 cm margin) and a sentinel node biopsy for staging purposes. Mr LB had a lymphoscintogram on the morning of his surgery and then proceeded to the operating theatres. The lymphoscintogram showed a single sentinel node in the right axilla.

Under general anaesthetic, Mr LB had 1 mL of Patent blue dye injected intradermally around the primary melanoma site. The wider excision was performed, then the sentinel node biopsy. The surgeon noted that there was a blue lymphatic channel passing into the sentinel node, and the node was blue stained and "hot" when measured with a gamma probe.

The pathology of the wider excision showed no further evidence of malignancy and the sentinel node showed no evidence of metastatic melanoma. Mr LB was advised to present for regular follow-up for the melanoma. He remains well 3 years later with no evidence of residual melanoma and no evidence of metastatic decrease. Regular skin checks have not found any new melanoma.

3. Metastatic Melanoma

Mr WM was a 66-year-old farmer. He had migrated to Australia from Germany when he was 12 years old. He was a diabetic, controlled on oral hypoglycaemics and was also on antihypertensive medication. He had had a melanoma on his left lower thigh treated with a wider excision only, 6 years earlier.

He visited his GP because he had noticed a lump in his left groin. The GP found a 4 cm firm mass in the left groin, below the inguinal ligament.

(continued)

(continued)

It was mobile and not tender. The previous melanoma scar on the left lower thigh appeared normal.

A fine needle biopsy of the mass showed cells consistent with metastatic melanoma. He was referred to a specialist surgical unit.

The surgeon recommended a left groin dissection and staging CT scans of the brain, chest, abdomen and pelvis. The CT scans showed no evidence of metastatic disease and Mr WM underwent a left lymph inguinal node dissection. Of 25 lymph nodes examined the pathology showed only one 4 cm node involved with metastatic melanoma.

Postoperatively, Mr WM had a prolonged lymphatic leak from his groin drain and went home with the drain still in-situ. The drain remained in for 1 month. He had no adjuvant therapy.

Mr WM failed to return for his regular follow-up visits but returned 18 months later when he found a 2-cm lesion, two 1-cm lesions and three smaller nodules in the skin of his right thigh and two small nodules in the skin just below his left knee. Needle biopsies confirmed the presence of melanoma cells in these nodules. Mr WM had no other symptoms. Staging CT scans of the brain, chest, abdomen and pelvis were again negative for tumour. No other lesions were detected.

He was advised that it was almost certain that there would be other undetected melanoma deposits elsewhere but especially in the left lower limb. He was advised that rather than having many operations with increasing difficulty to excise and control new lesions as they arose in the limb, one closed circuit infusion of concentrated chemotherapy to his limb would be likely to control the melanoma in his limb.

Mr WM agreed and a closed circuit infusion of his left lower limb was carried out. In this treatment a closed circuit was achieved using a tourniquet applied high around his left thigh and the chemotherapy agent was injected into the femoral artery. Blood was extracted from the femoral vein and reinjected with the femoral artery repeatedly for 30 min. The chemotherapy agent of choice was melphalan and the temperature in the limb was increased to 39°C.

Post infusion a marked red reaction of the whole lower limb accrued but slowly regressed. Over the next few weeks the tumour lumps also regressed and completely disappeared.

Mr MW remained well for 14 months but a routine chest X-ray then showed a suspicious mass in the right lung. New staging CT scans identified multiple liver metastases and multiple lung metastases, the largest of which corresponded to the lesion found on the chest X-ray.

He was referred to a specialist melanoma oncologist who offered treatment with another chemotherapeutic agent (DTIC) but there was little response and Mr WM died 5 months later from disseminated metastatic melanoma.

10

EXERCISE

Why is melanoma regarded as generally more dangerous than other skin cancers?

....

....

....

....

....

Lung Cancer (Bronchogenic Carcinoma)

11

In this chapter you will learn about:

> *Symptoms*
> *Investigations*
> *Pathology*
> *Treatments*
> *Mesothelioma*
> *Metastatic cancer in the lung*

Cancer of the lung has increased from being an uncommon disease 100 years ago to one that, in the Western world, now causes more deaths than any other cancer. Worldwide about 1 million cases are diagnosed every year and the reported death rates are about 90% of the diagnosis rates. This rapid increase in incidence is directly related to the widespread habit of cigarette smoking. The disease in smokers is eight to ten times more common than in non-smokers. With greater numbers of females smoking in recent years, the incidence of lung cancer in women is now approaching that of men. In the United States, other than skin cancer, lung cancer is now the second most common cancer in both sexes together. In fact, in the US, lung cancer now causes more cancer deaths than all colorectal, breast and prostate cancers combined (see Table 2.1). The increase in numbers of people with lung cancers has followed by 20 years or more behind the increase in tobacco consumption. Due to a slowly reduced incidence of smoking in men in many Western countries (including the US and Australia) over the last 30 years of the twentieth century lung cancer passed its peak incidence in men between 1985 and 1990. However it continues to rise in women, in whom smoking did not decline when it did in men.

Although tobacco smoking is by far the most significant cause of lung cancer, a number of other factors may also play a part in some cases. These include industrial and automobile pollutant gases. Workers in certain industries including chromium, arsenic and asbestos also have an increased incidence, especially if they are also smokers.

F. O. Stephens and K. R. Aigner, *Basics of Oncology,*
DOI: 10.1007/978-3-540-92925-3_11, © Springer-Verlag Berlin Heidelberg 2009

Diagnosis of lung cancers is most common in North America (especially in black males) and in New Zealand (especially in Maoris). It is also very common in the UK, Europe and Australia. It is least common in West and East Africa. It is extremely rare under the age of 30 years and is rarely diagnosed before the age of 40. Thereafter the incidence increases with increasing age. The median age of diagnosis is between 65 and 70 years. In Western countries it is more common in lower socio-economic groups than in higher socio-economic groups, probably because smoking is more common in lower socio-economic group.

Pathological sub-types of lung cancer. There are four major histological types of lung cancer. These are:

1. Small-cell lung cancer (SCLC)
2. Squamous cell cancer (SCC)
3. Adenocarcinoma and
4. Large-cell cancer

As the approach to clinical management of the last three cancer types is similar, they are grouped together as non-small-cell lung cancers (NSCLC). Thus for clinical and treatment purposes lung cancer is classified as either SCLC, or NSCLC.

SCLCs are generally more aggressive and patients have a median survival time of about 18 months. Five-year survival is rare.

Localised NSCLC is potentially curable in its early stages by surgical resection but SCLC has invariably spread beyond resectable tissues when first diagnosed.

Not only is lung cancer now showing an increase in incidence in women due to the relatively more recent uptake of the smoking habit by women, but women with lung cancer also have a rather poorer prognosis than men with lung cancer. This is because women have a higher proportion of SCLCs and adenocarcinoma than men. Men have a higher proportion of SCCs of lung that are relatively less aggressive and more likely to be resectable even though they are still potentially curable in less than 25% of cases.

11.1   Symptoms

During its early stages, lung cancer causes few problems, so that it is usually not diagnosed until it is quite advanced and usually incurable.

During its early stages, lung cancer causes few problems, so that it is usually not diagnosed until it is quite advanced and usually incurable. Perhaps this is partly because of the nature of the sufferer who, being a smoker, is adjusted to having a chronic cough and does not become aware of a change in the cough until the disease is advanced. A cough is the most common single symptom of lung cancer but other features are shortness of breath, coughing up blood or bloodstained sputum (haemoptysis), chest pain and attacks of chest infection or pneumonia that do not respond completely with treatment.

The first evidence of lung cancer can also be due to spread of the cancer causing metastases in lymph nodes, bone, brain or elsewhere. Sometimes lung cancers produce hormones or other substances that may affect the sufferer as a whole. These may result in changes in other parts of the body such as swelling of the breasts, changes in bones (osteoarthropathy), or fingernails (clubbing), or loss of nerve function often causing numbness or tingling sensations (neuropathies).

11.2 Investigations

Chest X-rays sometimes show a lung cancer that has not been causing symptoms but in most cases by the time symptoms are present, X-rays will show the cancer.

CT scans may also show more clearly the position and the size of a lung cancer and enlarged lymph nodes in the mediastinum.

Bronchoscopy (Sect. 7.4.5) will often allow the doctor to see a lung cancer and, if so, a biopsy may be taken. The biopsy specimen will be examined microscopically to confirm that cancer is present and to find out what sort of lung cancer it is, and therefore how best to treat it (Fig. 11.1).

Sometimes a cancer cannot be seen through a bronchoscope but sputum can be sucked out or coughed up and this can also be examined microscopically. This is called cytology and this test will often show cancer cells if a cancer is present. If a lump is seen on X-ray, sometimes it is possible to suck out cells for cytology from the lump through a needle inserted through the chest wall.

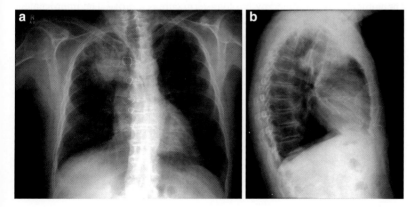

Fig. 11.1. (a, b) Anteroposterior and lateral chest X-rays showing a primary lung cancer as an increased white area in the apex of the right lung. Small metal sutures can be seen just to the right of anterior-midline. These sutures remain after previous cardiac surgery

11

11.3   Significance of Histological Findings

The several types of lung cancer are all usually smoking related but the distinction between the two main groups SCLC and NSCLC is convenient for planning treatment. SCLSs (about 20% of all lung cancers) are usually widespread when first diagnosed and are therefore not treated by surgery. NSCLCs are sometimes localised to their site of origin and some can be surgically excised with a chance of cure. They are usually not very sensitive to chemotherapy or radiotherapy.

11.4   Treatments

Unfortunately, most people with lung cancer do not go to a doctor until the disease has spread from the lung into surrounding structures, lymph nodes or other parts of the body. Most lung cancers are therefore probably incurable at the time of diagnosis. For those with NSCCS, who do present for treatment early and are diagnosed when their cancers are small, the best results are achieved by an operation to remove all or part of a lung. Yet even for people whose cancers appear to have been totally resected, only about 25% are cured in the long term.

Radiotherapy is sometimes used when surgery is unsuitable, but cure by radiotherapy alone is very uncommon.

Chemotherapy and immunotherapy have had disappointing results against lung cancer although newer anti-cancer drugs used in certain combinations and in certain treatment programs by experts, can produce worthwhile improvement for some types of lung cancer. SCLCs will often respond temporarily to chemotherapy or radiotherapy but long-term cure is a rarity. The improvement may last for several months or even a year or two.

Studies continue to try to improve results with combined treatment schedules. There is some hope that combinations of newer chemotherapy schedules used with radiotherapy and/or surgery may have more to offer in the future. Such combinations of drugs and other treatments are being investigated in a number of leading cancer treatment centres throughout the world.

CASE REPORT

Lung Cancer

Alex was a 57-year-old man who attended his doctor because his "cough would not settle down" and recently, after coughing, he had noticed blood in his sputum. Alex had been a smoker for almost 30 years, using 20 cigarettes/day. His wife stated that she had been aware of his cough for 2 or 3 years but it had become more persistent recently. He had lost weight and had little energy over recent weeks. He recently had "the flu" and in spite of taking antibiotics that were in the house the flu persisted with his productive cough.

On examination the doctor could hear moist noises in both sides of Alex's chest and noticed some dullness with little air entry over the lower right lung. An immediate chest X-ray showed a lesion in the lower right mediastinum and lung.

Alex was referred to a thoracic surgeon who arranged a bronchoscopic examination. A tumour growth was seen almost completely blocking the right lower bronchus. A biopsy of the growth proved it to be a squamous carcinoma.

The surgeon advised that he was prepared to attempt to resect the cancer but that would probably mean resecting the right lung and even then the chances of cure would be less than 20%. The alternative treatments would be radiotherapy or chemotherapy followed by radiotherapy with a good chance of improving Alex's symptoms for possibly a few months but unlikely to achieve long-term success.

Alex chose to have operation but it proved not possible to resect the cancer that had involved mediastinal lymph nodes. Alex was then given chemotherapy but developed nausea, loss of hair and bone-marrow depression (a fall in both platelets and white blood cells). Chemotherapy was suspended with the intention of treating the cancer with radiotherapy when Alex was well enough but Alex declined to have further treatment. He died 4 months after the cancer was first diagnosed.

11.5   Mesothelioma

Mesothelioma is a rare form of cancer that predominantly affects males over 60 years. There is a male to female ratio of about 3–1. Mesothelioma is well known to industrial workers because when it does occur it is often in people who have been exposed to asbestos in their work. Asbestos workers who are also smokers are particularly at risk. Protective industrial laws for asbestos workers have now made this a less common cancer although the cancer can develop years after the patient has stopped working with asbestos.

Mesothelioma is not truly a cancer of the lung; it is a cancer of the pleura surrounding and lining the lungs. It may rarely occur in other lining tissues such as the lining of the peritoneal cavity – the peritoneum. Mesothelioma may present with cough, chest infection, difficulty with breathing or chest pain. A tumour lump may be felt or seen on X-ray or CT studies.

Mesothelioma is difficult to diagnose and to treat. To confirm its diagnosis requires a panel of immuno-histochemical stains. It is usually too widespread and advanced to treat by surgery and it usually does not respond well to either radiotherapy or chemotherapy. Combinations of chemotherapy, radiotherapy and surgery are used but significant and worthwhile responses are uncommon.

Sadly the best treatment is often simply to give the patient best relief from symptoms while the tumour slowly progresses.

11.6   Metastatic Cancer in the Lung

The lungs are among the organs most commonly the site of metastatic growths spread from primary cancers that developed in other parts of the body. Cancers from almost any primary site are likely to spread through the bloodstream to the lungs, especially from cancers of the breast, kidney, bone, ovary or from a sarcoma or a melanoma. These usually show as a number of rounded opacities (white spots) seen in chest X-rays although sometimes, especially from the kidney or a sarcoma, a metastasis may be single showing as just one round white spot or lump resembling a "cannon ball" in the X-ray. Treatment depends upon the type of cancer that has spread to the lung A solitary metastasis can sometimes be resected with possible cure but solitary metastases are rare and in general anti-cancer drugs are likely to be more helpful than any other anti-cancer treatment. However, because cure is unlikely, treatment with risk of troublesome side effects may or may not be considered worthwhile (Fig. 11.2).

Sometimes primary or metastatic cancer in the lung will cause fluid to collect around the lung in the pleural cavity. This is a pleural effusion. Pleural effusion causes shortness of breath and difficulty with breathing due to pressure on the lung. Sometimes patients will achieve good, although temporary, relief if their

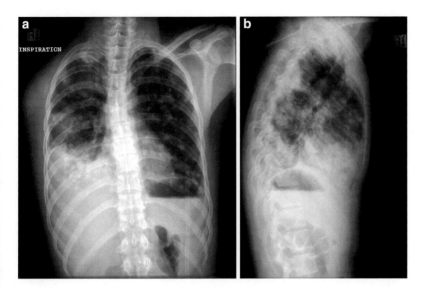

Fig. 11.2. (**a**, **b**) Anteroposterior and lateral chest X-rays showing multiple metastatic cancer deposits as scattered white areas in the otherwise dark lung tissue

doctor aspirates this fluid from the pleural cavity with a needle and syringe. After the fluid is aspirated an injection of an anti-cancer drug into the pleural cavity may slow the rate of further fluid accumulating.

EXERCISE

List reasons why lung cancer has such a poor prognosis.

Breast Cancer

12

Breast cancer became much more common in Western societies over the twentieth century. Apart from skin cancer it is now the most common cancer affecting women in most European countries, Britain, The United States, Canada, Australia and New Zealand (see Appendix).

In some of the above countries, the incidence of breast cancer appears to have levelled off but the incidence of lung cancer in women continues to increase, so that the incidence of lung cancer is now approaching the incidence of breast cancer. Because more women with breast cancer can be cured than women with lung cancer, in some countries, including the US, lung cancer is now responsible for more cancer deaths in women than breast cancer or any

F. O. Stephens and K. R. Aigner, *Basics of Oncology*,
DOI: 10.1007/978-3-540-92925-3_12, © Springer-Verlag Berlin Heidelberg 2009

other cancer (see Table 2.1). Not only did the incidence of breast cancer continue to increase during the twentieth century, was also diagnosed at an earlier stage, partly due to increased awareness and increased use of mamographic screening. This resulted in a greater likelihood of the cancer being diagnosed at a curable stage.

In North America, Northern Europe, Australia and New Zealand breast cancer is about five times more common than in women of most Asian or African countries. However, women of Asian or African ethnic origin who have lived all their lives in the US or other developed Western countries have a risk of breast cancer similar to other women of those countries. This suggests that the predominant influence is environment, social and other customs, or very likely diet of those countries rather than a racial or genetic influence. About one in nine American women will develop breast cancer during her lifetime, assuming a life expectancy of 80 years.

Although occasionally seen in women in their 20s or even rarely in teenagers, breast cancer is not common until after the age of 40 and becomes increasingly common with age. The average age for women first presenting with breast cancer is about 60 years.

The cause of breast cancer is unknown, but a number of associated factors have been noticed. Probably the one most significant factor is the age of a woman when she has her first baby. Having a baby at an early age seems to give some protection to a mother. Breast cancer is least common in women who had their first babies as teenagers and significantly more common in women who did not have their first baby until after the age of 35 years. Women who have not had any babies, such as nuns, have a greater risk of breast cancer.

The age of a woman when she experienced her first menstrual period and the age at menopause are also significant. Early menstruation and late menopause are both associated with increased risk of breast cancer. It does seem that the longer the woman's reproductive life cycle the greater the risk of development of breast cancer. This may be due to a more repeated and prolonged exposure to ovarian production of oestrogen.

A strong family history is a prominent risk factor for breast cancer. There may also be some protection in women who breastfeed their babies although the evidence for this is less clear. Women who live in undeveloped countries tend to breastfeed their babies for many months and have a low risk of breast cancer. However these women also usually have had their first baby at a young age and have a very different lifestyle including very different diets.

There is an association between breast cancer and being overweight, lack of exercise and smoking tobacco, although the association with tobacco smoking is not as strong as it is with lung cancer. Some studies have reported an association of breast cancer with a high-fat diet, particularly saturated animal fats, although this has not been found in all such studies. Breast trauma too has sometimes been suspected but it is really not known whether injury may cause a breast cancer. Although after injury some women first notice a lump that is found to be breast cancer, it is likely that in most cases the injury simply drew attention to a lump that was already present. Injuries may, of course, cause other types of lumps in the breast that are not cancer, for example a haematoma or a lump due to fat necrosis.

A strong family history is a prominent risk factor for breast cancer. The highest risk is related to having first-degree relatives with breast cancer, especially if pre-menopausal at the time of diagnosis. About 10% of breast cancers are considered familial, and of these *BRCA1* and *BRCA2* tumour suppressor genes (Chap. 2) account for about two-thirds. There are probably additional higher risk genes, as yet unidentified. Environmental influences including diet are also more likely to be similar in women of these families, so that genetic relationships are not always clear.

It was once believed that fibro-cystic disease (also known as fibro-adenosis-cystica, benign mammary dysplasia, hormonal mastopathy or "chronic mastitis") was a strong precursor of breast cancer but more recent studies have found a modest increased risk only. However if there are histological features of *atypical hyperplasia* the risk is substantially increased. Because both fibro-cystic disease and breast cancer are common, making a diagnosis of breast cancer in a woman who already has lumpy breasts from other causes may present difficulties.

After the atomic bomb explosions at Hiroshima and Nagasaki, an increase in numbers of women with breast cancer was reported but the increase was not apparent until some years after the event.

Tobacco smoking has also been associated with an increased incidence of women with breast cancer but the increase is usually apparent only in women who have been smoking for 20 or 30 years.

In practical terms, other than regular self-examination, routine mammography every 2 years for women over 50, (or more often in women who belong to special risk groups), remains the best early detection measure against breast cancer at the present time. An annual mammogram may be advisable for women with a previous history of breast cancer, or a strong family history of breast cancer. Increasingly, in some countries, breast cancer is being diagnosed by screening mammography before a lump can be felt and before the onset of discomfort or other local feature. Ultrasound of the breast is mostly useful for patients with a palpable mass that is not seen in mammograms or to help determine whether a lump is solid or cystic. It is also more likely to help screening in pre-menopausal women and safe to use in pregnancy. It is far superior to mammography or physical examination in evaluating lymph nodes for possible metastases and can be helpful in directing a needle into a suspected lesion for needle biopsy.

12.1 Hormone Replacement Therapy (HRT)

Using oestrogen or oestrogen-progesterone medication to relieve menopausal and postmenopausal symptoms, has been incriminated as increasing the risk of breast cancer. The increased risk of small doses of hormones is small but nevertheless significant in most women, and considerable for women with predisposing factors. Therefore HRT is reserved for women who experience severe menopausal or postmenopausal problems that cannot be relieved in any other way and even then, small doses are usually given for a limited period only and the woman kept under regular monitoring. Meanwhile studies continue to try to find something equally effective, but without risk, to relieve these menopausal symptoms. One study under investigation is with the use of naturally occurring hormones, the phytoestrogens which are present in all plant foods but especially in legumes such as soybeans.

There is a reduced risk in women who have a high intake of fruit, vegetables, nuts, grains and other plant foods, especially if they are complete vegans (see Sects. 2.5 and 2.12 in Chap. 2).

12.2 Symptoms

Breast cancer is usually first noticed by a woman finding a painless lump in one breast. The most common situation is in the upper outer quadrant of the breast (Fig. 12.1a).

The majority of breast lumps are not cancer, but when a lump is first noticed in a breast the woman should seek medical advice without delay. Usually she should be sent for further investigation or a specialist opinion.

As a general rule a solitary breast lump first noticed in a woman under 50 is rather more likely to be benign but a solitary lump first noticed in a woman over 50 is likely to be malignant. However any lump in a breast or any other change in a breast should be checked out.

A reddish nipple that looks rather like an abrasion of the nipple may be early Paget's disease of the nipple and this may be an indication of an underlying breast cancer (Fig. 12.1b).

Women with breast cancer may be aware of a change in the position or shape of a nipple (called retraction or inversion) (Fig. 12.1c); redness, and puckering or ulceration of skin over the breast (especially if over a lump).

These are sometimes features of breast cancer noticed either by the woman herself or by her doctor. Other features may be discharge of blood from a nipple or discharge of other fluid from a nipple not associated with a pregnancy or lactation, redness of a nipple or a change in size of one breast.

Occasionally breast cancer may first be discovered after finding a lump in an axilla or a metastasis in another organ such as the lungs (seen in a chest X-ray), liver or bone.

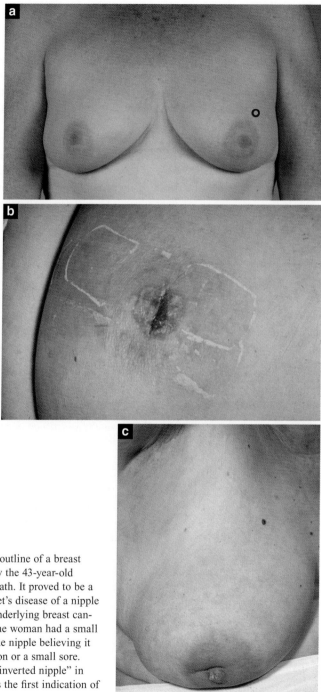

Fig. 12.1. (a) An outline of a breast lump noticed by the 43-year-old woman in the bath. It proved to be a cancer. (b) Paget's disease of a nipple indicating an underlying breast cancer. Typically the woman had a small dressing over the nipple believing it to be an infection or a small sore. (c) A recently "inverted nipple" in this woman was the first indication of an underlying breast cancer

12.3   Inflammatory Breast Cancer

Occasionally the first indication of breast cancer is a red inflamed breast very like acute mastitis (Fig. 12.2). If this change develops for no apparent reason or does not settle down after a week or 10 days of appropriate treatment (including antibiotics), the possibility of an underlying cancer must be considered and a biopsy taken.

Inflammatory breast cancer is an uncommon but aggressive form of cancer. The diagnosis is more obvious when it occurs in older women not associated with pregnancy or lactation but can be very difficult to diagnose in pregnant or lactating women because it can easily be confused with mastitis. Treatment needs to be aggressive as for other advanced breast cancers but the outlook must be very guarded.

12.4   Cancer of the Male Breast

Less than one per cent of all breast cancers are in males, but when they do occur they show up and behave in a similar way to cancer in female breasts. The outlook for breast cancer in males is usually worse than for females, possibly because men are more likely to delay seeking medical advice.

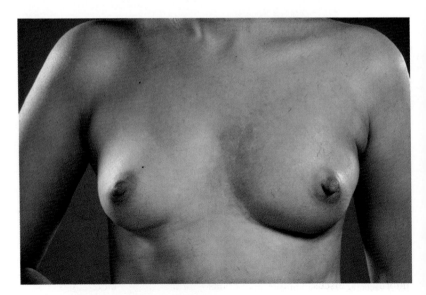

Fig. 12.2. Photograph showing an "inflammatory" cancer in the left breast of a young woman. If it occurs during or after a recent pregnancy it can easily be confused with mastitis

12.5   Signs

Typical features of breast cancer are a lump that is hard, often irregular in outline and possibly fixed to skin, muscle or other tissue. Other signs include retraction of a nipple, Paget's disease of a nipple, nipple blood stained discharge or a dimpling of the skin over a lump (there may be multiple small dimples in an area of skin like orange peel and known as peau d'orange). These may have first been noticed by the patient herself or first detected by her doctor. Lymph nodes in the axilla or elsewhere must be examined for evidence of enlargement. Examination will include examination of the chest and abdomen for possible evidence of lumps or spread into other organs such as lungs, liver, ovaries or bone.

Typical features of breast cancer are a lump that is hard, often irregular in outline and possibly fixed to skin, muscle or other tissue.

12.6   Investigations

Screening tests for breast cancer have been discussed in Chap. 7.

For a woman who presents with a breast lump, a number of investigations may be arranged to discover whether it is cancer. Mammograms may show the size, position and type of lump and the general condition of the breast. Ultrasound and CT scans usually give little further information unless cysts are present. Ultrasound is safer to use in younger and pregnant women. Ultrasound is also better at demonstrating lesions in the more dense breasts of younger women and it better demonstrates the presence of cysts.

If a breast lump is thought to be cancer from the initial examination, and especially if it is an advanced cancer, other general investigations may be needed. These may include chest X-rays, liver CT or scan and bone scan to look for evidence of possible spread to lungs liver or bone. Results should be known before any major breast surgery is carried out. Involvement of any of these organs may sometimes indicate the need for some form of treatment other than removal of all or part of the breast, because cure would not be achieved by removing the breast.

The most important investigation is a biopsy. In many cases a pathologist will perform a needle biopsy on an outpatient basis. Sometimes it is better for a surgeon to take a larger biopsy specimen taking a core of tissue with a special instrument or even cutting out a piece of the lump in an operating theatre. This is the most reliable method of diagnosis. If a surgical biopsy is carried out and frozen-section pathology technique confirms a diagnosis of cancer, the surgeon can operate without further delay provided the patient has been appropriately prepared. However this approach is becoming less common. In most clinics it is preferred to establish a diagnosis and staging of the cancer and, with this information, discuss appropriate options with the patient before any treatment intervention is started.

12.6.1   Breast Cancer Staging

Clinicians depend on skilled pathologists to classify cancers and to decide on likely prognosis and which treatment option is most likely to achieve a best result. Information that may be supplied by the pathologist has been discussed in Chap. 6.

To make a final determination of tumour staging after tumour removal the pathologist should also provide the dimensions of the cancer removed, and whether the surgical margins are clear of the edge of the tumour. The pathologist will also provide the oestrogen-receptor and progesterone-receptor findings. These may indicate the likelihood of hormone sensitivity of the cancer.

Stage 1 breast cancer is a small lump that is confined to the breast and should be eminently curable by removal of the breast or the part of the breast in which it is located.

Stage 2 breast cancer is when the primary cancer is less than 5 cm in diameter and has spread into adjacent lymph nodes that are still mobile but there is no evidence of spread beyond.

Stage 3 breast cancer is when there is a large cancer in the breast and/or involvement of overlying skin and/or involvement and adherence to underlying muscle and/or axillary lymph nodes are adherent to surrounding tissues, but there is no evidence of spread into more distant organs or tissues.

Stage 4 breast cancer is when there is metastatic spread into more distant organs or tissues. These cancers are clearly not curable by treatment of the breast alone (Fig. 12.3).

12.7   Treatments

Treatment of breast cancer will largely depend upon whether the cancer was detected early and is likely to be cured by surgery or surgery with radiotherapy and other local treatment, or whether it is so advanced that cure by treatment of the breast alone is impossible.

12.8   Prevention

There is no known practical way of preventing breast cancer. However studies of the use of the anti-oestrogen hormone compound Tamoxifen, given in small doses over a prolonged period of years, will reduce the risk of breast cancer developing in women at special risk. It may be recommended in women with a high incidence of the disease in their immediate family or those who have already had cancer in one breast. However the final results of such trials and any possible long-term risks of this treatment are not yet fully known. Long-term use of

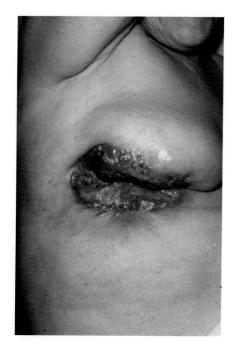

Fig. 12.3. An advanced and neglected fungating breast cancer. The patient was a 55-year-old woman who had not previously sought medical help due to fear of having confirmed what she suspected but had been trying to deny that she had a breast cancer. Such seemingly irrational behaviour is not uncommon even in very intelligent people who might appear to be well adjusted in every other way

Tamoxifen has been shown to be associated with an increased development of cancer in the uterus and also a possible risk of thrombosis. More recent studies have shown that a new drug raloxifene, (Evista), has similar cancer prevention properties apparently with less risk of these long-term side effects.

EXERCISE

What local features of a breast might be suggestive of breast cancer? (Fig. 12.4)

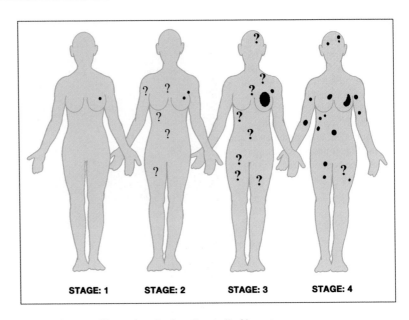

STAGE: 1   STAGE: 2   STAGE: 3   STAGE: 4

Fig. 12.4. Diagrams illustrating the four "stages" of breast cancer

Treatment of breast cancer will largely depend upon whether the cancer was detected early.

Further studies are based on the fact that women in Asian countries have a lower incidence of breast cancer, other breast problems and post-menopausal syndrome, than women in Western societies. As previously mentioned, Asian women have a diet high in certain leguminous plants that contain relatively high quantities of phytoestrogens. Studies are underway to determine whether the phytoestrogens, and especially the isoflavones in phytoestrogens, reduce the risk of breast diseases including cancer (see Sect. 2.13 in Chaps. 2 and Sect. 3.5 in 3).

Lycopene (Chaps. 2 and 3) is another "natural" agent being studied for possible anti-cancer or cancer-preventive potential. At the time of writing this book it is too early to speculate whether this or other agents will develop a place in cancer-prevention therapeutics but encouraging studies continue.

12.9   Pathology

There are two main types of breast cancer depending upon whether the cancer developed in breast ducts (duct carcinoma), or in the breast lobules at the end of the ducts (lobular carcinoma). Although either may present in a non-invasive in situ stage before becoming invasive, lobular carcinoma is more likely to become invasive at an earlier stage and is more likely to be bilateral, especially in younger women.

Fig. 12.5. Diagram
showing phases of
development of breast
cancer

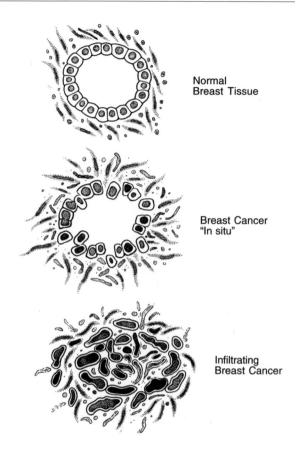

Normal
Breast Tissue

Breast Cancer
"In situ"

Infiltrating
Breast Cancer

Duct carcinoma, which is more common, may remain in situ for a period
before it develops into invasive cancer (Fig. 12.5).

12.10   Early Breast Cancer

12.10.1   Surgery and/or Radiotherapy

There has been much controversy in deciding the best treatment for early breast
cancer. For years, surgeons believed that for stage 1 or a small stage 2 breast cancer,
the best chance of cure was by total removal of the breast and all draining axillary lymph nodes. This operation, radical mastectomy, used for many years,
undoubtedly cured many women of breast cancer but it was probably unnecessarily radical for many women.

Later studies showed that for early breast cancer, results of treatment were just as
good if the breast only was removed and lymph nodes were treated by radiotherapy.

A number of non-radical breast saving treatment options can now be offered for treatment of early breast cancer (stage 1 and 2) with equally satisfactory prospects of cure.

For small in situ breast cancers local removal of the lump with some surrounding tissue and followed by radiotherapy to the breast is good treatment.

If a breast cancer is showing early evidence of becoming invasive then either removal of that segment of the breast or total breast removal will give equally good results. Radiotherapy is given post-operatively in case there is further cancer in the breast.

With invasive breast cancer, which shows no clinical evidence of lymph-node involvement, it is important to investigate lymph nodes in case there is microscopic cancer cell invasion, even though the nodes are not enlarged. This is now done by removing one or more "samples" of the closest axillary nodes and having them examined microscopically. If no cancer cells are found in the lymph nodes then no further lymph-node treatment may be indicated. But if cancer cells are found in the nodes then total removal of all axillary lymph nodes is recommended. The cancer is then classified as a pathology stage 2 cancer and adjuvant treatment with chemotherapy or hormone therapy is usually indicated (as discussed below).

More recently the technique of sentinel node biopsy is often used to detect and examine the most likely lymph nodes to contain tumour cells. (This was discussed in relation to melanoma Chap. 10, Sect 10.4.)

For treatment of possible or proven involvement of axillary lymph nodes, surgical excision is now usually regarded as the preferred option. Although radiotherapy is generally used as follow-up treatment to the breast area, radiotherapy to the axilla is better avoided after surgery to the axilla because of the high incidence of impairment of shoulder movement and of subsequent lymphoedema of the arm that can follow.

Thus there are now different options for treatment without total mastectomy that have been shown to have equally good prospects of cure in most patients. Patients should be offered a choice of the treatment options.

In most cases long-term results are equally good if only that part of the breast, which contains the lump, is removed and radiotherapy is administered following the surgery.

It is important to learn of the woman's personal attitude to her breasts and to her cancer. Some women regard their breasts as being crucial to their self-image and femininity. For such women, if equally satisfactory results can be offered without removing the whole breast, this would be preferable. To other women, a breast is not so important and if a breast has a cancer in it they would prefer to have the breast totally removed. Because in most cases long-term results have been equally satisfactory, the patient's wishes should be discussed with her and taken into consideration.

Most women do not wish to lose an entire breast unless the surgeon can assure them that this is essential in order to achieve best prospect of cure. In most cases no such assurance can be given. In fact, most women can be assured that their prospects of cure would be just as good with partial breast removal provided radiotherapy is administered to remaining breast tissue and all axillary draining lymph nodes are removed if there is pathology evidence of node involvement.

12.10.2 Adjuvant Chemotherapy

Whatever the initial form of treatment given, in a number of women with breast cancer apparently confined to the breast and possibly nearby lymph nodes, there will also be early but undetectable spread of some cancer cells to other parts of the body. Adjuvant chemotherapy will improve the outlook for these women.

The most common sites for such spread are the lungs, distant nodes, liver, ovaries and bones but almost any tissue may be a site for a secondary cancer. If chemotherapy is given at this stage, the very small clumps of scattered cancer cells, if present, are more likely to be destroyed than if they are allowed to get bigger before any potentially effective treatment is given. In women who have had an early breast cancer removed but the cancer has also been found in the axillary lymph nodes, or the cancer is histologically anaplastic and high grade, or is greater than 2 cm diameter, especially in a young woman, or it is a hormone receptor negative poor prognosis cancer, there is a real chance that it has spread. Although there may be no proof of spread, the risk that it may have spread is significant, therefore a program of adjuvant chemotherapy is usually given after the operation just in case there are still some cancer cells somewhere (see Sect. 8.3.4). Women given adjuvant treatment are up to 10% less likely to have future metastatic cancer and are therefore more likely to be cured. Adjuvant chemotherapy, must be given skilfully and the effects watched closely as side effects are common.

> Radio-therapy to the axilla is better avoided after surgery to the axilla because of the high incidence of impairment of shoulder movement and of sub-sequent lymphoedema of the arm that can follow.

12.10.3 Hormone Sensitivity Tests

Not all breast cancers will respond to hormone therapy. Nowadays, when a breast biopsy is taken and found to be cancer, a small piece is usually tested for hormone sensitivity (called the oestrogen and progesterone receptor or ER and PR tests). These tests will give an indication as to whether the cancer is likely to respond to hormone manipulation. If not then some other form of treatment, as for example cytotoxic chemotherapy, may be more appropriate.

In general patients with ER^{-ve} tumours should be treated with adjuvant chemotherapy as their cancers are unlikely to respond well to hormonal management. Patients with ER^{+ve} tumours are likely to get a favourable response to hormonal management and are usually better treated with tamoxifen if their tumour is of intermediate or high risk. Adjuvant chemotherapy is also better tolerated by younger rather than older women. In older age groups tamoxifen is unlikely to be toxic and is better tolerated so that for elderly and frail women tamoxifen may be the preferred adjuvant treatment regardless of hormone receptor findings.

Recent trials have indicated that another group of agents, called *aromatase inhibitors* (anastrozole, arimidex, letrozole, exemestane) are even more effective than tamoxifen for postmenopausal women with metastatic cancer or women who have had their ovaries removed as treatment for metastatic breast cancer.

12.10.4   Options in Management of Early Breast Cancer

There is no one best management of early breast cancer. Depending on circumstances the options for integrated management are as follows:

- Removal of the breast or that part of the breast containing the cancer.
- This to be followed by irradiation of the remaining breast tissue or chest region from which the breast was removed.
- Sentinel node biopsy.
- Total excision of axillary nodes if tumour was found in any lymph node or if the primary cancer was large and/or infiltrating and aggressive.
- Adjuvant chemotherapy if there was cancer in any lymph node, or if the primary cancer was infiltrating and aggressive or greater than 2 cm diameter, or if ER/PR^{-ve} (especially in younger women).
- Hormone management (usually with Tamoxifen) if the cancer was ER/PR^{+ve}.

Studies continue to determine more precisely which combinations of therapy should be recommended for treatment of a particular cancer in a particular patient.

12.11   Locally Advanced and Metastatic Breast Cancers

For women who present for treatment with advanced breast cancer, such as cancer fungating (ulcerating) through the skin or cancer adherent to underlying muscles or cancer with distant metastatic spread to other tissues or organs, cure cannot be achieved by standard local surgery alone. Sometimes chemotherapy or radiotherapy or both may be given first to reduce the tumour size. Sometimes this may be followed by surgical removal of the breast to prevent further local growth or fungation. (Chemotherapy given before planned surgery and/or radiotherapy is a form of induction or neoadjuvant chemotherapy. See Chap. 8.) If the cancer was clinically a stage 3 cancer without evidence of metastatic spread sometimes a cure can result from this form of combined, integrated treatment. But in case there is undetected metastatic spread further follow-up adjuvant chemotherapy is also given.

However for such advanced local cancers with distant metastases in other tissues, the best palliation may often be achieved by some form of hormonal treatment or by chemotherapy alone or with radiotherapy (as discussed in Chap. 8). In many cases metastases will respond well to localised radiotherapy giving at least temporary pain relief. This is especially appropriate for isolated painful metastases in bones.

Two further treatments may be helpful for pain relief from bone metastases. These are bisphosphonates or with radio-isotopes strontium 89 or samarium 153 (see Sect. 8.6.2 Treatment of Complications).

Strontium 89 is a beta-emitting radioisotope that becomes incorporated in bone metastases causing local tumour cell destruction and pain relief. Being poorly penetrating irradiation it is unlikely to cause damage to other tissues other than nearby bone marrow. Before the treatment can be safely repeated care must be taken to ensure that any blood count depression, and especially platelet depression, has fully recovered. Samarium 153 is used similarly to Strontium 89.

In addition to pain relief, treatment of other complications may be required. Such treatment may include using a syringe to aspirate fluid from the chest (pleural cavity) blood transfusions to relieve symptoms of anaemia and always psychological or spiritual support.

Real progress is being made in three new approaches in breast cancer treatment, including development of various anti-enzymes involved in cancer-cell development. These include enzymes called signal-transduction inhibitors, related to relevant breast cancer growth factors.

Herceptin (Trastuzumab) is a prototype of successful development of therapeutic monoclonal antibodies (See Sect. 8.4.2 in Chap. 8). Herceptin has already been shown to improve survival, possibly by 30%, when given in combination with chemotherapy. It is now under study as adjuvant therapy. Other treatments under investigation are the tyrosine-kinase inhibitors such as Gleevec, Iressa, OSI 774; farnesyl transferase inhibitors; and angiogenesis inhibitors.

Another new approach is with gene therapy in which abnormal genetic material in cancer cells is replaced with non-malignant genetic material. At the time of writing techniques being developed to make gene therapy clinically effective are causing a great deal of research interest.

12.12 Physical and Emotional Needs

12.12.1 Breast Prostheses and Breast Reconstruction

After loss of a breast, many women feel quite depressed and even humiliated and require sympathetic help and understanding. Emotional depression to a greater or lesser degree is almost inevitable after breast cancer treatment and further depression following radiotherapy is common. Fortunately the most severe stage of depression is usually temporary and improvement is usual after treatment has been completed but it may take longer.

One obvious aid is the provision of a breast prosthetic padding to wear in a brassiere or in a swimming costume. Many good appliances are now available that allow normal activity, even swimming, without detection. This is good for the woman's morale.

In other cases, reconstructive surgery may be considered to form a new breast. In the past these procedures were usually not advised until at least a couple of years after mastectomy, in order to be as sure as possible that no further local tumour recurrence was likely, but more recent studies suggest that immediate reconstruction does not present any long term disadvantage. Some surgeons are now offering immediate reconstructive surgery to replace the breast immediately after its removal, with equally satisfactory results.

Some women do not choose to have any further surgery but to others breast reconstructive procedures offer considerable emotional support and very good cosmetic results can now be achieved (see Figs. 12.6a, b).

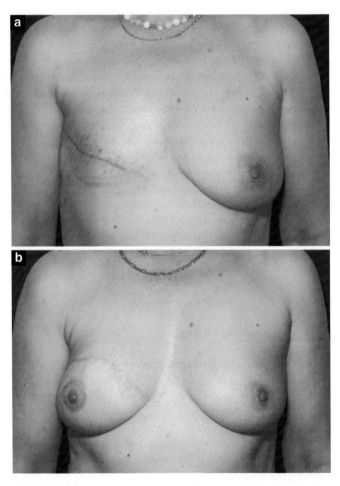

Fig. 12.6. Photographs (**a**) before and (**b**) after breast reconstruction surgery. The reconstructed breast can be of very good appearance and will give the patient considerable mental, physical and emotional support

12.12.2 Breast Clinics

Because of the high incidence of breast cancer in Western Societies and the broad range of skills needed to best detect, manage and follow up patients often needing integrated treatments for both clinical, emotional and supportive care, specialised "Breast Clinics" have become widespread throughout most Western countries. These involve not only diagnostic facilities and clinical medical specialists but also special breast care nurses, physiotherapists and social workers in a team approach.

12.12.3 Cancer Societies and Breast Cancer Support Groups

Emotional support and understanding of family and friends is essential for most women who have had a breast cancer especially after a mastectomy. As breast cancer is one of the most common cancers in Western Societies many cities will have a breast cancer support club (previously called a mastectomy club). Women who have lost a breast are welcome to join. The companionship and advice from fellow club members or from experienced professionals of a Cancer Society can be of great help in coping with both physical and emotional needs of patients (Sects. 8.6.3–8.6.5 and Chap. 9).

CASE REPORT

Early breast cancer

Sylvia is a 52-year-old lady who has had three children. She breast-fed all three. She is otherwise fit and well and went through the change of life at 46 years of age. She was placed on hormone replacement therapy for post-menopausal symptoms and has been attending the Breast Screen Unit annually from the age of 50. She regularly self-examines herself and there is no family history of breast cancer. She is on no regular medications.

She attended the Breast Screen Assessment Unit, where a screening mammogram with two views showed an area of spiculation in the upper outer quadrant of the left breast at the 2 o'clock position, 4 cm from the nipple. When she was examined by the surgeon in the breast-screening unit she was found to have some thickening of the breast in the left upper outer quadrant. The rest of the left breast was normal to examination with no tethering or peau d'orange. Her right breast was normal to examination. She had no evidence of axillary or supraclavicular lymphadenopathy and no bony tenderness. An ultrasound was performed of both breasts especially concentrating on the area in the left upper outer quadrant and

(continued)

(continued)

she was noted to have a hypo-echoic (solid) lesion with an irregular margin. Clinically and radiologically, she had a lesion that was graded most likely to be breast cancer so she underwent core biopsy. The core biopsy returned a grade 2 invasive ductal carcinoma, which was ER and PR+ve.

The surgeon discussed management options for her disease. He recommended wide local excision followed by 6 weeks of adjuvant radiotherapy. To stage the axilla, he recommended a sentinel lymph node biopsy. Adjuvant hormone therapy and chemotherapy would be considered once the surgery had been performed.

A bone scan showed no evidence of any bone metastases. She was booked in for her surgery and had a wide excision and sentinel lymph node biopsy. The margins of excision were clear and the sentinel lymph node was negative for any micro-metastases and negative for cytokeratin staining for epithelial cells. The final tumour pathology was a 21 mm, grade 2, invasive ductal tumour that was ER/PR+ve and HER 2−ve (see Chap. 6).

She was seen at the Multidisciplinary Clinic by the radiation oncologist and medical oncologist, where there was discussion of the use of adjuvant chemotherapy, in addition to Tamoxifen. In view of her young age, the infiltrating nature of the ductal cancer, the cancer was more than 2 cm in diameter and her expressed wish to have any treatment that might help her outcome she underwent 6 weeks of radiotherapy and this was followed by four cycles of adriamycin and cyclophosphamide chemotherapy over 3 months. Following this, Tamoxifen was commenced for the next 5 years.

Sylvia will be followed-up in the first instance every 3 months to exclude local recurrence and then 6 monthly for 2 years. Thereafter an annual examination will be recommended for the rest of her life.

CASE REPORT

Breast cancer

Asha is a 40-year-old woman who was admitted to hospital after finding a lump in her left breast. She is the mother of two children. Her menarche was at 13 years. Her personal and family histories were unremarkable but she had used oral contraceptives for several years. Mammography revealed a 2.5 cm speculated lesion of left breast and the ultrasound confirmed the presence of an irregular solid lesion. A needle biopsy confirmed the presence of malignancy.

She underwent a surgical excision as recommended. This consisted of excision of the quadrant of breast containing the cancer (quadrantectomy) and axillary node dissection. The final histology showed an infiltrating ductal carcinoma, measuring 2.6 cm. Hormone receptive studies showed the tumour to be oestrogen positive (ER+) and progesterone receptor negative (PR−). Tumour margins were clear She was given radiation therapy to the left breast followed by six cycles of chemotherapy (anthracycline-based) with good tolerance.

An adjuvant chemotherapy program was decided because axillary lymph nodes were found to be positive for malignancy, Radiotherapy to the axilla was avoided because of the high risk of impaired shoulder movement and of subsequent lymphoedema of the arm that can follow.

As the ER test was positive, she was given hormone therapy consisting of tamoxifen for 5 years, after completion of radiation therapy.

She is kept under close and regular surveillance, which will be a life-long recommendation.

EXERCISE

Why is it so important to "follow up" breast cancer patients for virtually as long as they live?

. . . .

. . . .

. . . .

. . . .

. . . .

Cancers of the Digestive System (Alimentary Tract)

13

13.1   Cancer of the Oesophagus

Cancer of the oesophagus is a comparatively common disease in Eastern Asia, especially China, and some African countries, particularly Southern African countries, including South Africa. It also has a relatively high incidence in males in France and Eastern Europe, especially Hungary (see Appendix). Although less common in Britain, America, Canada, Australia, New Zealand and the white population of South Africa the incidence is rising in some of these countries, particularly in Britain. The reasons for this difference in incidence are not fully understood although consumption of alcohol and perhaps different diets play a part. In those parts of China and Africa that have a high incidence, a fungus that grows on stored food may be at least partly responsible. Oesophageal cancer is more common in men than in women especially in the middle and lower thirds of the oesophagus but in the upper end, it is more common in women. Oesophageal cancer, like cancers in the mouth and throat, is more common in smokers and especially in smokers who are heavy drinkers.

Cancer of the lower end of the oesophagus is most often seen in people who have a history of inflammation or degeneration (metaplasia) or an ulcer in the lower oesophagus caused by long standing regurgitation of stomach contents. Such an inflammatory degeneration with metaplasia in the lower oesophagus is

F. O. Stephens and K. R. Aigner, *Basics of Oncology,*
DOI: 10.1007/978-3-540-92925-3_13, © Springer-Verlag Berlin Heidelberg 2009

now called a Barret's oesophagus but if an ulcer develops it is known as a Barret's ulcer. The conditions were first described by Dr Barret, an Australian surgeon working in London. Barret's ulcer is becoming more common in Western countries, so too is cancer of the lower oesophagus.

13.1.1   Pathology

Most cancers of the upper and middle regions of the oesophagus are of the flat pavement or squamous-cell type, having developed in the squamous mucosal lining. At the lower end of the oesophagus, where there may be glandular mucosa similar to that of the stomach, increasing numbers of cancers are of glandular-type cells. That is, adenocarcinoma is more common and increasingly so in association with long-standing Barret's ulcer.

13.1.2   Symptoms

Cancer of the oesophagus is usually well established before it is diagnosed.

Unfortunately, cancer of the oesophagus is usually well established before it is diagnosed. The most common symptom is dysphagia (difficulty with swallowing). First, there is difficulty in swallowing solid foods that seem to get caught in the throat or chest. Later, there is difficulty in swallowing liquids. A person with cancer of the oesophagus thus soon loses weight and may become quite wasted and even dehydrated.

13.1.3   Signs

The earliest sign of oesophageal cancer is for the doctor to observe the patient having difficulty with swallowing. A later sign will be evidence of weight loss and even dehydration.

13.1.4   Investigations

Barium swallow or barium meal X-rays (described in Sects. 7.3.2–7.3.3) will usually show an obstruction to swallowing in the oesophagus. An irregular, "apple-core" shaped, narrowing is a common feature at the site of this cancer.

Oesophagoscopy is carried out (described in Sect. 7.4.6) and, through the oesophagoscope, the doctor can usually see an irregular tumour mass or an ulcerated tumour. A biopsy will establish the diagnosis microscopically.

Cancers of the oesophagus have usually spread up and down and under the mucous membrane lining of the oesophagus and into lymph nodes and other structures in the chest before the patient notices much in the way of symptoms. Thus they are very often incurable when first diagnosed.

13.1.5 Treatment

Very early intramucosal adenocarcinoma in Barret's oesophagus can sometimes be treated effectively by endoscopic resection. However, long-term cure of well-established or invasive oesophageal cancer is all too infrequent but the best hope of cure is by operation. The oesophagus is removed and either the stomach or a section of bowel is used to make a new oesophagus for passage of food.

Radiotherapy is also used to treat this cancer. Although it often makes a cancer smaller for a period, and relieves symptoms temporarily, it does not often cure the cancer.

Even when radiotherapy and surgery are used together results have been disappointing.

Chemotherapy alone has also been disappointing in treating this cancer.

The earliest attempts to improve results by using chemotherapy first to reduce the cancer and then surgery to remove the remaining cancer did not improve patient outcomes. However, more recently some encouraging results have been reported using different drug combinations in integrated treatment programs in which chemotherapy has been integrated and synchronised with radiotherapy and possibly followed by surgery. Further studies are needed before a change in standard practice can be recommended with confidence.

Sometimes attempts at removing an oesophageal cancer are not possible and the most helpful treatment is for the surgeon to pass a plastic tube through the oesophagus and past the cancer into the stomach, to allow the patient to swallow food through the tube. Otherwise, some alternative food passage, possibly by putting a feeding tube directly into the stomach or another method of feeding, like intravenous nutrition may be required.

Screening. Because of the increased risk of cancer of lower oesophagus and upper stomach associated with Barret's metaplasia or Barret's ulcer, it is recommended that people with persistent or uncontrolled reflux or a known Barret's oesphagus be regularly screened by oesophagoscopy or endoscopy for early detection of any malignant change.

13

CASE REPORT

Lower oesophageal cancer

Michelle is a 63-year-old nurse.

She was 59-years old when she first complained of reflux and "burning" in her lower oesophagus. It had been troubling her for some months or possibly a year when she first consulted her family doctor. Her doctor arranged oesophagoscopy that confirmed gastric reflux and some mucosal irritation suggestive of Barret's oesophagus. The doctor advised Michelle to avoid bending, to lose some weight, to elevate the head-end of her bed and sleep with extra pillows under her head. He also prescribed an antacid medication. He asked Michelle to return for consultation in 3 months. Michelle explained that she was committed to working in an African mission for 2 years. The doctor then proscribed a "proton pump" medication for Michelle to take with her in case her symptoms were not distinctly better in 3 months. He advised Michelle to return to Brussels or another major centre for reassessment in no longer than 6 months.

Initially Michelle got some relief from the antacid medication but symptoms returned so she took a course of the "proton pump" medication. It too gave her initial relief but symptoms returned and worsened. She continued with her work but eventually had trouble swallowing and lost a great deal of weight. After 13 months she returned to Brussels where her doctor arranged a further gastroscopy. An ulcer with raised edges was seen in the gastro-oesophageal junction. Biopsies showed it to be an adenocarcinoma. Chest X-rays and CT scans did not show any evidence of tumour spread.

Possible treatments were discussed with Michelle. She was advised that surgery alone would offer her no more than a 20% chance of cure. Radiotherapy alone would probably give her temporary relief with but an even less chance of cure. The specialist involved advised that his oncology group was taking part in a clinical trial using either pre-operative (induction) chemotherapy followed by radiotherapy or preoperative chemotherapy followed by surgery to determine whether better results could be achieved.

Michelle agreed to take part in the study. After five treatments with chemotherapy at weekly intervals her cancer had become significantly smaller. Surgical resection of lower oesophagus and proximal stomach with draining lymph nodes was then performed and the residual oesophagus was anastomosed to the remaining stomach in the chest.

After initial trouble with eating and some anaemia, Michelle is now taking smaller nutritious meals more frequently, some treatment for anaemia and is beginning to gain some weight. To date, 6 months post-operatively, she feels relatively well but has reduced energy. So far there is no evidence of cancer recurrence.

13.2 Cancer of the Stomach

Stomach cancer is uncommon before the age of 40 but thereafter the incidence increases with age, reaching a peak between the ages of 60 and 65. For some unknown reason, in most countries males are affected about two or three times more commonly than females.

In the past, cancer of the lower or middle stomach was one of the more serious and more common cancers affecting mankind but fortunately, over recent years, it has become less common.

Stomach cancer has distinct racial, geographic and dietary associations. It is about seven times more common in Japan and Korea and three or four times more common in Eastern Europe than in the US (see Appendix).

Epidemiological studies suggest it has a direct close and relationship to diet. People who have a diet that is high in animal fats, (especially chemically preserved meats) and low in fresh fruit and vegetables have a greater risk of developing stomach cancer. It may be related to a high intake of chemical food preservatives and other methods of food preparation, curing, storage and preservation. For example the high intake of smoked fish in Japan has been incriminated. There is also a high incidence among people of northern Iceland who eat large amounts of crude smoked fish as opposed to a lower incidence in the people of southern Iceland who have a different diet. In Korea, the custom of eating a great deal of red pepper and possibly other irritating spices in food is thought to be significant.

It has been suggested that a reason for the decreasing incidence of stomach cancer in modern industrialised societies is the greater availability of fresh fruit and vegetables due to modern transport and the greater use of refrigeration to store foods rather than chemical preservatives and additives.

Medical conditions that increase a person's risk of developing stomach cancer are pernicious anaemia (six times the normal risk), chronic gastritis, polyps in the stomach and gastric ulcers that may be due to *Helicobacter pylori* infection. Smokers also have an increased risk and the risk is greater in smokers who are also heavy consumers of alcohol.

13.2.1 Pathology

Having developed in gastric mucosa, most gastric cancers are glandular type (adenocarcinoma). In the past, gastric cancer was much more common in the lower stomach but the pattern is now changing. It is now becoming less common in the lower stomach and increasingly more common in the upper end, especially about the gastro-oesophageal junction. This change in pattern is at least partly due to effective treatment of the Helicobacter pylori bacillus that commonly caused ulceration and other mucosal changes in the lower stomach. Effective treatment of this infection appears to have reduced the incidence of cancer in the lower stomach.

13.2.2　Symptoms

Like cancer of the oesophagus, cancer of the stomach is usually quite advanced before pain or other symptoms cause most patients to seek medical attention. The earliest symptom is usually vague indigestion that gradually becomes worse and more persistent. Persistent indigestion occurring for the first time in someone over the age of 40 must always be considered with suspicion. Sometimes an early feature is loss of appetite especially for certain foods. Loss of appetite for meat is common. Other symptoms may be of fullness or even feeling "blown up" in the stomach after eating small amounts of food, or vomiting after food. Vomiting may become frequent, regular or blood-stained. If a cancer has blocked the stomach, vomiting becomes persistent. Pain is sometimes the first symptom noticed but when pain is persistent the cancer is often quite advanced. Sometimes a patient has not been aware of any symptoms but has found a lump in the upper abdomen. Other patients feel weak and tired due to anaemia, or have experienced recent unexplained weight loss that may be the reason they seek medical attention, rather than any particular indigestion or abdominal complaints. Occasionally the first evidence of trouble is due to the cancer having spread to other organs or tissues, for example an enlarged liver or jaundice or back pain from the pancreas or other tissues behind the stomach.

13.2.3　Signs

Clinical examination may detect one or more of the following features: a swelling or lump in the upper abdomen; evidence of enlarged liver or lymph nodes; evidence of spread into the pelvis or onto an ovary (felt on vaginal or rectal examination); or evidence of fluid in the abdominal cavity (ascites). Evidence of anaemia or weight loss should also be checked. A palpable involved lymph node just above the medial end of the clavicle, and usually on the left side, is called a Virchow's node and is often a feature of advanced intra-abdominal cancer, especially stomach cancer, because these nodes drain lymph from around the thoracic duct which comes up from the abdomen.

13.2.4　Investigations

Blood tests for anaemia or other abnormalities and examination for blood in the faeces are standard investigations for possible cancer of stomach or bowel.

Endoscopy (or gastroscopy as described in Sect. 7.4) is a very useful test. Endoscopy may allow a cancer to be seen (as an ulcer with raised edges, a cauliflower-like mass or rigid abnormal distortion of the stomach wall) and a biopsy to be taken. Present-day endoscopy is now so readily practised and without stress to the patient that it is usually performed before barium meal X-ray studies.

A CT scan may be useful to determine the size and exact position of a cancer. It may show, for example, that the cancer has spread into the pancreas or liver or enlarged adjacent lymph nodes.

Barium meal X-rays (Sect. 7.3.2) may show an ulcer (usually with raised, rounded edges), or they may show a lump on the stomach wall looking something like a small cauliflower. The X-rays and screening may show a blocked stomach, a change in its shape or size (bigger, or shrunken and smaller), or a more rigid and stiff-walled stomach.

13.2.5 Treatment

The only present curative treatment of cancer of the stomach is surgery: to remove all of the stomach (total gastrectomy), most of the stomach (sub-total gastrectomy), or part of the stomach (partial gastrectomy). Because of the high risk of lymph-node involvement, draining lymph nodes are removed with the gastric resection.

The only present curative treatment of cancer of the stomach is surgery.

If a cancer has already spread beyond the stomach region surgical cure may not be possible but it may still be possible to relieve symptoms for example a gastro-enterostomy to relieve stomach obstruction.

After total gastrectomy the small intestine is anastomosed (joined) to the oesophagus or, in the case of a sub-total or partial gastrectomy, the small intestine may be anastomosed to the small remaining part of the stomach to allow food to pass through normally. After surgery the patient can eat only small meals and therefore needs to eat frequently to avoid too much weight loss. Without a stomach, the patient will also be given treatment to prevent anaemia. Anaemia may be a macrocytic anaemia due to loss of gastric intrinsic factor or a microcytic iron-deficiency anaemia due to inadequate iron absorption or, possibly, blood loss.

In the past results of surgery alone in treating apparently resectable stomach cancers have been disappointing (about 25–30% cures) but in general, the smaller a cancer is at surgery the better the chance of cure. For this reason, endoscopy and other diagnostic tests may be used to look for evidence of cancer as soon as a patient complains of early symptoms. If the patient is a male over the age of 40 years there is a greater risk that persistent symptoms of indigestion, lack of appetite and local epigastric pain and discomfort are due to a cancer. In some countries, and especially Japan, screening tests are often carried out in people at risk even though they may have no symptoms. When stomach cancers are found whilst they are small and in the early stages of the disease (as is now often the case in Japan), surgery results are good with a high rate of cure (more than 80% cure rates have been reported). However this is not often the case in Western countries where stomach cancer is less common and is not often diagnosed until troublesome symptoms have developed, by which time the cancers are more advanced and less likely to be cured by surgery alone.

Presently available anti-cancer drugs do not cure this cancer but they may be useful in treating people whose cancers cannot be cured by operation. The drugs will often make the cancers smaller and may give the patients good but temporary relief.

More recently, anti-cancer drugs have been given to some patients before the operation is carried out (see Sect. 8.3.4). Some reports have shown that if the cancers are made smaller by the drugs and then the operation (gastrectomy) is carried out, the results will be better and the chances of cure improved. The most effective way of giving the anti-cancer chemotherapy before operation may be by giving drugs directly into the coeliac axis artery that supplies blood to the stomach. After 5 or 6 weeks of this therapy, the cancer is usually smaller and, with following surgery, better results have been reported. These studies continue but as yet there has been no agreement about the most effective plan for integrated treatment.

More studies of these techniques are needed but there is some hope of better results with treatment of stomach cancer in the future. Firstly, by earlier diagnostic tests to detect cancers at an earlier and more curable stage and secondly, by the use of induction or neoadjuvant chemotherapy followed by surgery for those people who present for treatment with established, invasive, but removable cancers.

Studies in the use of postoperative adjuvant chemotherapy are in progress but at the time of writing, although some positive results have been reported there is no agreement on the benefits of adjuvant chemotherapy.

After gastrectomy it is important to carefully follow-up these patients not only for possible tumour recurrence but for general nutrition and to avoid both microcytic anaemia (possibly a feature of poor nutrition and iron deficiency) and macrocytic anaemia (due to loss of gastric intrinsic factor).

EXERCISE

List predisposing factors that may be associated with cancers of the stomach and the oesophagus.

13.3   Cancers of the Liver

Cancers in the liver are either cancers that began in the liver cells (primary) or cancers that have spread to the liver from another primary site (secondary or metastatic).

13.3.1   Primary Liver Cancer (Hepatoma or Hepatocellular Carcinoma)

Cancer starting in liver cells (primary cancer) is uncommon in European races but is common in Africans, South-East Asians, Chinese and Japanese (see Appendix). It ranges as high as half of all cancers in African Bantu men. The reasons for this difference in incidence are not completely understood although differences in diet and food storage and preparation are probably important. Long-standing liver infection with hepatitis B and hepatitis C and parasitic infestation, particularly by the liver fluke, are responsible for much of the increased incidence in some Asian countries. Certain fungi that commonly contaminate food in parts of Africa and Asia may also play a part whereas food stored by refrigeration in Westernised societies should be free from fungus contamination.

In Western Countries primary liver cancer is more likely in people with long-standing cirrhosis of the liver, whether the cirrhosis is the result of excessive alcohol consumption, post hepatitis or other causes.

13.3.1.1   Features of Primary Liver Cancer

The first evidence of primary liver cancer may be deterioration in general health (loss of appetite, lassitude, malaise, weight loss, weakness and debility) or features of liver enlargement with pain in the upper abdomen, swelling, jaundice or fluid in the abdominal cavity (ascites).

13.3.1.2   Investigations

Investigations that may help include CT scans, MRI scans, ultrasound, sometimes arteriography, but especially liver biopsy (see Sect. 7.3). Also, blood tests for liver function, anaemia and biochemical changes are often helpful. The tumour marker alpha-foeto-protein is usually raised in people with this cancer and should fall to normal levels if the cancer has been successfully treated. Progressive alpha-foeto-protein tests may give a useful indication of the effectiveness of treatment. Other serological tests for hepatitis B surface antigens (HBsAg) or antibodies for hepatitis C (anti-HCV) may also be positive in liver cancer.

13.3.1.3   *Treatment*

Treatment of primary liver cancer is successful only if the disease is detected whilst it is confined to a part of the liver that can be surgically resected. Because the cancer has usually spread widely in the liver when first detected, cure is usually not possible.

Chemo-embolisation can sometimes reduce tumour size and achieve palliation of symptoms. This treatment, in which anti-cancer agents are combined with a clotting agent and injected into the hepatic artery feeding the cancer mass, is commonly used in Japan. Another form of treatment now widely practised in Japan and other Eastern countries is to infuse chemotherapy into the hepatic artery together with different materials (often Lipiodol or microspheres) that slow the rate of the anti-cancer agents in their flow through the liver. The slower liver circulation increases the uptake of anti-cancer drugs by keeping the liver and cancer cells exposed to them for longer periods. Several reports of improved results are now well documented. In some trials immunological agents have also been incorporated to make the chemo-embolic materials or other liver circulation slowing agents even more effective.

Another treatment in suitable patients is cryosurgery (Sect. 8.5) or percutaneous alcohol injections to destroy all visible cancer. Some patients have repeated treatments and some gain long-term relief.

Tamoxifen is sometimes used in patients with poor performance status who wish some form of active treatment. This may give temporary relief and is unlikely to cause toxicity.

Meanwhile the most hopeful way of dealing with the high incidence of primary liver cancer is by more intense and widespread hepatitis B immunisation programs to prevent this cancer-prone liver disease. Although much needed there is, at the time of writing, no effective hepatitis C vaccine.

CASE REPORT

Hepatoma (primary liver cancer)

Henri was a 70-year-old retired winemaker who had become a heavy consumer of his wine product for many years. He had not felt well for some months with loss of appetite for food, weight-loss and loss of energy but unfortunately no loss of appetite for his wine.

He had developed abdominal discomfort and pain, especially pain in his right shoulder, when he consulted his family doctor.

His doctor found him to be a thin, wasted man with slight jaundice, some abdominal swelling with some ascites. Some petechial spots were noticed on the skin of Henri's abdomen. He felt an enlarged liver, with a distinct mass protruding downwards from the right liver lobe. When he put his stethoscope over the mass he could hear a vascular bruit.

Ultrasound, angiography and CT scans confirmed the appearance of a vascular liver mass consistent with a primary liver cancer. Blood count showed the presence of anaemia with a reduction in platelets. There was no evidence of a stomach, bowel or lung cancer that might have suggested the liver mass could be a secondary cancer so that a primary liver cancer was assumed without a biopsy. Biopsy was not performed due to the risk of haemorrhage.

Henri was given a transfusion of whole blood but was otherwise treated symptomatically only. He died 1 month later and autopsy confirmed a primary liver cancer (hepatoma) in a cirrhotic liver.

Comment

In Henri's state of health there would have been no question of resecting this cancer even though it appeared to be confined to the right lobe of the liver and was not involving the vena-cava. There was also no possibility of improving his outlook by systemic chemotherapy alone. However had Henri been well enough, consideration might have been given to treating his liver cancer by chemotherapeutic embolisation. In such treatment a chemotherapeutic agent together with a "blocking agent" (such as lipiodol or microspheres), is infused into the hepatic artery. The blocking agent slows the arterial blood flow in the liver thus allowing a longer period of exposure of the cancer cells to the chemotherapy. Such treatment is often worthwhile in younger, fitter patients with liver cancer.

13

13.3.2   Secondary (Metastatic) Liver Cancer

The liver is one of the most common sites of secondary cancer in Western races.

The liver is one of the most common sites of secondary cancer in Western races. Cancers of the digestive tract, especially the stomach, pancreas, colon and rectum commonly spread via the bloodstream to the liver. Cancers of almost any other tissue may also metastasise to liver, especially breast cancer, lung cancer and melanoma.

Once involved with metastases, the liver enlarges. It may become uncomfortable or even painful. Jaundice often develops and ascitic fluid may accumulate in the abdominal cavity. A person with secondary liver cancer sooner or later usually notices a general malaise, loss of appetite, loss of weight and loss of energy. Breathlessness may also develop.

13.3.2.1   Investigations

The most helpful investigations are usually the CT or MRI scan, ultrasound, sometimes arteriography and laparoscopy. Liver isotope scans, once a standard investigation, have largely been replaced by more helpful MRI scans. If needed, a liver biopsy may be required to confirm the diagnosis but very often the diagnosis is obvious from the known previous history of a cancer.

Liver biopsy can be carried out under local anaesthesia with a special needle through the lower chest or abdominal wall. Alternatively it may be carried out at laparoscopy or open operation.

If the site of a primary cancer that has spread to the liver is not known, investigations may be required to discover where the metastatic cancer in the liver originated (i.e. the primary cancer site) (Fig. 13.1 and 13.2).

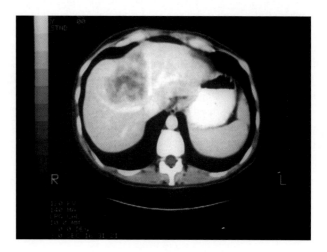

Fig. 13.1. CT of liver showing a metastasis from a colon cancer

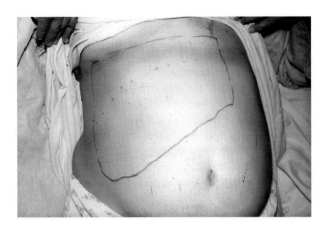

Fig. 13.2. Photograph of abdomen of a 63-year-old jaundiced woman with a big liver and ascites. The liver contained many metastatic lumps from a primary breast cancer treated 6 years previously

13.3.2.2 Treatments

Metastatic cancer in the liver is usually incurable. The best hope of cure is when there are only one to four metastases that are in a part of the liver that can be removed by surgical operation. However provided all metastases are in one resectable section, surgical removal may be worthwhile even if more than four metastases have been identified. This is uncommon. In most people, the secondary cancers are spread throughout both sides of the liver.

Although there is no cure for most patients, some metastatic cancers are sensitive to anti-cancer drugs, especially those that have come from primary cancer of the colon or rectum, stomach or breast.

Although the drugs do not totally cure them, metastases may be reduced sometimes giving the patient good relief for some months.

The simplest method of giving such anti-cancer drugs is either by mouth or intravenous injection. However, a more effective method is by direct chemotherapy infusion into the hepatic artery either intermittently through a catheter placed into the hepatic artery or by a continuous infusion using a continuous infusion pump.

Intermittent intra-arterial infusion chemotherapy can usually be given only in a hospital and the patient returns for treatment at intervals as necessary. There is now evidence that a larger dose and more effective treatment (using

5FU) is better tolerated if systemic protection with low dose folinic acid is first administered.

Some years ago a small pump was developed in America to continuously pump anti-cancer drugs into the hepatic artery. A surgeon implants this pump under the skin of the anterior abdominal wall where it stays without discomfort. It allows patients who are having continuous intra-arterial infusion chemotherapy to go home and lead relatively normal lives, returning for re-filling of the pump once every week or two. Although such pumps are expensive and suitable only for certain patients using certain drugs, most patients with pumps live comfortably for several months or even 2 years or more. For many of these patients, their survival time has been increased with good quality of life. Other studies are aimed at developing less expensive and more easily available methods of giving similar relief to greater numbers of patients using the principle of intra-arterial chemotherapy.

Implantable infusion pumps are expensive but can often be used with good effect. All methods have shown encouraging results as far as improving the patient's quality of life and possibly life expectancy are concerned but, as yet, with few exceptions, infusion chemotherapy is unlikely to achieve long-term survival or cure. Studies of each technique continue.

Different combinations of anti-cancer drugs given in different treatment schedules with or without infusion pumps are under study in many world cancer centres. Although good results can be achieved when the drugs are given into the hepatic artery, as yet there are a number of difficulties and problems to be solved before this form of treatment can be recommended for general use other than in specialised cancer clinics.

Destruction of obvious liver metastatic masses by cryosurgery or by alcohol injection under laparoscopic control is used in some specialised centres, usually with good effect. Some patients obtain considerable benefit, and in some the treatment can be repeated with reasonably good long-term control. In some highly specialised clinics this treatment is sometimes combined with hepatic-artery infusion chemotherapy with good long-term control in suitable patients. Over 70% long-term survivors have been reported from some clinics. Such studies are continuing but this sort of treatment does require a dedicated team of specialists.

Some encouraging results are also being reported from implantation of radio-active "seeds" into liver cancers.

Radio-frequency ablation (RFA) is another new approach under study for treating some cancers in the liver.

CASE REPORT

Metastatic liver cancer

Kiri was a 62-year-old Maori woman who attended her doctor for her regular follow-up having had a bowel cancer resected 3 years previously.

Over the last 6 months, since her last attendance she had had a reduced appetite and lost some weight. She said that she had little energy.

The surgeon could feel a lump protruding from her liver edge below the right costal margin. He arranged CT scans and three distinct masses were seen in the liver, three in the right lobe and a smaller lump in the left lobe. A needle biopsy confirmed the presence of metastatic cancer of large bowel origin.

Resection of these tumours was out of the question so that Kiri was offered the option of systemic chemotherapy, chemotherapy infusions into her hepatic artery on a monthly basis or cryosurgical injections into the liver metastases. Although more complex to administer she was advised that hepatic arterial chemotherapy would be more likely to achieve a tumour response than systemic chemotherapy. She chose this treatment as her preferred first line of therapy. She was treated on a monthly basis with chemotherapy (5-FU infused over 8 h into the hepatic artery). On each occasion a vascular radiologist inserted a cannula into the hepatic artery via one of her femoral arteries.

Over the next 7 months the tumour masses were first reduced in size but they then began to increase in size so that the surgeon proposed treatment by cryotherapy to which Kiri agreed.

Under a general anaesthetic, with laparoscopic visual control, the surgeon inserted a probe into each tumour mass and injected a measured amount of liquid nitrogen into each mass.

In subsequent weeks the tumour masses reduced in size but after 5 months further masses had developed in the liver.

The cryosurgery was repeated on one more occasion and although there was an initial good response for 3 months further masses developed in the liver. With this Kiri's general health had deteriorated with development of jaundice and ascites. Kiri was thereafter treated symptomatically.

Comment

Life expectancy after first diagnosis of colon cancer metastases in the liver is about seven or 8 months. Kiri and her family were grateful that she had survived to attend her granddaughter's wedding 1 year after the liver metastases were first treated and she survived 19 months in all.

13

List the reasons why in Eastern and developing countries primary cancers in the liver are more common than metastatic cancers but metastatic cancers in the liver are much more common in Western and developed countries.

13.4   Cancer of the Gall Bladder and Bile Ducts

These are uncommon cancers in Western countries although quite common in some countries such as South India. In Western countries, cancer of the gall bladder is usually associated with gallstones that have been present for many years. It is most common in older women. Cancer of the bile ducts, on the other hand, is rather more common in men.

A cancer may develop as a result of years of irritation with gall-stones.   One reason for advising removal of gall bladders with gallstones, especially in young women, is that there is a risk that over the years a cancer may develop as a result of years of irritation with gallstones.

Early cancer may occasionally be found unexpectedly and incidentally on examination of the gall bladder after it has been removed for other reasons. In such cases, cure of the cancer may have been achieved simply by the operation of cholecystectomy.

13.4.1   Symptoms

If not diagnosed early, cancer of the gall bladder may cause persistent pain in the upper right side of the abdomen, with inflammation of the gall bladder. It may cause a swelling or lump felt in the upper abdomen under the ribs on the right side.

13.4.2   Signs

Cancer of the gall bladder and more especially cancer of the bile ducts may present with jaundice due to obstruction of the flow of bile from the liver. The jaundice is often accompanied by a severe itch of the patient's skin.

13.4.3 Pathology and Treatment

Cancer of the gall bladder tends to invade the liver as well as nearby lymph nodes. Once this has happened it is virtually incurable by surgery and does not respond well to radiotherapy. It also does not respond well to chemotherapy although good response to more concentrated intra-arterial chemotherapy (see Sect. 8.3.4.6) and cure with subsequent surgery has been reported. In advanced cases jaundice and itch if present, can usually be relieved by a surgical operation in which the obstruction to bile flow is bypassed allowing the bile to flow into the bowel by another route. Alternatively a rigid stent is sometimes inserted surgically through the obstruction in the bile duct to allow passage of bile and so relieve the jaundice.

13.5 Cancer of the Pancreas

Cancer of the pancreas has become increasingly common in Western Countries over recent years. It is now the fourth leading cause of cancer death in middle-aged males in the US. It is more common in males than females (see Appendix), but the reason for this is unknown. It is becoming increasingly common in smokers and is also more common in heavy drinkers of alcohol. Diabetics and people with a history of chronic pancreatitis also have an increased risk of pancreatic cancer. Questionable associations of pancreatic cancer with consumption of coffee have been reported but not confirmed however tea drinking may even be protective (possibly due to anti-oxidants in tea).

13.5.1 Presentation

Cancer of the pancreas often involves the common bile duct causing bile duct obstruction and often first presents as obstructive jaundice As the obstruction continues, the jaundice becomes a deeper yellow. The jaundice may be painless although there is often pain felt deep in the upper abdomen and passing through to the back. The jaundice may cause the patient's skin to become very itchy (*pruritus*). As obstructive jaundice develops, the gall bladder and the liver may become enlarged and palpable. Sometimes a pancreatic tumour mass can be felt.

Most patients with cancer of the pancreas have vague malaise, anorexia and weight loss, in fact these may be the first features of the disease. Diarrhoea may also be a feature. Sometimes patients first present with a painless jaundice with no otherwise obvious cause.

13.5.2   Investigations

Because the pancreas lies across the back of the upper abdomen, behind the stomach and other organs, it has been one of the more difficult organs to feel or to investigate. With the improved methods of investigation now available, abnormalities including cancer are now more often diagnosed in earlier stages.

Ultrasound and CT scans have been of some help in detecting earlier cancers although early detection of the smallest cancers at a potentially curable stage is still difficult.

A tumour marker, CA19-9, is often elevated in patients with pancreas cancer. A low level might suggest a resectable cancer but a level of more than 2,000 usually indicates a non-resectable cancer.

Endoscopic retrograde cholangio-pancreatoscopy (ERCP discussed in Sect. 7.4.10), has allowed pancreatic secretions to be examined for cancer cells and X-rays to be taken of the duct. These may be helpful in detecting evidence of some pancreatic cancers at an early stage.

An isotope material suitable and specific for scanning the pancreas has not been found but work continues in the search for such a substance. When PET scans become more readily available (see Sect. 7.3.12) this is one area where it is hoped they will help significantly in early detection as well as diagnosis and monitoring response to treatments.

Needle biopsy of any lump in the pancreas is the most useful method of establishing a diagnosis but this procedure is not always reliable and does have risks. It depends very much on getting the needle into exactly the right part of the pancreas. A significant risk is that the needle tract might cause pancreatic juices to leak into the peritoneal cavity and possibly establish a fistula that will cause further problems.

13.5.3   Treatment

When first detected, cancer of the pancreas has usually spread to lymph nodes and the liver and cure by surgery is usually not possible. However, some small early cancers can be resected by a major surgical operation with fair prospects of cure.

The operation is known as a Whipple's operation.

To date, treatment by radiotherapy or chemotherapy has been disappointing although more effective anti-cancer drugs and combination therapies are constantly being investigated. Downgrading some cancers by radio/chemotherapy prior to surgical resection has been successful in some studies with some long-term cures reported but further studies are needed before such treatment can be more widely accepted.

Present studies include more effective use of intra-arterial chemotherapy as the first measure of an integrated treatment program with radiotherapy and surgery but a number of difficulties need to be solved and further studies are needed before this can be recommended as safe or effective treatment.

For most pancreatic cancers, some hope of temporary palliation of symptoms is usually the best that can be achieved.

Relief of jaundice due to pancreatic cancer obstructing the bile duct can usually be achieved by surgery to bi-pass the obstruction. Alternatively, a rigid stent passed through the lumen of the bile duct at the site of obstruction might give temporary relief of bile-duct obstruction.

CASE REPORT

Advanced cancer of pancreas

Boris was a 54-year-old Russian factory worker. He had been a smoker for more than 30 years.

His wife had noticed a change in colour of his skin for 3 or 4 weeks and that he had not been eating well and seemed to be losing weight, when she convinced him to consult a doctor. By the time he saw his doctor an obvious jaundice was present. He confessed to his doctor that he had had some upper abdominal and back pain and discomfort for 5 or 6 weeks.

On examination the doctor felt the liver was enlarged below the right costal margin. No abdominal mass could be felt but a CT showed a mass, in the region of the head of his pancreas. He explained that this was likely to be a cancer and that a laparoscopy was recommended to confirm this.

At laparoscopy a cancer in the head of the pancreas was confirmed and the presence of a dilated gallbladder was noted.

A laparotomy was recommended. It was explained to Boris that the fixed cancer mass was unlikely to be resectable but his jaundice could be relieved by anastomosing his gall bladder to his small bowel, so bypassing the obstructing mass in the head of his pancreas.

Boris agreed to surgery and the presence of a cancer fixed to the posterior abdominal wall with several firm enlarged adjacent lymph nodes was confirmed. The gallbladder and common bile duct were dilated.

The cancer was clearly not resectable so the surgeon anastomosed the dilated gall bladder to small bowel to bypass the obstruction.

Over the next 2 or 3 weeks the jaundice resolved. Boris was then commenced on a course of chemotherapy (5-FU) given by intravenous infusion.

After 6 weeks when CT examination showed the mass to be a little larger and his white cell and platelet count had fallen to dangerous levels the chemotherapy was stopped.

Thereafter all but palliative treatment was withdrawn. Boris required increasing doses of morphine and eventually a morphine drip to get pain relief.

Boris failed to eat, lost weight and his condition deteriorated until she died 10 weeks after his operation.

EXERCISE

Using as examples case reports in this chapter and other chapters of this book, construct a case report of a typical patient presenting with and being investigated and managed for an operable cancer of pancreas.

13.6   Cancers of the Small Intestine

Metastatic cancers, especially melanoma, sometimes involve the small intestine and the small intestine is sometimes involved from cancers of other nearby organs, especially colon and ovary, but primary cancer of the small intestine is rare.

The most common of the rare primary malignant tumours of small intestine are adenocarcinoma (a glandular cancer), a lymphoma (as described in Chap. 19) and a tumour called a carcinoid (cancer-like) tumour. These are rare causes of abdominal pain, bowel bleeding or small bowel obstruction. They are usually treated by a surgical resection.

13.6.1   Carcinoid Tumour

Carcinoid tumours may occur anywhere in the alimentary tract between the mouth and anus. The most common site is in the appendix. Most carcinoids in the appendix, and in fact most small carcinoids, are benign. Sometimes when an appendix has been taken out for appendicitis, a small carcinoid tumour may be found in it. In most such cases the tumour has been cured by removal of the appendix. Further treatment is usually not necessary.

When a carcinoid tumour is found in the small intestine, rather than the appendix, it is more likely to be larger (2 cm diameter or more) and more likely to be malignant.

Treatment is by resection of the section of bowel and draining mesenteric lymph nodes but it may have already metastasised to the liver. Carcinoid metastases in the liver may release certain biochemical substances that can cause wheezing, bouts of diarrhoea, flushing of the skin of the face. Treatment can be given to control these episodes but once this tumour has spread into the liver, complete cure is unlikely.

13.7   Cancer of the Large Bowel (Colon and Rectum)

In most Western societies the large bowel is the third or fourth most common site of primary cancer although in the Australian and New Zealand populations, in both sexes combined, large bowel cancer is the most common after skin cancer. In the adult population of the US lung cancer is by far the most common cause of cancer death followed by colorectal cancer then breast cancer and prostate cancer.

Bowel cancer is a glandular cancer (adenocarcinoma). Although occasionally seen in young adults (and even in children) it is not commonly seen until after the age of 40. Thereafter the incidence rises with age, reaching a peak between 60 and 75 years.

Cancer of the large bowel is most common in Western societies where the food intake is relatively high in meat and animal fats, relatively high in refined foods and relatively low in fibre such as in wholemeal grains, nuts, legumes, fruit and vegetables (as discussed in Chaps. 2 and 3). It is a relatively uncommon cancer in Asian countries except Japan and Singapore where "Western" diets are now widespread. Colo-rectal cancer is uncommon in developing countries and in vegetarians.

Polyps in the large bowel often predispose to cancer and should be removed to avoid the risk of malignant change. People who have had polyps removed should be kept under regular observation in case further polyps develop.

The most useful screening tests for bowel polyps and bowel cancer are chemical tests for occult blood in the faeces and regular colonoscopy, particularly for people in higher risk groups. The higher risk groups include anyone who has previously had a bowel cancer, anyone with a strong family history of bowel cancer and in fact anyone over 55 who has been living on a traditional Western diet.

Colorectal cancers in total are more common in males (especially rectal cancers) but cancers in the right side of colon are rather more common in females. Smoking, obesity and a sedentary occupation are risk factors.

A highly pre-malignant condition is the uncommon hereditary condition *familial polyposis coli*, in which about half of the members of an affected family are likely to develop multiple polyps. Those who have these polyps should have all large bowel surgically removed otherwise they will develop bowel cancer usually before the age of 40. All close blood relatives in an affected family should be kept under regular observation. If polyps are found, these people too should have a total colectomy.

A villous papilloma, less common than polyps, sometimes occurs in the rectum. It has considerable propensity to become malignant in its base and should be surgically removed when detected (Figs. 13.3 and 13.4).

Other conditions with an increased risk of large bowel cancer are the inflammatory bowel disease ulcerative colitis and to a lesser extent granulomatous (Crohn's) colitis. The longer ulcerative colitis has been present and the greater the severity of the disease and length of bowel affected, the greater is the risk of cancer developing. About 10% of people with continuing ulcerative colitis

Polyps in the large bowel often predispose to cancer and should be removed to avoid the risk of malignant change.

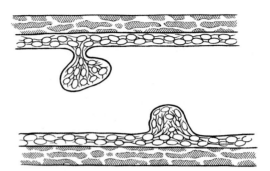

Fig. 13.3. Diagram of bowel polyps

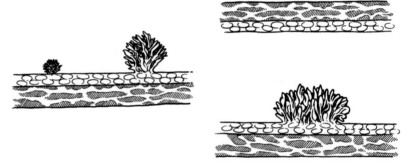

Fig. 13.4. Diagrams of a benign bowel papilloma and a previously benign papilloma developing into a large malignant villous papilloma

What are the differences between bowel polyps and bowel papillomata?

will develop colon cancer after about 10 years. People with long-standing and extensive ulcerative colitis must be kept under close and regular observation and in some circumstances may be well advised to have the colon removed as a precautionary measure.

Apart from familial polyposis coli, close relatives of a patient with any large bowel cancer have a slightly increased risk of developing a similar cancer. Whether this is mainly a genetic factor or due to similar diet and other habits is uncertain. Although the majority of patients successfully treated for bowel cancer do not develop a second tumour they do have an increased risk so that regular "follow-up" checks are important.

13.7.1 Clinical Features

The most common symptoms of large bowel cancer are a change in bowel habits (constipation or diarrhoea or sometimes alternating constipation and diarrhoea), bleeding from the bowel, and a feeling of incomplete evacuation after going to the toilet. In some cases patients are not aware of any symptoms until the cancer has caused partial or complete bowel obstruction. The first symptoms may thus be of bowel obstruction with intermittent griping abdominal pain (colic), constipation and abdominal distension.

Other features of large bowel cancer may be of general debility, weight loss, tiredness and lassitude (sometimes due to anaemia) or features of liver enlargement or jaundice due to liver metastases.

It may be possible to feel an abdominal lump or localised swelling or on anal examination with a gloved finger, a mass in the anus or lower rectum can sometimes be felt. There may be evidence of blood in the faeces. In obstructive bowel cancer, colic with abdominal distension or swelling is likely.

13.7.2 Investigations

Investigations include sigmoidoscopic or colonoscopic examinations (described in Sect. 7.4.2). About half of large bowel cancers are in the rectum or lower sigmoid colon. These can be seen and biopsied through a sigmoidoscope.

Barium (or Baryum) enema screening and X-rays may reveal a cancer, especially if an air-contrast barium study is used (see Sect. 7.3.2).

If there is no evidence of bowel obstruction and especially if a cancer is suspected in the first part of the large bowel (the caecum or ascending colon), barium meal studies and X-rays may help outline a tumour mass but colonoscopy with biopsy is still the most helpful method of diagnosis.

Sigmoidoscopic examination, barium enema and barium meal studies can all be done on an outpatient basis without anaesthesia but colonoscopy requires good sedation or in some cases a general anaesthetic. Colonoscopy will allow the

Colonoscopy will allow the whole length of the large bowel to be examined visually and for biopsies to be taken

whole length of the large bowel to be examined visually and for biopsies to be taken from any part of the length of the colon.

A day in hospital is sometimes required for this examination although increasing numbers are now performed on a short stay basis of half a day or so. In some modern clinics the procedure can be carried out with the patient being mildly sedated and even able to watch the procedure on a TV monitor.

Blood studies are used to detect anaemia or changes in biochemistry of the blood or impaired liver function. Carcino-embryonic antigen (Sect. 7.5.5) is a tumour marker that is usually strongly positive in people with large bowel cancer and becomes negative after successful treatment. If it becomes positive again at a later stage after treatment this suggests a recurrence of the cancer.

CT scans are used in detecting evidence of liver metastases.

13.7.3   Treatment

In good hands an early operation will cure about half the patients with large bowel cancer. The only way of curing a large bowel cancer is by a surgical operation in which the part of the bowel containing the cancer is excised together with its draining lymph nodes, into which the cancer may have spread. In most cases, cut ends of bowel are joined (anastomosed), so the patient can return to normal life. The place of chemotherapy or radiation therapy as adjuvant treatment before or after surgical resection is still under study. Some studies have suggested that there may be a place for pre-operative radiation for some advanced rectal cancers but the use of radiotherapy is somewhat controversial. Several studies have shown some improvement in long-term results using adjuvant chemotherapy after surgical resection of more advanced colo-rectal cancers with or without radiotherapy. Adjuvant chemotherapy (often with *5-FU and leucovorin)* is now standard practice in many modern clinics when the cancer has involved local lymph nodes.

Recent studies using an angiotoxic substance "Avastin" are showing encouraging results in enhancing the cytotoxic properties of chemotherapy for bowel cancer.

When the cancer is in the lower rectum it may be necessary to remove the anus as well as the rectum and a *colostomy* bowel opening is made in the abdominal wall for passage of faeces. The patient learns to wear a bag over the colostomy and the bowel empties at regular intervals into the bag. The patient learns to empty the bag at convenient times and gradually learns to live an active and virtually normal life.

A *colostomy club* has been established with branches in many large cities. Membership is open to all people who have a colostomy. This club is a meeting ground for people with similar problems and has been a great help in assisting many patients to adjust to the new circumstances of living with a colostomy. Mutual support and advice help people to learn to live with a colostomy and to cope with necessary social adjustments.

In good hands an early operation will cure about half the patients with large bowel cancer. With adjuvant chemotherapy in appropriate patients, even better results are reported. With or without a colostomy, most people then return to normal life. The cure rate depends on the degree of penetration of the cancer into the bowel wall and the involvement of nearby or more distant lymph nodes.

If a cancer first presents with bowel obstruction it may be necessary to make a *temporary colostomy* to relieve the obstruction. Usually the cancer is resected 3 or 4 weeks later and the colostomy is subsequently closed, resulting in a return to normal passage of bowel actions.

13.7.4 Follow-Up Care

As for all patients who have had a cancer treated, regular "follow up" consultations and care are required for patients who have had a bowel cancer resected. There is always a risk of metastatic cancer showing up in the liver or elsewhere and there may be a risk of another bowel cancer developing that can be effectively treated if detected while still small. In the case of bowel cancer any metastatic cancer usually shows up within 2 years. It is uncommon for recurrence to first show up after 5 years.

Treatment for patients with metastatic cancer in the liver using surgical resection, intra-arterial chemotherapy, cryotherapy or alcohol injections has already been discussed in this chapter (*liver cancer*).

13.8 Cancer of the Anus

13.8.1 Presentation and Pathology

Cancer of the anus is not common but may present as a lump, an ulcer, bleeding, or pain in the anal region. Sometimes it may develop in a pre-existing lesion such as a papilloma (possibly caused by the human papilloma virus (HPV)), a patch of leukoplakia (white patch) or in a long-standing anal fissure (a crack in the wall of the opening of the anus).

Most cancers of the anus are similar in type to squamous cell cancer of skin but behave more aggressively. A minority of anal cancers are adenocarcinomas of the glandular mucosa of the upper anal canal.

Most anal cancers tend to spread to lymph nodes in the groins or in the pelvis at an early stage and often require radical treatment to achieve the best chance of cure.

13

CASE REPORT

Colon cancer

Bruce was a 59-year-old former smoker and a little overweight. He had had coronary bypass surgery 4 months previously when he mentioned to his cardiologist that he had noticed a little fresh blood in his bowel motions on three or four occasions recently. He had no other bowel symptoms and had made a good recovery from his cardiac surgery.

The cardiologist could not detect any mass or other abnormality on either abdominal or anal examination. She referred Bruce to a gastroenterologist who did not detect any significant abnormality but arranged a colonoscopy examination. Blood and liver biochemistry tests were normal.

At colonoscopy the doctor found a polypoid lesion with a 2 cm diameter ulcer with raised edges in the sigmoid colon. Biopsy showed it to be an adenocarcinoma.

CT scans of abdomen, liver and chest did not show any evidence of cancer spread.

Bruce was advised to have a surgical resection of left colon including descending colon, sigmoid colon and upper rectum. The draining lymph nodes were also resected with the specimen.

No tumour involvement of lymph nodes was detected.

Bruce enquired as to whether he needed to have adjuvant chemotherapy but it was explained to Bruce that there appeared to be no need for him to be given adjuvant chemotherapy because no lymph nodes were found to have cancer involvement, the liver was not involved and the cancer had not penetrated the bowel wall.

Regular follow-up examinations were carried out, including annual colonoscopies for 5 years but no residual tumour and nor any polyps were detected.

After being relatively well for 8 years further cardiac problems resulted in Bruce's death 11 years after colon surgery. His bowel function had been normal with no evidence of any residual bowel or cancer problem.

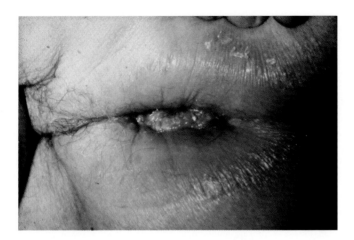

Fig. 13.5. An advanced cancer of the anus of a 67-year-old man

An increased risk of anal cancer has been correlated in people who practice anal sex. This increase may be associated with the HPV or HIV infection (Fig. 13.5).

13.8.2   Treatment

First a biopsy is taken to confirm the presence and type of cancer.

Treatment may then be by local surgery or radiotherapy for small early cancers with the objective of preserving the anal sphincter. Radical surgery, including excision of the rectum and anus was standard practice for rather more advanced cancers until reports of good results from combined use of integrated chemotherapy and radiotherapy, and this has now become standard practice in most modern centres. Radical surgery may still be required for cancers that have not responded to chemo/radiotherapy. Radical excision of draining lymph nodes from the groin will be required if these nodes appear to be involved.

Head and Neck Cancers

14

In this chapter you will learn about:

> Cancers of the lips
> Cancers of the mouth, anterior tongue and buccal mucosa
> Cancers of the posterior tongue, tonsillar region and pharynx
> Cancers of the post-nasal space
> Cancer of the larynx
> Salivary gland cancers
> Cancers of the thyroid gland

Cancers of the lips, mouth, tongue, nasal cavity, the paranasal air sinuses, throat, larynx and pharynx constitute about 5% of all cancers recorded in the US and the incidence is similar in most developed and developing countries. Most of these cancers are of squamous cells lining the mucosal epithelium. They are similar in type to squamous cell carcinoma (SCC) of the skin. However they tend to behave in a more malignant and more aggressive fashion than SCCs of skin. As a rule the further the cancers are away from the lips, the more aggressively they behave. Cancers of the lips are more aggressive than skin cancers. That is, they tend to grow more rapidly locally and have a greater tendency to spread to draining lymph nodes at an earlier stage. Cancers of the floor of the mouth, the anterior two-thirds of the tongue, and palate are more aggressive than cancers of the lips. Cancers of the back of the tongue, in the region of the tonsils and pharynx and upper air passages are the most aggressive. Cancers of the vocal cords of the larynx are an exception to this rule. Possibly because the vocal cords are poorly vascularized, these cancers tend to remain localised to the vocal cords with no evidence of spread when they first cause symptoms. The majority are readily curable at that stage.

These cancers are all much more common in smokers than non-smokers and are most common in males over 50. It has been estimated that cancers in the mouth and throat are about six times more common in smokers than in non-

The further the cancers are away from the lips, the more aggressively they behave.

F. O. Stephens and K. R. Aigner, *Basics of Oncology,*
DOI: 10.1007/978-3-540-92925-3_14, © Springer-Verlag Berlin Heidelberg 2009

smokers and this is increased to about 15 times if the smokers are also heavy drinkers of alcohol. Other pre-malignant conditions that predispose to cancer in the mouth include leukoplakia, papillomata, and chronic irritation from such causes as ill-fitting dentures or jagged teeth (see Chap. 1).

14.1   Cancers of the Lips

Cancers of the lips being more obvious than cancers further back in the mouth or throat are usually diagnosed at an earlier and more curable stage. They may develop as a thickening in an area of hyperkeratosis (sun damage) – most commonly on the lower lip. They tend to ulcerate and possibly bleed or may form a lump. They may then metastasise to lymph nodes under the jaw and in the sides of the neck that may be felt as enlarged and usually firm or hard lymph nodes.

A biopsy is taken to confirm the diagnosis and thereafter treatment is usually by surgical excision. Good results, both cosmetically and clinically are usually achieved. Radiotherapy can also be used with good results.

For larger cancers of the lips, either radical surgery, (removing a large part of the lip with some form of plastic or reconstructive surgery to fashion a new lip), or radiotherapy may be used, and the chances of cure are still good.

If hard, enlarged lymph nodes are present either when the patient is first seen or at a later follow-up visit to the doctor, these are best treated by surgical block dissection to remove all local lymph nodes.

Occasionally, a patient first consults a doctor when the cancer is very large. Possibly the whole of the lip is involved with cancer. In these patients, considerable success can be achieved with induction (neoadjuvant) chemotherapy to first reduce the cancer then following this treatment with radiotherapy or surgery or both. If special facilities for intra-arterial chemotherapy are available, the chemotherapy may be best given regionally by infusion into the arteries that supply blood to the cancer region but such treatment should be done only in specialist clinics with special experience, equipment and skills. It is not necessary to use this more complicated combined treatment for smaller cancers that can be readily cured by operation or by radiotherapy (Figs. 14.1–14.2).

14.2   Cancers of the Floor of the Mouth (Under the Tongue), Anterior Two-Thirds of the Tongue, and Buccal Mucosa (Inside the Cheek)

These cancers are more aggressive than lip cancers. Lymph nodes are involved in about 30% of cases.

These cancers are usually first noticed as an ulcer or a lump either by the patient or sometimes by their dentist before symptoms develop. Other common features are bleeding or localised soreness. These cancers tend to be on the

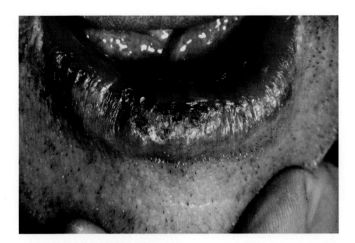

Fig. 14.1. A squamous cell carcinoma developing in sun induced hyperkeratosis of the lower lip

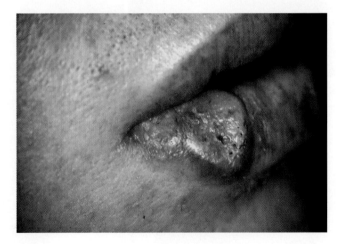

Fig. 14.2. A localised SCC of lower lip

surface at first but soon invade locally with firm induration surrounding the lump or ulcer. They usually become quite tender. Diagnosis is confirmed by taking a small biopsy for microscopic examination.

Cancers in the buccal mucosa of the cheek pouch are most common in India, Pakistan, New Guinea and The Solomon Islands due to the common practice of chewing betel nut. After initial chewing, the nut is often stored in the cheek pouch where its carcinogenic properties take effect.

Most cancers are well treated by surgical excision or radiotherapy. Involved lymph nodes are best treated by block dissection of all lymph nodes in the region. Sometimes reconstructive surgery may be required to replace resected tissue.

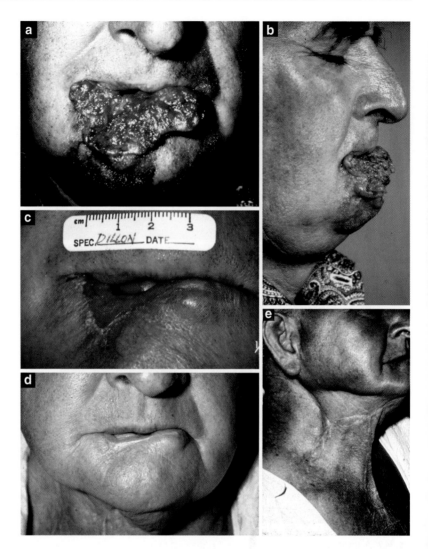

Fig. 14.3 (a, b). Anteroposterior and lateral photographs of a man who first presented with this very advanced SCC of his lower lip. The swelling under the jaw was a mass of metastatic cancer in lymph nodes. (**c**) Photograph of the same lip after treatment with chemotherapy (given over 5 weeks by continuous intra-arterial infusion). Three weeks after completion of chemotherapy "follow-up" treatment with radiotherapy was started. Right sided cervical nodes and submental nodes were resected 4 weeks after completion of radiotherapy. They included a small residual node mass containing some cancer cells. (**d**) The end result. This photograph was taken 2 years after completion of treatment. (**e**) Lateral view of the end result. This man was well and without evidence of cancer when last seen 12 years after treatment

For larger cancers in the floor of the mouth, anterior two-thirds of tongue, or the cheek, treatment by prior induction chemotherapy followed by radiotherapy or surgery, may give the best results. In some specialised clinics such induction chemotherapy is given by intra-arterial infusion more directly to the tumour site.

By these combined treatment methods, cures can now be achieved in patients with advanced cancers, which, until recently, were considered incurable or possibly only curable by the most radical surgery. Such treatments do require special skills, equipment and experience and should be carried out only in experienced cancer centres (Chap. 8) (Fig. 14.4–14.6).

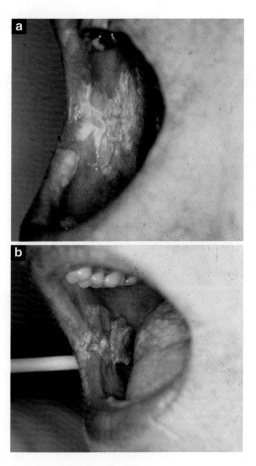

Fig. 14.4. Photographs showing (**a**) leukoplakia in the buccal mucosa of a 54-year-old heavy smoker and heavy alcohol drinker; (**b**) the same mucosa 2 years later. It had developed into a papillary squamous carcinoma

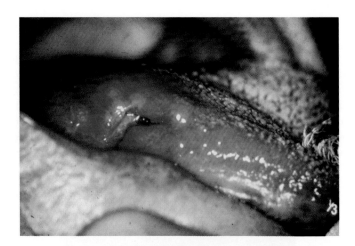

Fig. 14.5. An ulcerating SCC of the side of the tongue

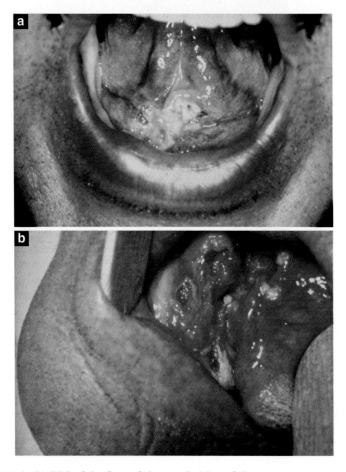

Fig. 14.6. (**a**, **b**) SCC of the floor of the mouth. Most of these cancers are associated with smoking

CASE REPORT

Squamous cancer of the tongue

Tony was a 70-year-old Italian migrant enjoying his retirement in Sydney, Australia. He had generally good health despite a smoking history of 40 years duration. He had rolled his own cigarettes (ten daily for 40 years) but had stopped smoking 5 years before his first consultation. After stopping smoking he continued to enjoy beer and wine, having up to five alcoholic drinks daily.

Two months prior to presentation, Tony had noticed a small lump on the side of his tongue. This was initially painless, so he ignored it thinking he must have bitten his tongue in his sleep. However the lump progressively enlarged. After a few weeks, he felt pain in his tongue, jaw and left ear. Eventually the lump came to interfere with his speech and swallowing. He reported the problem to his family doctor

His doctor recognised a large cauliflower-like tumour on the left side of his tongue. He was promptly referred to a Head and Neck Surgeon. Tony was then advised that he had developed a cancer of the side of his tongue

A small biopsy was performed in the surgeon's office under local anaesthesia. Within 24 h it confirmed an invasive SCC.

Neither his family doctor nor the surgeon could feel any involvement of lymph nodes in the neck. For confirmation, Tony underwent a CT scan. There was no evidence of nodal metastasis. A chest X-ray showed some emphysema, but no sign of spread to the lungs.

The tongue cancer was defined as Stage II (T2N0M0). However, because of the tumour's size and depth of invasion, there was still a 25% chance of spread to the neck. He was advised to have surgical excision of both the primary tumour and the lymph nodes at risk in the left neck.

Tony underwent excision of the left side of his anterior tongue. His tongue was repaired primarily. A total of 45 cervical lymph nodes were removed. Of these, one proved to contain metastatic cancer. As a result, he also required post-operative radiation therapy to the mouth and neck.

The treatment for his tongue cancer took almost 3 months. Swallowing was particularly difficult during the radiation therapy He lost a total of 18 kg in weight. His speech remained surprisingly good. After 1 year, he continues to gradually recover from his ordeal. His mouth is very dry due to irradiation involving his salivary glands but some taste has returned and he has managed to regain some weight. He will remain under surveillance for head and neck cancer for several years to come.

14

14.3   Cancer in the Posterior Third of Tongue, Tonsillar Region and Pharynx

These cancers may present as an ulcer, a lump in the throat or tongue or sometimes a constant sore throat that has not responded to conservative treatment
including antibiotics. Sometimes patients will first notice a lump in the side of the
neck that is, in fact, an enlarged, hard lymph node containing metastatic cancer.
Diagnosis may appear to be obvious but must be confirmed by biopsy.

Except for small cancers in this region, most cannot be cured by surgery other
than extensive radical surgery and tissue reconstruction and even then long term
results have all too often been disappointing. Radiotherapy too is likely to cure
only small cancers although it may offer good temporary palliation to people
with large cancers.

Unfortunately, most people with these cancers do not attend a doctor or clinic
until the cancer is advanced and the chances of cure by surgery or radiotherapy
are not good. Most of these patients are heavy smokers and many are alcoholics

EXERCISE

What are the most significant causes or predisposing features of cancers in
the lips, mouth and throat?

EXERCISE

Using as examples case reports in this and other chapters of this book,
construct a case report of a typical patient presenting with and being
investigated and managed for a cancer of the floor of mouth.

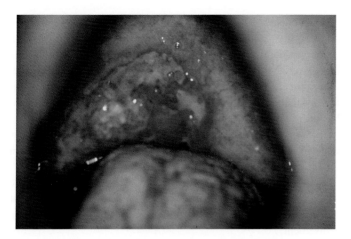

Fig. 14.7. A SCC of palate and oropharynx

and often do not notice symptoms until the tumours are advanced. In any case, these cancers are aggressive and tend to grow and invade locally and metastasise into lymph nodes in one or both sides of the neck at a relatively early stage. There is a greater than 50% risk of lymph-node involvement.

Although radical surgery will cure some of these patients and radiotherapy may cure some and offer palliation to the majority, combined treatment using chemotherapy (preferably given by regional intra-arterial infusion) followed by radiotherapy with or without surgery, may offer the best prospect of success (Fig. 14.7).

14.4   Cancers of the Post-Nasal Space
(The Air Passage at the Back of the Nose)

These cancers are most common in adult Chinese people, especially those from the Quantong province of China, Hong-Kong and Singapore (see Appendix). Sons and daughters of people from Quantong and Hong-Kong regions also have an increased incidence of this cancer even though they may have never lived in China.

Blood tests show that this cancer is most common in people who have been infected with the Epstein-Barr virus. Their blood usually has a high level of Epstein-Barr virus antibodies. If the Epstein-Barr virus titre is high before treatment and returns to normal after treatment, it does indicate that treatment has been effective and the patient has probably been cured.

14.4.1 Presentation

People with post-nasal space cancer may present with symptoms of a blocked nose.

People with post-nasal space cancer may present with persistent symptoms of a blocked nose, nasal or post-nasal discharge of mucus, pus or bloodstained material or, alternatively, they sometimes first notice a lump in the side of the neck. The lump is due to metastatic cancer in a lymph node. Sometimes lymph nodes on both sides of the neck are involved.

The cancer may sometimes be seen with a mirror in the back of the throat, but diagnosis is made by taking a biopsy from the back of the nose or sometimes by biopsy of an enlarged lymph node in the neck.

Occasionally the cancer invades bones at the base of the skull or the cranial nerves that pass from the brain through the base of the skull and into the neck. Special X-rays (tomograms) or CT scans may be taken to look for evidence of bone involvement.

14.4.2 Treatment

Cancer in the back of the nose is not accessible to surgery. It is usually treated by radiotherapy. With small cancers and no lymph node involvement 80% are cured by radiotherapy. For larger cancers with involved lymph nodes in the neck, the prospects of cure by radiotherapy alone are not good. The possibility of improving results by first giving induction (neo-adjuvant) chemotherapy (usually three courses) by intravenous injections prior to radiotherapy has now been proven. Such combined integrated chemotherapy and radiotherapy is now achieving better results in the treatment of advanced cancers even when lymph nodes are involved (see Sect. 8.3.4.8–8.3.4.9, Treating Cancers).

If bone at the base of the skull is invaded by cancer, the chance of cure by any means is poor.

14.5 Cancer of the Larynx

Laryngeal cancer is also a cancer most common in smokers and especially in smokers who are also heavy drinkers.

This, too, is a cancer most common in smokers and especially in smokers who are also heavy drinkers. It is more common in men than women. The most common site for cancer in the larynx is on a vocal cord. Cancers of the vocal cord usually cause a hoarseness or change in the voice when they are quite small and are therefore usually diagnosed early. They can be seen and biopsied through a laryngoscope and if treated early either by radiotherapy or by surgery (in which the cord is removed), the results of treatment are good. Approximately 90% are cured either by radiotherapy or by surgery.

If neglected until the cancer has spread from the vocal cord into surrounding tissues, the chances of cure by simple surgery or radiotherapy are much reduced. In some cases, partial removal of the larynx can be curative. However for more advanced laryngeal cancers that have spread onto the walls of the larynx or metastasised into lymph nodes in the neck, or cancers that have recurred after previous radiotherapy, the best chance of cure is by radical surgery. In radical surgery the larynx is totally removed, possibly together with removal of all draining lymph nodes (an operation called a radical laryngectomy).

Cancers in the larynx that develop above or below the vocal cords (supra-glottic or sub-glottic respectively) are usually more advanced when they are first diagnosed than cancers on a vocal cord. They also tend to be more aggressive and for this reason are often treated by combined radiotherapy and laryngectomy. Treatment using combinations of chemotherapy and/or radiation therapy and/or surgery are also under study to try to produce better results. By using chemo-therapy with radiotherapy it seems that equally good long-term results can be achieved without surgical removal of the larynx.

If laryngectomy is necessary and is expertly performed the chance of cure is reasonably good but the patient (usually a male) is left with an opening of his trachea in the lower neck (tracheostomy). Without a larynx he cannot speak normally but most patients learn a form of oesophageal speech. By this method they can be taught to swallow air and use regurgitated air from the stomach to

CASE REPORT

Cancer of larynx

Alex is a 67-year-old man who first consulted with his family doctor about increasing hoarseness of his voice for 3 months.

He was a heavy smoker (20 cigarettes/day for 50 years) but was other-wise healthy. No enlarged cervical nodes were detected.

Consultation with an ENT surgeon was arranged. A thorough exami-nation was carried out including examination of the larynx with an en-doscope.

Under general anaesthetic an endoscopic examination revealed an ir-regular wart-like lesion on the right vocal cord. Biopsy showed this to be a squamous carcinoma that appeared to be confined to the right vocal cord.

He was referred for radiotherapy. External beam radiation therapy was given and 3 months after treatment there was no evidence of residual tu-mour.

Now 6 months after treatment he has now stopped smoking but has some minor residual hoarseness of his voice. He will be kept under regular observation but has been advised that this cancer is unlikely to recur.

14

make sounds and words. Alternatively, a mechanical vibrator powered by a small battery can be applied to the throat muscles to make speech that sounds rather like the artificial voice of a robot or computer.

14.5.1   The Lost Cords Club

The Lost Cords Club is a club of people who have lost their larynx by surgery and support each other in learning to speak as well as their endeavours to cope with other social, health and mechanical problems. Like the Colostomy Club (for patients with a colostomy) and breast cancer support groups, there are branches in many big cities. The mutual social support offered to members is a great help for people who have had a laryngectomy and need to re-adjust to their changed circumstances and learn to live a relatively normal life again.

14.6   Salivary Gland Cancers

The salivary glands are located about the mouth and secrete saliva into the mouth especially during eating to prepare food for digestion. Most salivary gland cancers are adenocarcinomas but some that develop in the duct lining are SCCs. There are three major and many minor salivary glands on each side of the face.

The largest salivary gland is the parotid gland, which is situated partly in front of and below the ear and behind the jaw. This is the salivary gland in which both benign and malignant tumours most commonly develop. Cancers in the parotid gland are usually first noticed as a lump just in front of or below the ear. As the cancer grows it commonly invades and destroys the facial nerve passing through it, causing facial nerve palsy. Facial nerve palsy causes weakness of the muscles of that side of the face resulting in inability to close the eye or to properly move the corner of the mouth. There may be obvious loss of facial expression due to paralysis of the muscles on that side of the face. These cancers usually develop in middle-aged or older adults. They enlarge locally and tend to spread to local lymph nodes in front of the ear and in the upper part of the neck. Occasionally cancers develop from a pre-existing benign tumour in the parotid gland (a pleomorphic adenoma or mixed parotid tumour) that may have been present for years.

Treatment of cancers of the parotid gland is usually by surgical resection. With small cancers it may be possible to save the facial nerve but with larger cancers it is likely that the facial nerve will be involved and will need to be sacrificed. If lymph nodes are enlarged they are usually removed in the same block of tissue with the parotid gland. Post-operative radiotherapy is often given because of the risk of local recurrence of these cancers.

Cancers in the second largest salivary gland, the sub-mandibular gland under the jaw, and the third major salivary gland, the sublingual gland in the floor of the mouth under the tongue, are less common. However when present they tend to spread early to lymph nodes and are best treated by surgical excision of the whole of the gland together with any likely involved lymph nodes.

Salivary gland tumours occasionally occur in minor salivary glands either in the tongue, in the cheeks, lips or elsewhere. Wide surgical excision is required for treatment otherwise the chances of local recurrence are high. If there is any doubt that the cancer has been totally removed, post-operative radiotherapy is usually given.

The use of chemotherapy in the treatment of salivary gland cancers is not yet established. It has been used with limited success in the treatment of cancers that have recurred after surgery. The use of induction (or neo-adjuvant) chemotherapy prior to surgical excision of salivary gland tumours is under investigation. This is one site where preoperative induction chemotherapy can be more concentrated given by infusion into the external carotid artery but although some success has been experienced as yet it is uncertain whether results will be consistently improved by this combined, integrated technique (Fig. 14.8–14.10).

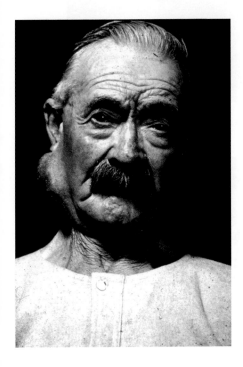

Fig. 14.8. Photograph showing a large pleomorphic adenoma (benign mixed parotid tumour) of a parotid gland of an elderly man

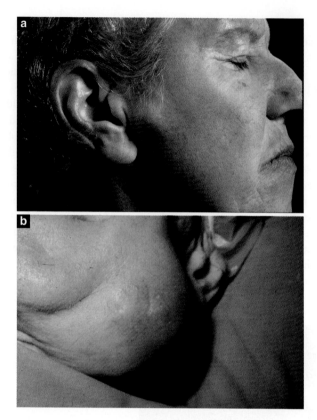

Fig. 14.9. Photographs showing small (**a**) and large (**b**) cancers in the parotid gland

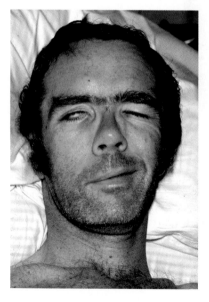

Fig. 14.10. A man with a right-sided facial palsy from a cancer in his right parotid gland

14.7 Cancers of the Thyroid Gland

The thyroid gland lies across the lower part of the neck with one lobe on either side of the trachea on the lower part of the larynx. The thyroid gland uses iodine to make the hormone thyroxine, which is essential for basic metabolism.

14.7.1 Causes and Presentation

Cancer of the thyroid gland is usually first noticed as a single lump in the gland. The lump is most often just to one or other side of the midline in the lower anterior part of the neck but cancer may occasionally develop as one lump that enlarges and becomes more obvious and harder in a multinodular goitre. Lumps in the thyroid move up and down when the patient swallows due to movement of the tongue that elevates the hyoid bone and the larynx, to which the thyroid gland is attached.

Cancer of the thyroid gland is usually first noticed as a single lump in the gland.

General enlargement of the thyroid gland is called a goitre, and multiple cysts and other lumps may develop in some goitres. This process is usually due to a shortage of iodine in the food. A lumpy goitre is known as a multinodular goitre.

CASE REPORT

Cancer of parotid gland

Akira, a 63-year-old retired Japanese businessman, first presented to his doctor with a 3-month history of a lump just in front of his left ear. He thought the lump had been slowly increasing in size.

The doctor found a 3 cm subcutaneous lump anterior to the left ear but no other lumps or other abnormality was detected. Facial nerve function was normal. The doctor referred Akira to a Head and Neck Surgeon who performed a needle biopsy of the lump.

Biopsy showed the lump to be a pleomorphic adenoma (mixed parotid tumour).

Parotidectomy was performed with care to preserve the facial nerve. Final pathology examination showed the presence of an area of malignant cells in the tumour.

Although apparently completely excised the tumour margin had been close to the facial nerve. In order to reduce the risk of recurrence, post-operative external radiation therapy was given.

Twelve months after treatment there is no evidence of residual disease. He remains well, his facial nerve function is normal and his voice is normal but he still has dryness in his mouth.

Akira has been advised that his prognosis is good but it is still important for him to be kept under regular observation.

Occasionally one of the lumps in a multinodular goitre will become malignant and develop into a cancer although more often when a cancer develops in the thyroid gland it begins as a single lump in an otherwise apparently normal thyroid gland. Most thyroid cancers, especially those that occur in young people, are generally characterised by slow growth with a relatively good long-term outlook compared to other cancers.

14.7.2   Accidental Irradiation

Increased numbers of people with thyroid cancer have been one of the most serious long-term consequences of atomic irradiation as seen in survivors of Hiroshima and Nagasaki atomic bombs and again after the Chernobyl atomic energy plant disaster.

14.7.3   Investigations

An isotope scan is a useful investigation for thyroid cancer. In this procedure a scan of the thyroid is taken after injection of a very small dose of radioactive iodine into a vein (as described in Sect. 7.3.8). The cancer will usually show as a *"cold nodule"*, that is, part of the thyroid gland that is replaced by cancer, does not concentrate the iodine and appears non-functional and clear on the scan. Most cold nodules are benign cysts or benign adenomas but about 10% of solitary cold nodules are cancer. However as cysts and some other lumps also show up as "cold nodules", to make a diagnosis the lump should be biopsied. This is usually done by needle aspiration of fluid or cells from the lump. Alternatively the diagnosis is more certain if the lump is surgically excised and examined microscopically. Frozen section examination (described in Sect. 7.6.5) may then allow the surgeon to proceed with further surgery if the lump proves to be a cancer. Occasionally a "hot nodule", that is a functioning thyroid lump, may be found to be a cancer.

14.7.4   Types of Thyroid Cancer

There are four broad types of thyroid cancer.

14.7.5   Papillary Cancer

Papillary carcinoma constitutes about 60% of thyroid cancers and is three times more common in women than men. It is more common in young adults, occasionally in teenagers or even children but fortunately it is the least malignant of thyroid cancers.

Papillary cancer may be present in different parts of the thyroid gland at the same time and may spread to nearby draining lymph nodes, but usually does not spread further until very late in the disease. For this reason, removal of the whole of the thyroid gland together with any enlarged lymph nodes will usually cure the patient. After total removal of the thyroid gland the patient thereafter must take thyroid or thyroxine tablets by mouth because thyroxine is essential for normal body function.

14.7.6 Follicular Cancer

The second most common type of thyroid cancer more commonly affects adults of middle age and is called follicular carcinoma. It too, usually presents as a lump in the thyroid gland and is usually not diagnosed with certainty until the lump has been removed surgically and examined microscopically.

These cancers tend to be present in one lobe of the thyroid gland only and have a greater tendency to spread by the bloodstream to bone, lungs or liver rather than by lymphatics to lymph nodes. These cancers often more closely resemble normal thyroid tissue than do the other thyroid cancers and although they usually appear as "cold nodules" in radio-iodine scans, they may sometimes scan as normal thyroid tissue or even rarely as hyperactive "hot nodules".

Because of their tendency to involve one lobe of the thyroid gland only they are usually treated by removal of the involved half of the thyroid gland, leaving the other half to carry out normal thyroid function and production of thyroxine.

Metastases may be treated by surgical excision (if in lymph nodes) by radiotherapy or by radio-active iodine being injected intravenously so that it becomes concentrated in thyroid tissue where it irradiates and destroys cells, including the cancer cells wherever they are. Again thyroxine tablets must be taken thereafter to maintain normal endocrine body function. Chemotherapy is also sometimes effective in the treatment of metastases.

14.7.7 Medullary Cancer

This type of thyroid cancer arises from the calcitonin-producing cells in the thyroid gland. It may be familial and it may be associated with other endocrine disturbances or with an adrenal gland tumour called pheochromocytoma. *Calcitonin* levels can be elevated with this cancer and will fall to normal if treatment has been successful. Total removal of the thyroid gland usually results in cure.

14.7.8 Anaplastic Cancer

The fourth broad type of thyroid cancer is anaplastic cancer. This is the most dangerous form of thyroid cancer and is usually rapidly growing. It is fortunate that it is also the least common. It tends to affect older people and may grow rapidly presenting as an enlarging lump or enlarging swelling of the whole of the thyroid gland. It may press on the trachea and make breathing difficult. This cancer is virtually incurable by surgery and is best palliated by radiotherapy or sometimes by chemotherapy.

14.7.9   Other Types

The thyroid gland is occasionally the site of other primary malignant tumours such as lymphoma, sarcoma or even secondary cancers from a primary cancer elsewhere, but these are uncommon.

CASE REPORT

Metastatic thyroid cancer

James was a 43-year-old schoolteacher when he first consulted his family doctor about a lump in his right upper neck that he had first noticed 6 months ago. His doctor did not find any other significant abnormality so James was referred to a Head and Neck Surgeon.

A needle biopsy showed the lesion to be metastatic papillary cancer of the thyroid in a lymph node.

James had previously been well with no history of thyroid disease and no other palpable lumps or nodes were detected but a thyroid ultrasound showed the presence of multiple small nodules throughout both lobes of the thyroid gland. The largest nodules were one measuring 17 mm in the right lobe and one measuring 15 mm in the left lobe.

When his larynx was examined his vocal cords were symmetric with normal mobility.

James was advised that although he had a thyroid cancer and that a lymph node was involved most such cancers were eminently curable by surgery. Total thyroidectomy (surgical resection of his thyroid both lobes and isthmus) together with all nearby lymph nodes in the right side of his neck was advised and carried out without any complication. James made an uneventful recovery.

A total of 23 lymph nodes were found in the resected tissue but no other nodes were found to contain cancer. Pathology examination of the thyroid gland showed it to contain multi-focal papillary thyroid cancer within the right lobe.

James was commenced on thyroid hormone replacement therapy (thyroxin by mouth) and was advised that he would need to take thyroxin for the rest of his life.

After 3 months James is well and has returned to his school-teaching profession. He will be kept under regular observation but a long-term cure is expected.

Cancers of Female Genital Organs

15

In this chapter you will learn about:

> *Cancers of the uterus*
> *Cancer of the ovary*
> *Cancer of the vagina*
> *Cancer of the vulva*

15.1   Cancers of the Uterus

There are two distinct types of cancer of the uterus. Squamous cell carcinoma (SCC) of the cervix or opening of the uterus is the more common. The other type is an endometrial or glandular cancer (adenocarcinoma) of the lining of the cavity of the uterus (the body of the uterus).

15.2   Cancer of the Cervix

15.2.1   Presentation and Risk Factors

Cervical cancer can occur in any woman especially over the age of 40 but there are particular risk factors in some groups of women, for example it is more common in smokers and erosions and inflammation of the cervix are predisposing factors Infection with a sexually transmitted virus, the human papilloma virus (HPV), has become a very significant factor. The HPV, being sexually transmitted, is more common in women who have had multiple sexual partners, particularly if sexual activity started early in life. Prostitutes are at particular risk. Cervical cancer is significantly more common in women in lower socio-economic groups and in recent years has been seen to be one of the cancers that more commonly develops in women with HIV infection or AIDS.

An annual routine cervical smear test (the Pap test) will usually detect these cancers early and at a very curable stage.

F. O. Stephens and K. R. Aigner, *Basics of Oncology,*
DOI: 10.1007/978-3-540-92925-3_15, © Springer-Verlag Berlin Heidelberg 2009

The earliest changes associated with this cancer are most often present in women between the ages of 30 and 40. Usually at this age there are no symptoms but there may be a little blood staining from the vagina between periods, especially after intercourse, or there may be a watery discharge.

Cancers of the cervix tend to develop slowly but can usually be detected by routine cervical screening examination (the Papanicolaou or cervical smear test described in Sect. 7.2.1) in which abnormal (*dysplastic*) or frankly malignant cells may be found. An annual routine cervical smear test (the Pap test) will usually detect these cancers early and at a very curable stage.

15.2.2   Investigations

Sometimes the cancers cannot be seen on visual examination of the cervix but at other times a cancer may be seen as a reddish, eroded ulcerated or possibly bleeding lesion. Modern colposcopes are now often used to better visualise the inner lining of the cervix and uterus. In any case a biopsy is taken for pathological examination to confirm the diagnosis.

15.2.3   Treatment

Very small early cancers may be treated by surgical removal of the lining of the cervix only, especially in women who wish to have more babies. Larger invasive cancers are best treated by removal of the uterus (total hysterectomy). Cancers that have begun to spread from the cervix onto the adjacent vagina present more of a problem. They often respond well when initially treated with a combination of chemotherapy/radiotherapy given together as concomitant treatment and sometimes followed by hysterectomy.

If cancer of the cervix has not been diagnosed until it is quite advanced, there is a risk of metastatic spread to lymph nodes, especially lymph nodes in the pelvis. This situation is more likely in women of more than 40 years of age who have not had regular Pap tests. These women often complain of some bleeding and discharge between menstrual periods or after intercourse. If an advanced, ulcerating or fungating cancer is present it should be obvious on examination of the cervix. Surrounding tissues such as the ureters or the rectum may become involved as well as the local draining lymph nodes in the pelvis. CT scans will help detect the extent of the cancer. Such advanced cancers are usually treated by radical surgery or by radiotherapy or both or by radiotherapy and chemotherapy concomitantly followed by radical surgery.

Early use of chemotherapy alone was disappointing with this cancer. It has been given as induction treatment both systemically and by regional infusion as part of an integrated treatment program and although early results were disappointing studies have been continued in some centres using different treatment schedules in different combinations with more encouraging results. However programs of chemotherapy (using the anti-cancer agent cisplatin) and radiotherapy, given together as concomitant treatment, have given best results in several studies. Chemotherapy is also sometimes given as palliative treatment for widespread cancer but substantial prolonged benefit is not common.

15.2.4 Prevention

In recent years the association of the HPV with cancer of the cervix has been more intensely investigated with a view to introducing more effective preventive measures. Types 16 and 18 of this virus are considered to be the most pathogenic and attempts at developing a vaccine against the virus are more than encouraging. A successful preventive vaccination trial in a large study group has recently been reported. National vaccination programmes are now being established in several countries to 12–13-year-old girls.

CASE REPORT

Cervical cancer

When she first presented Dianne was 46 years of age and had previously been in good health. She was married with three children. She had not had regular Pap smears, the last possibly some 5 years previously. On presentation she had recently experienced some menstrual cycle irregularity and post-coital bleeding. Her general practitioner initially treated her with progesterone agents to control what was thought to be dysfunctional bleeding.

She returned some 3 weeks later with reduced but ongoing irregular bleeding. She was then referred to a gynaecologist who on vaginal pelvic examination confirmed an obvious malignant growth involving her cervix. A biopsy in the clinic confirmed an invasive SCC.

Dianne was then referred to a specialist gynaecological oncologist. An examination under anaesthesia (EUA) was arranged, meanwhile an abdominal and pelvic CT scan confirmed a large cervical lesion measuring 5 cm in diameter without obvious extension and no radiological evidence of involvement of lymph nodes. The EUA, which included a cystoscopy, sigmoidoscopy, vaginal speculum examination and bimanual recto-vaginal pelvic examination, confirmed a large "barrel-shaped" cervical tumour approximately 5 cm in diameter without para-metrial or vaginal extension. She was then staged (officially according to the international system) as a stage 1b2 cervical cancer, meaning a large locally invasive cancer but apparently limited to the cervix).

(continued)

15

(continued)

At the post-operative consultation, the gynaecological oncologist discussed with Dianne and her husband the options for management. The first option was for an abdominal radical hysterectomy and pelvic lymph node dissection. Advantages of such an approach is the removal of the tumour and a formal assessment of the pelvic lymph nodes rather than relying on radiological evidence of apparent disease spread. Disadvantages of such an approach is that the majority of patients with large barrel shaped tumours have pelvic lymph node metastases and the majority of patients also then need to undergo additional treatment comprising concurrent chemo-irradiation treatment. The second and largely favoured option was to treat with definitive chemo-irradiation therapy and avoid surgery. Advantages of such an approach would be an identical survival rate but significantly reduced morbidity, as surgery has not been undertaken.

Dianne considered her options and opted for the latter approach. She underwent 6 weeks of external pelvic irradiation therapy with weekly chemotherapy (using low dose cisplatin). Towards the end of her external beam treatment she was given additional treatment by internal or brachytherapy.

Now 3 years post treatment Dianne remains well without clinical evidence of disease. She has undergone menopause, probably related to the effects of therapy on her ovaries. Her only ongoing morbidity is narrowing of the vagina requiring regular vaginal dilator treatment.

EXERCISE

Consider the reasons why there has been an increased incidence of cancer of the cervix over the latter part of the twentieth century and why this pattern is now likely to be reversed.

15.3   Cancer of the Body of the Uterus (Endometrial Cancer)

15.3.1   Presentation

These cancers are most commonly seen in older women. It is believed that change in female sex hormones, and especially an imbalance of hormones, may contribute to development of this cancer, which is becoming rather more common, because more women are living longer. It is now recognised that endometrial cancer is sometimes associated with long-term post-menopausal oestrogen therapy or long-term use of tamoxifen to treat or prevent of breast cancer.

The most common feature of endometrial cancer is bleeding and bloodstained discharge after the menopause but sometimes a watery discharge is the only feature.

15.3.2   Investigations

The uterus is usually enlarged and, to establish a diagnosis, curettage is performed. The scrapings from the curette are sent for pathology examination.

15.3.3   Treatment

Treatment of cancer of the body of the uterus is usually by radical surgery. The surgeon performs a total hysterectomy as well as removal of ovaries, fallopian tubes and removal of draining lymph nodes. For advanced cancers, radiotherapy is sometimes given before or after hysterectomy.

Like most cancers, treatment at an early stage can achieve good results but for more advanced cancers, results of treatment are often disappointing.

If endometrial cancer has spread to other tissues or organs it will often respond to hormone treatment (for example large-dose progesterone therapy) but a long-term cure is unlikely. Studies are being made of combined integrated treatment using intra-arterial chemotherapy first as "induction" treatment followed by radiotherapy and/or surgery (see Sects. 8.3.4.8–8.3.4.9). Chemotherapy and radiotherapy are sometimes given concomitantly as induction treatment. Whether these programs of treatment will achieve significantly better results is as yet uncertain.

15

CASE REPORT

Corpus cancer

On presentation Lynne was a 63-year-old obese woman with multiple medical complaints. She had been constantly in attendance at her general practitioner's surgery with various complaints. Apart from her obesity, she was also diabetic and hypertensive. She had undergone menopause at age 51 and although she had subsequently been on combined oestrogen replacement therapy for 5 years, she was not on any hormonal treatment when she presented. Lynne had experienced 2–3 episodes of bright vaginal spotting over the preceding 3 months. Her general practitioner performed a speculum and vaginal pelvic examination and a Pap test. The cervix appeared normal and the Pap test was subsequently also reported as normal. A trans-abdominal and trans-vaginal ultrasound was arranged confirming a bulky uterus and an endometrial lesion measuring 13-mm in thickness. She was referred to a gynaecologist and subsequently underwent a hysteroscopy and dilation and curettage (D&C). A fundal polypoid tumour was seen at hysteroscopy and curettage confirmed a carcinoma (classified as grade 2 endometrioid adenocarcinoma).

Lynne was referred to a specialist gynaecological oncologist. Management options were discussed with Lynne and her husband including radiation therapy and surgery. As the survival of patients treated with pelvic irradiation is inferior to those treated with definitive surgery, the latter was chosen as the preferable treatment option. Through a vertical midline incision an abdominal hysterectomy and bila-teral salpingo-oophorectomy was performed. There was no apparent extra-uterine spread. As frozen section histology confirmed evidence of myometrial invasion a pelvic lymph node dissection was then performed to define the extent of disease.

Lynne recovered from surgery without major morbidity. There was no evidence of lymph node invasion in any of the 22 pelvic nodes examined. Likewise pelvic cytology was negative for malignant cells and no malignancy was found in an omental biopsy. Lynne was not given further treatment as her disease had been confirmed surgically to be confined to the uterus.

Her post treatment surveillance comprised regular attendances to her gynaecological oncologist, pelvic examination, and vaginal vaults smears. Now 5 years post treatment Lynne remains without clinical evidence of disease.

15.4 Choriocarcinoma

Although a choriocarcinoma starts and grows in the uterus, it is strictly not a cancer of the uterus. A choriocarcinoma is best considered as a cancer of an abnormal pregnancy.

This is one of the success stories of chemotherapy.

After conception, very occasionally an abnormal growth of tissue develops instead of a normal foetus and placenta. If the foetus does not develop and the placenta grows as a group of cyst-like structures something like a bunch of grapes, this is called a *hydatidiform mole*.

Sometimes cells of an hydatidiform mole develop into an invasive cancer called a choriocarcinoma. Occasionally choriocarcinoma will develop in association with a foetus, usually an abnormal foetus, which is aborted spontaneously, or rarely even with an otherwise normal pregnancy. However, most in fact are in association with a hydatidiform mole with no foetus, usually in women over 40 years of age.

In the past, choriocarcinoma spread widely and rapidly through the mother's body and was a fatal form of cancer. Nowadays the condition is treated by emptying the uterus of its contents, (curettage), and giving cytotoxic chemotherapeutic drugs. This is one of the success stories of chemotherapy as choriocarcinoma has been changed from a cancer approaching 100% fatality 30 or 35 years ago to a cancer that is curable in 80% or more cases with modern chemotherapy.

15.5 Cancer of the Ovary

The ovaries are the source of a greater variety of tumours, both benign and malignant, than any other body organ. This is probably because of the multicellular and changing nature of the ovaries, as organs with a function of undergoing monthly cyclic changes to prepare one of the eggs (ova) in the ovaries for potential development into new tissues, i.e. a foetus. Not only does the ovary produce a variety of tumours ranging from benign (the majority) to low-grade malignancy and to highly malignant cancers, they may also produce tumours that excrete hormones that may affect body development and function. Some ovarian cancers are germ-cell cancers not unlike some cancers of the testis.

The ovaries are the source of a greater variety of tumours, both benign and malignant, than any other body organ.

Cancers of the ovary may be solid or cystic or they may contain a mixture of solid and cystic elements. They tend to cause no symptoms early in their development and so they are often advanced when first diagnosed.

There is no known cause of ovarian cancers but there are some genetic associations. The *BRCA1* and *BRCA2* tumour suppressor genes are known risk factors and there is sometimes a strong family history of ovarian cancer (see Sect. 2.4). These same genes are more commonly recognised as risk factors in premenopausal breast cancer and there is an increased risk of women who have had a breast cancer before menopause to later develop ovarian cancer.

15.5.1 Presentation

Cancers of the ovary develop insidiously. Cancers of the ovary develop insidiously. They usually cause a gradually increasing swelling in the pelvis and lower abdomen. The swelling may have been noticed by the patient or may be found on examination by a doctor who may sometimes find a symptomless pelvic mass during a general examination. They may sometimes cause a "heavy feeling" or local discomfort or pain. Some produce hormones, in which case the first evidence may be due to hormonal changes such as premature menopause and the woman may notice loss of feminine features and the development of male characteristics such as growth of hair on the face or deepening of the voice. Sometimes too, generalised abdominal swelling may be noticed due either to a huge tumour or to fluid in the abdominal cavity (ascites).

Any rapidly enlarging swelling on an ovary, especially if it is solid or contains a mixture of cystic and solid elements, must be regarded with suspicion as likely to be malignant.

15.5.2 Investigations

Examination of the pelvis and pelvic structures by abdominal, vaginal or rectal examination without anaesthetic may not be adequate and EUA may be required.

Abdominal X-rays or CT scans may help but ultrasound examination is the least harmful examination, especially in young women, and is often the most helpful because cystic changes in the ovary and cystic tumours are best detected by ultrasound.

Laparoscopy or culdoscopy (Sects. 7.4.12–7.4.13) may allow the surgeon or gynaecologist to see the contents of the pelvis, especially the ovaries.

A tumour marker, CA125, can be useful in assessing not only the presence of cancer but response to treatment and risk of recurrence after treatment. Similarly germ-cell tumours, like germ-cell tumours of the testis, usually produce the tumour markers alpha-foeto-protein (AFT), human chorionic hormone (HCG) and lactate dehydrogenase (LDH). Measuring the levels of these may give a good indication of the presence of this cancer and its response to treatment.

Usually a diagnosis of cancer cannot be established with certainty until an operation (laparoscopy or laparotomy) has been carried out and a biopsy specimen of any suspicious lesion has been examined microscopically.

15.5.3 Treatment

The best treatment of ovarian cancer, especially if not advanced, is by total surgical removal of the ovaries and fallopian tubes. Because the other ovary and other pelvic organs may also be the site of cancer, it is usual to remove both ovaries as well as the uterus and tubes and any other involved tissue. However in a young woman with early and localised ovarian cancer, sometimes one ovary can be spared. The operation is sometimes followed by radiotherapy to the pelvis or chemotherapy. If the cancer is advanced chemotherapy and radiotherapy may be used together with good effect. Even if the cancer cannot be removed, results are better if the tumour is "debulked", that is, as much of the cancer as possible is removed. The patient is often then treated by radiotherapy. Adjuvant chemotherapy after surgical removal also improves survival rates.

Chemotherapy is often effective in controlling widespread metastases for a worthwhile period (possibly some years) but long-term cure is unlikely.

Combinations of local chemotherapy (intra-arterial infusion and/or intra-peritoneal) with radiotherapy and/or surgery, are presently under study in some special clinics but it is not yet certain whether these techniques of integrated treatment will achieve significantly better results with safety.

Studies are also being carried out on the use of pre-operative chemotherapy given as induction treatment to reduce locally advanced cancers. The surgery that follows is then hopefully more likely to be curative but even if it is not curative "debulking" the cancer mass by removing most of the residual cancer does improve the patient's quality of life for a longer period. In some clinics, where appropriate and facilities are available, pre-operative induction chemotherapy is given by intra-arterial infusion with a greater concentration and apparently greater local tumour impact. To date results have been encouraging but long-term results of clinical trials are awaited with interest (see Chap. 8).

15.5.4   Prevention

Because cancers sometimes develop from benign tumours of the ovary it is usually advisable to remove both ovaries in treating any woman over 40 years for a benign ovarian tumour. In some women whose families have strong associations with breast and/or ovarian cancer or women known to have *BRCA1* or *BRCA2* genes, oophorectomy should be considered as an effective cancer prevention measure. Also, gynaecologists often advise removal of ovaries as a preventive measure when they perform hysterectomy in women over 40.

A slightly lower incidence of ovarian cancer in women who use modern oral contraceptives has been reported.

15.5.5   Metastatic Cancer of the Ovary

The ovaries are commonly a site of secondary metastatic cancer from a primary cancer elsewhere. Advanced cancer of the breast, stomach, bowel and melanoma frequently metastasise to ovaries. Sometimes a cancer of the ovary that appears to be a primary ovarian cancer has come from an unknown and symptomless primary cancer in another organ or tissue. When stomach cancer was much more common that it is today, it was not uncommon to find an apparently primary cancer of the ovary was composed of gastric cancer cells and was in fact a secondary gastric cancer. This was first described by a Dr Krukenberg and became known as a Krukenberg tumour.

The ovaries are commonly a site of secondary metastatic cancer from a primary cancer elsewhere.

CASE REPORT

Ovarian cancer

Mary was a 63 year-old woman who had been unwell for 3 months when she noticed increasing non-specific gastrointestinal upsets and abdominal swelling. While her complaints were initially attributed to a minor gastrointestinal upset, she returned to her GP with progression of symptoms. On physical examination shifting dullness confirmed clinical ascites. A CT scan of the abdomen and pelvis confirmed a large complex pelvic mass, gross ascites and thickening in the omentum, consistent with an ovarian cancer.

She was referred directly to a specialist gynaecological oncologist. (A CA125 tumour marker test was ordered and noted to be grossly elevated at 1,200 U/mL; the normal being < 35 U/mL). A pelvic examination confirmed a large fixed pelvic mass.

The options for management discussed with Mary were for initial induction (neoadjuvant) chemotherapy for three cycles to assess the chemosensitivity of the tumour followed by debulking or cytoreductive surgery. This would be followed by another three cycles of chemotherapy. The second and more commonly employed management of patients with suspected ovarian cancer was for initial surgery, again to confirm the diagnosis, secondly to debulk or remove as much tumour load as possible and then follow this with six cycles of combination chemotherapy.

Mary subsequently underwent exploratory surgery via a midline abdominal incision. Three litres of clear ascites fluid was drained. Operative findings included a large pelvic mass arising from the left ovary and involving the recto-sigmoid colon. There was also a large omental tumour mass, (sometimes referred to as "cake"), replacing both the infra and supra-colic omentum. Successful tumour de-bulking was accomplished but this required resection of the pelvic mass en bloc including the uterus and recto-sigmoid. A primary end-to-end anastomosis was performed to restore functional integrity of the bowel.

Final pathology confirmed a high-grade serous ovarian cancer.

Mary completed six cycles of combination chemotherapy (comprising Carboplatin and Taxol) and was in clinical, biochemical and radiological remission for 22 months. At one of her surveillance visits her CA125 level, which had become normal with treatment, was again rising from a baseline of 20–120 U/mL. She remained asymptomatic and no disease was initially seen on CT scanning but she was given Tamoxifen for 3 months. However a PET scan 3 months later confirmed widespread recurrence of cancer. Her CA125 level had risen to 400 U/mL and she was now developing further non-specific gastrointestinal symptoms.

(continued)

(continued)

She was again treated with chemotherapy but despite having initial improvement in her symptoms and her CA125 level, she suffered another further relapse some 9 months later and was commenced on second line palliative chemotherapy. Further response was not achieved despite receiving a number of other chemotherapy agents. Lynne died of disease causing further bowel obstruction 42 months after her initial surgery.

CASE REPORT

Ovarian cancer

A 55-year-old woman was admitted to hospital with abdominal pain and vomiting. She had surgery 10 years previously for a right ovarian cyst. She was the mother of one child and had been menopausal for 5 years. Since menopause she had been taking hormone replacement therapy.

Her family history included breast cancers in her mother and a maternal aunt and a colon cancer in her father. Rapidly, Investigations were immediately arranged, including abdominal CT scan and tumour marker tests. The CT scans showed a right ovarian tumour with ascites and enlarged retroperitoneal lymph nodes. Tumour markers were CEA (carcinoembrionic antigen) with a high level of 50 ng/mL and most significantly a CA125 of 1,200 U/mL.

A laparotomy was carried out both to establish a diagnosis and to remove as much of the tumour as possible. This is called "de-bulking surgery". It included removal of both ovaries and fallopian tubes, the uterus and most of the omentum, as well as pelvic lymph nodes.

The tumour was an undifferentiated adenocarcinoma of the ovary, with bilateral ovarian, peritoneal and lymph nodes involvement. Cancer cells were also in the ascitic fluid.

After surgery, the CA125 level fell to 500 U/mL and the CEA to 20 ng/mL.

Adjuvant chemotherapy has been shown to improve survival rates with metastatic ovarian cancer so the oncologist arranged six cycles of a taxane-based chemotherapy. After completing the six cycles of chemotherapy a CT-scan showed no evidence of a residual cancer and the tumour markers were normal. No further surgery was performed but the patient was kept under regular surveillance.

Less than 2 years later, the patient faced an increasing swelling in the pelvis and lower abdomen and the diagnosis of local recurrent disease was

(continued)

(continued)

made (ascites and peritoneal carcinomatosis). Another combination of cytotoxic agents was administered over 6 months without success. Abdominal pain and discomfort developed so that a program palliative care commenced first by her oncologist and subsequently by a specialist palliative care team. Much needed symptomatic, physical, psychological and emotional support and care were achieved until the patient's final death.

As the history of breast cancer in her family and her personal ovarian cancer, the oncologist proposed to investigate the status of the patient's daughter for genetic mutations in BRCA1 and BRCA2 genes was advised as a possible preventive measure. Some women with mutations in these genes elect to have a double mastectomy to prevent risk of cancer.

EXERCISE

Consider why cancers of the ovary are of so many and varied types
and why cancers of the ovary are so often not diagnosed
until the later stages of the disease.

Metastatic cancers in an ovary are best treated by removal of the ovaries if there is no apparent cancer anywhere else, otherwise the treatment will depend upon the best treatment for the type of cancer concerned wherever else it may be and from where it originated.

15.6   Cancer of the Vagina

The vagina is occasionally the site of a cancer. Most are squamous cell cancers in middle aged or older women. However some cases of adenocarcinomas of the vagina have been reported in adolescent girls and young women. Some of these have been associated with stilboestrol which was once given to their mothers, in the early stages of the mother's pregnancy, to prevent spontaneous abortion.

Cancers of the vagina usually present as bleeding and discharge. Pain on passing urine and pain with intercourse (dyspareunia) are often features that most trouble the patients.

Most small cancers can be cured by surgical excision but larger cancers are treated with radiotherapy with about a 50% cure rate. Care must be taken to treat groin lymph nodes if they show evidence of involvement either at the time of treatment of the primary cancer or in the follow-up period.

15.7   Cancer of the Vulva

Like cancer of the anus, cancer of the vulva is a rare but rather aggressive form of skin cancer usually of the squamous cell type. Most occur in women of post-menopausal age. Cancer of the vulva is often preceded by a long history of irritation, discomfort or inflammation of the vulva and possibly with a local bloodstained discharge. There may be a pre-malignant condition of leukoplakia or a chronic rash. Previous infection with the sexually transmitted HPV is responsible for some cases.

Cancer of the vulva is often preceded by a long history of irritation, discomfort or inflammation of the vulva.

In the more advanced stages there may be an ulcer, a lump or a cauliflower-like growth. Metastatic spread to lymph nodes in one or both groins is likely in about half of the patients at the time of diagnosis.

Diagnosis is established by biopsy and treatment is usually by wide and radical surgical excision, and most patients are cured. Pre-malignant papillomas or a localised patch of leukoplakia are best treated by surgical excision as a cancer preventive measure.

For very advanced cases, radiotherapy offers palliative relief but integrated treatment using chemotherapy and radiotherapy or intra-arterial induction chemotherapy followed by radiotherapy and/or surgery, are presently under study in specialised centres. As yet it is not established whether better long-term results will be achieved by these techniques.

Cancers of the Male Genital Organs

16

In this chapter you will learn about:

> *Cancer of the penis*
> *Cancer of the testis*
> *Cancer of the prostate gland*

16.1 Cancer of the Penis

Penile cancer is uncommon, particularly in Western societies. It is almost unknown in Jewish males who are circumcised soon after birth but is a little more common in Muslim males who are circumcised at about 10 or 12 years. Most that are seen are in uncircumcised men. Lack of genital hygiene and cleanliness may be a factor or sometimes this cancer is associated with the sexually transmitted human papilloma virus.

It is essentially a squamous cell cancer similar to the common skin cancers but somewhat more aggressive. It tends to spread rather more readily to draining lymph nodes in the groins than is usual for other squamous cancers of skin.

Most cases are first seen when a small crusty, papillomatous or small ulcerated skin lesion is present and these can usually be well treated by surgical removal of the lesion, keeping a close watch on draining groin lymph nodes thereafter. Occasionally very advanced cases are seen, usually in men living in remote places or undeveloped communities. These usually respond well to induction chemotherapy especially if given by intra-arterial infusion. Involved lymph nodes should be surgically resected. A series of quite spectacular responses of very advanced cancers on the penis have been reported from Taiwan using intra-arterial infusion chemotherapy, followed by surgery or radiotherapy. A high incidence of cure was reported.

F. O. Stephens and K. R. Aigner, *Basics of Oncology,*
DOI: 10.1007/978-3-540-92925-3_16, © Springer-Verlag Berlin Heidelberg 2009

16.2   Cancer of the Testis

Testicular tumours are not common but when they do occur they are almost always malignant. Most occur in young adult males between the ages of 18 and 40. They are almost all classified as "germ cell" tumours. Germ cells are embryonic type cells capable of developing into different cell types. Germ cell cancers are uncommon, but they occur most often in a testis. Occasionally they occur in midline structures like the mediastinum or retro-peritoneum or pineal gland usually in children or young adults. Some cancers of the ovary are also germ cell cancers.

There are no known causes of testicular cancer. They are more common in developed than developing countries but the reason for this is not known. They are distinctly more likely to occur in undescended testes. Cryptorchidism is a condition in which the testes have not descended from the abdomen, where they develop, into the scrotum where they should be present at birth. If one or both testes are not present in the scrotum of infant boys, they are retained in the abdomen or the inguinal canal or somewhere nearby. Surgical operation (orchidopexy) should be performed before the age of 8 or 10 to place the testes into their normal position. This will reduce the risk of development of testicular cancer sometime later in life, after puberty. It is postulated that the warmer temperature of the testes in the abdomen may be responsible for the increased risk of testicular cancer in undescended testes.

Similarly there is an increased risk in men with *Klinefelter's syndrome*. This is an abnormal genetic condition in which rather than having XX or XY sex chromosomes, the affected individuals have three chromosomes, XXY. This gives some female characteristics in otherwise apparently tall, thin underdeveloped males with small underdeveloped testes that are more prone to malignant change.

16.2.1   Presentation

Cancer of the testis is usually found as a painless and non-tender swelling of a testis. Cancer of the testis is usually found as a painless and non-tender swelling of a testis although occasionally the swelling is tender and possibly painful. Occasionally no swelling is noticed in the testis until there is evidence of metastatic spread of a cancer. Metastases may be noticed as a mass of enlarged and sometimes tender lymph nodes in the abdomen, enlarged lymph nodes in the neck, usually the left side known as Virchow's nodes (Sect. 5.4) or as metastases in lungs seen in chest X-rays. Occasionally the first evidence of a testicular cancer may be swelling of a man's breasts due to hormonal changes. In other patients the first evidence may be of general debility, anorexia (loss of appetite) and weight loss.

16.2.2 Investigations

If a swelling is detected in a testis, ultrasound of the testis will help confirm if a solid tumour is present. If found it is almost always a cancer. In such cases investigations are carried out to look for evidence of metastatic spread. CT scans and excretory urograms (IVP X-rays described in Sect. 7.3.2) and these may be helpful in detecting any enlarged lymph nodes in the abdomen. Chest X-rays may help detect metastases in lungs or in lymph nodes in the chest (mediastinal lymph nodes).

An operation is recommended to confirm the diagnosis and allow the testis to be examined and removed if a tumour is clearly present.

16.2.3 Pathology

There are two broad types of testicular cancer, of about equal incidence, *seminomas* and *non-seminomas* most of which are *teratomas*. Seminomas tend to occur in slightly older age groups (mean 35 years) and are very sensitive to radiotherapy. Non-seminomas, or non-seminoma germ cell tumours (NSGCT), often contain a mixture of histologies including embryonal, yolk sac, choriocarcinoma, teratomas and seminomas. They are most often in younger age groups (mean 25 years) and are less sensitive to radiotherapy but are highly responsive to chemotherapy.

A number of tumour markers in the blood will help detect and classify testicular cancers and so indicate most appropriate treatment and help assess response to treatment. Alpha-feto-protein (AFP), human chorionic gonadotropin (HCG) and lactate dehydrogenase (LDH) can all be useful testicular cancer markers. If the level of a tumour marker is elevated, it helps establish a diagnosis of tumour type and if the level falls to normal after treatment it indicates a good response to treatment and probably a cure.

> A number of tumour markers in the blood will help detect and classify testicular cancers.

16.2.4 Treatment

Cancer of a testis is treated by surgical removal of the testis (through an inguinal approach) and radiotherapy is given to draining lymph nodes in the abdomen or to any other lymph nodes likely to be involved, especially if seminoma was diagnosed.

In the case of teratoma even if the cancer is widespread into the lungs or elsewhere, good results, with a high proportion of long-term cures, are achieved with chemotherapy.

From being among the cancers with a poor prognosis a few years ago, with present-day integrated and combined treatment programs using surgery, radiotherapy and chemotherapy, testicular cancers are now among the most curable cancers.

Patients should be advised that it is still possible to lead a normal sex life and to father children with only one testis.

16

Drawing on case reports in this chapter and other chapters of this book, construct a case report of a typical patient presenting with and being investigated and managed for a testicular cancer.

16.3   Cancer of the Prostate Gland

Cancer of the prostate is uncommon before the age of 45 but in Western countries, other than skin cancer, it is the most common cancer in men over the age of 65 and became increasingly common during the twentieth century, especially in the latter part of the twentieth century.

This rapid rise in recorded incidence is due in part to the use of the prostate specific antigens (PSA) test for detecting early subclinical prostate cancers or "latent" prostate cancers that might not have otherwise progressed to a clinical stage. The rise in apparent incidence of prostate cancer after the common use of PSA as a screening test is somewhat similar the increased numbers of early breast cancers in the 1980s and 1990s after common use of mammography as a screening test. However the PSA test is much less specific for prostate cancer, a raised index simply indicates increased prostate cell activity that may be due to benign prostate disease, latent prostate cancer or established prostate cancer. Evidence suggests that early breast cancers are unlikely to remain "latent" for any length of time but "latent" prostate cancer may well remain non-invasive indefinitely.

Almost all men over the age of 90 have microscopic evidence of at least early prostate cancer. The cause of prostate cancer is largely unknown but its association with old age is illustrated by the fact that in Western countries almost all men over the age of 90 have microscopic evidence of at least early prostate cancer.

There is a familial association of prostate cancer especially in younger men (below 55 years) and some of these are linked to mutations of the *BRCA2* gene (see Sects. 2.4 and 2.5). The increased familial association is greater if male relatives have had prostate cancer but there is also some increase in families with a high incidence in men on the mothers' side of the family.

There is also an increased risk in men with a history of prostatitis.

Prostate cancer is now the second most common cancer in males in Western countries, after skin cancers, and it is second only to lung cancer as a cause of cancer death in men. In stark contrast epidemiological studies show that Asians,

Africans and native-Americans living in their traditional lifestyles have a low incidence of prostate cancer (see Appendix and Table 1).

The highest incidence is in black males in the USA followed by white males in the USA, Europe, and other Western countries. The lowest incidence of prostate cancer is in men in India and South East Asia and also in black males living in Africa. Men of Asian or African ethnicity who have lived all their lives in Western Countries have a high risk, and in Afro-Americans an even higher risk, than in white males of those countries. This suggests that causes are more closely related to environmental factors rather than racial or genetic factors. It is likely that differences in diet may play a part because prostate cancer is less common in communities that have predominantly vegetarian diets.

Recent studies have indicated that diets with a high content of legumes, such as soybeans, may be protective and it could be that the high content of phytoestrogens is at least partly responsible. Results of studies of the possible preventive or clinical use of lycopene are similarly being awaited with considerable interest. Laboratory studies with lycopene indicate that its apparent anti-cancer protective activity is synergistically enhanced if used together with beta-carotenes or vitamin D (Sects. 2.8, 2.13 and 3.5.1). Each of these alone has been shown to have some cancer protective activity but used together the total anti-cancer activity is greater than the sum of the activity of each used alone. Whether a similar symbiotic activity might result from phytoestrogens used with lycopene is presently under study.

There have also been reports of a protective factor in tea, possibly by virtue of anti-oxidants in tea, but this is as yet unconfirmed. Other anti-oxidants that may have some protective effect are selenium, and vitamin E as well as lycopene, possibly by interfering with the pathway towards cellular mutation. It has also been reported that men taking Statins (used for lowering blood cholesterol) have been incidentally found to have a reduced incidence of aggressive metastasising prostate cancers. Fish and fish oils in diet also give some protection against prostate cancer.

Oboesity with lack of exercise and a high animal fat intake are increased risk factors.

16.3.1   Presentation

The most common presentation of prostate cancer is frequency, hesitancy and other difficulties in passing urine. Non-malignant enlargement of the prostate (prostate hyperplasia) is very common in late middle-aged and older men and is most often the cause of urinary difficulty, but prostate cancer is also a common cause of this trouble, especially in older men.

Occasionally the first evidence of cancer of the prostate is due to metastases either in bone (causing bone pain or fractures) or in the liver (causing liver enlargement). Metastases in the lower vertebral column or pelvis may cause pressure on a sciatic nerve before it passes into the leg, but causing severe pain in the back and leg called sciatica. Sciatica is sometimes the first evidence of prostate cancer but more often there is another physical cause such as a "slipped vertebral disc".

16.3.2   Investigations

The prostate gland can be felt by an examining finger in the rectum. This is called a digital rectal examination (DRE). With a gloved finger passed through the anus into the rectum the prostate gland can be felt in front of the finger. Cancer in the prostate usually feels like a hard lump or lumps in the prostate or sometimes the whole of the prostate gland may feel hard and rigid. A biopsy may be taken with a needle passed via the anus through the anterior rectal wall or it may also be taken with a needle passed through the skin in front of the anus and guided by a finger in the rectum.

Ultrasound is now used with special equipment that is passed through the anus into the rectum. Ultrasound will show any lumps in the prostate and any general prostate enlargement. Biopsies are usually now best taken with a special punch or needle during ultrasound examination to discover whether any of the lumps are cancer.

X-rays will be taken for evidence of metastatic spread into bones. These may show as dark eroded areas in bone or as sclerotic (dense white) areas in the bone if, as is often the case, they contain calcium. Chest X-rays may show metastases in the lungs, in lymph nodes in the chest, or even in the ribs. Isotope bone scans are also valuable in showing evidence of bone metastases (Sect. 7.3.8) (Fig. 16.1).

Blood studies may show anaemia if bone metastases have developed and are destroying the blood-forming cells in bone marrow. Cancer of the prostate may also cause an elevation of a serum enzyme, *acid phosphatase*, and, if bone is destroyed by metastatic cancer, an enzyme released from the bone called *alkaline phosphatase* may also be elevated.

Obstruction by the cancer to the flow of urine may result in infection in the bladder and possibly in the kidneys. The urine and blood are examined for evidence of infection in urine or damage to the kidneys.

16.3.3   Screening Tests: The PSA (Prostate-Specific Antigens) and the DRE (Digital Rectal Examination)

Nowhere in the field of cancer treatment is there more controversy and confusion than is the case with prostate cancer.

In recent years the PSA blood test has been developed which indicates whether there is likely to be an abnormality in the prostate. PSA is a special tumour marker that is now commonly used as a screening test in men over the age of 55 to help find those with early prostate cancer that might be effectively treated. A raised PSA does not necessarily indicate cancer is present but it may indicate the need for further investigations, possibly including ultrasound study and biopsies. However DRE is a very helpful prostate cancer detection test that

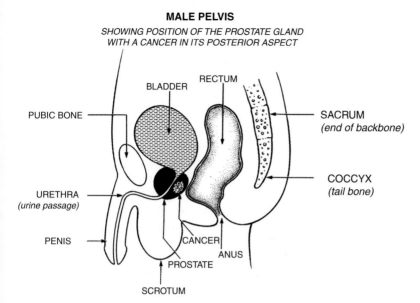

Fig. 16.1. Diagram showing a common site for cancer in the prostate gland

can be easily and safely carried out in a doctor's rooms. If a prostate is found to be hard or lumpy then biopsies should be taken to determine whether a cancer is responsible. A raised PSA must certainly indicate the need for a DRE if a DRE has not already been carried out. If the PSA is significantly raised and a DRE indicates a hard or lumpy prostate, the chance of prostate cancer is high.

16.3.4   Controversies in Management of Men with Prostate Cancer

Nowhere in the field of cancer treatment is there more controversy and confusion than is the case with prostate cancer.

Some bias is inevitable in trying to compare survival statistics in men with prostate cancer. Elective screening will usually detect this cancer before it becomes symptomatic. It is therefore inevitable that men with prostate cancer detected before it is symptomatic will generally live longer than men whose cancer was causing symptoms before being detected. This is called "lead-time bias".

Similarly more slowly developing cancers are more likely to be detected at an earlier phase by routine screening than rapidly growing cancers so giving a bias so that post treatment survival time will be biased in favour of those detected by PSA screening. This is called "length-time bias".

Another inbuilt bias in comparing treatments is known as "selection bias". Radical surgery will not proceed if a patient is found to have extensive cancer whereas radiotherapy is more likely to have been given to a proportion of patients who already have extensive cancer. Thus these potentials for inbuilt bias make it difficult to compare management protocols.

However the PSA screening test has led to investigation and diagnosis of prostate cancer in increasing numbers of middle aged and elderly males. Yet even if a biopsy diagnosis of cancer is confirmed it is estimated that only about one in four or five prostate cancers will grow in a malignant fashion to become life threatening by spreading to tissues beyond the prostate during the patient's otherwise expected lifespan. There is as yet no way of determining those cancers that are likely to spread. Most prostate cancers are slow growing and even after some years may show no evidence of spread beyond the prostate, but some will spread to such places as lungs, liver and especially to bones where they are likely to form painful metastases and lead to the death of the patient. Appropriate treatment of early cancers will cure most patients but all treatments have serious side effects and it is not possible at this stage to determine which patients will benefit from treatment and who might be better left untreated. A PSA found to be rapidly rising is more likely to be associated with metastasising prostate cancer.

A most common and distressing side effect of treatment is erectile dysfunction causing impotence. This occurs in the majority of patients whether treated by surgical removal of the whole prostate gland or by radiotherapy. Other side effects can be prolonged incontinence or occasional stress incontinence, especially after radical surgery, or some damage to the bladder or rectum after radiotherapy. Irradiation damage to bladder or rectum can leave the man with long-term urinary scalding or frequency or with precipitous diarrhoea. When hormones are used to treat metastases, either by giving feminising hormones or anti-male hormones or by castration or a combination of treatments, loss of libido and impotence are also usual (see Sect. 8.4.1).

Whether or not to use the PSA or any other attempt at screening for prostate cancer in asymptomatic men in the age group most at risk remains controversial. If cancer is detected, especially a small area of "latent" or "in situ" cancer, it is often impossible to know whether the cancer is likely to cause the man any significant problem during his otherwise expected lifespan. Thus it is a matter of controversy as to whether anxieties should be raised about a cancer being detected that may never cause him any serious trouble. Yet if left undetected or untreated one in four or five will advance to an incurable stage likely to cause a painful and miserable death but for some, who opt for treatment (and its inevitable side effects), life expectancy will not have changed.

Whether to treat or not to treat will depend on many factors. These will include whether there is evidence of progressive disease (e.g. rising PSA or enlarging cancer or increasing biopsy changes), the family history, the family circumstances and social circumstances of the patient, the age and general health of the patient, his otherwise life expectancy, and especially his personal priorities in life. For example. he may not think life would be worth living if he were impotent or alternatively sexual activity may no longer be of any interest to him but he has a lot of other interests in life. It should always be explained to these men that in most cases there is now effective treatment for impotence be it with prostaglandin penile injections, Viagra or similar medications, a special vacuum pump device to engorge the penis or other techniques.

One of the greatest needs in medical research is a test to determine whether low-grade prostate cancer cells detected by biopsy are likely to become aggressive. The pathologist can help in this by indicating the relative aggressiveness and local invasion of cancer cells in the prostate by estimating a "Gleason score". The Gleason score, ranges from 1 to 10; Gleason 1, being very early evidence of local (in situ) malignant cells, and Gleason 10 indicating highly anaplastic invasive cancer likely to have spread beyond the prostate.

16.3.5   Treatments

Although at present controversial and uncertain as to whether treatment should be recommended, the following are standard treatments that should be considered and discussed between a patient and his medical advisers.

For small cancers apparently confined to the prostate, total surgical removal of the prostate gland, possibly with removal of adjacent lymph nodes, should result in cure. Radical prostatectomy (total removal of the prostate gland and adjacent lymph nodes) is most-often performed by an open surgical operation but like several other abdominal operations it can now be performed by a robot assisted laproscopic technique.

Alternatively, obstruction to the flow of urine may be relieved by a TUR (transurethral resection) in which an instrument (resectoscope) is passed into the urethra through the penis and some of the enlarged prostate is cut away to relieve obstruction. Specimens of the resected tissue are sent for microscopic examination to look for the presence of cancer.

Cancer of the prostate will respond to radiotherapy that is often used to treat both the primary prostate cancer and a limited number of painful metastatic deposits in bone. In suitable patients local external radiotherapy and/or brachytherapy with radioactive "seeds" implanted into the prostate and the cancer, can now give results virtually matching results of radical surgery (Sect. 8.3.3). Although there are still risks of similar side effects, they are less likely than after radical prostatectomy. More locally advanced cancers are often better treated by radiotherapy as the field of irradiation can extend beyond the local prostate region. Sometimes after radical surgery for locally advanced cancer, when there is doubt as to whether all the cancer-involved tissues were removed, follow-up radiotherapy is also recommended.

High Intensity Focused Ultrasound (HIFU) is a more recently studied treatment for some cancers not extending outside the prostate gland. From different sources high-energy ultrasound waves are directed into the prostate tissue by means of a rectal probe. The whole prostate tissue is destroyed by the heat created, leaving a small remnant of scarred remnant. Advantages of this treatment are that it can be repeated and it is less likely to cause troublesome side-effects. However more studies are needed before the most appropriate use of this treatment will be known.

When American doctors, Charles Huggins and Clarence Hodges, discovered that prostate cancers would often respond to stilboestrol, stilboestrol then became standard treatment for prostate cancer. Most patients had some benefit with symptom relief and some increased life expectancy but not a cure in the long term. Stilboestrol is no longer the preferred hormone therapy but other forms of hormone therapy are now used.

Prostate cancer is androgen (testosterone) dependent; that is, without any androgen the cancer cells will not grow although eventually some aggressive prostate cancers will continue to grow in the absence of androgens. Most but not all androgen in men comes from the testes but the testes can produce testosterone only if they are stimulated by gonadotrophic hormone. One way of reducing the growth of prostate cancer therefore is by castration – a treatment not at all popular with most men. Another way of reducing the effects of androgen is to use an anti-hormone, either an anti-testosterone or an anti-gonadotrophin.

The modern alternatives to stilboestrol, Lutenising Hormone Releasing Hormone (LH-RH) analogues have long been used in treatment for advanced prostate cancer when cure by surgery or radiotherapy has not been possible. More recently anti-androgens have been used but (LH-RH agonists) are now becoming more commonly used because they are equally effective and less likely to have troublesome side effects. With stilboestrol and some other agents, some patients reported feeling nauseated, many developed some enlargement and tenderness of the breasts and there was an increased risk of deep-vein thrombosis. Desire for sexual activity was reduced and there may have been complete impotence. With modern hormone treatments these side effects are still often a problem but less common and less severe. Eventually aggressive prostate cancers will become androgen resistant and will grow in the absence of androgens.

There have been few studies of the use of cytotoxic chemotherapy in treatment of prostate cancer. In general, early cancers can be well treated by operation, slightly bigger localised cancers are often well treated by radiotherapy, and metastatic cancer usually responds well, possibly for some years, to hormone treatment. Radiotherapy can be given to a limited number of bone secondaries. Prostate cancers are slowly growing so that palliative chemotherapy, with all its side effects (more toxic than hormone therapy), is usually not advised, as first treatment in these older age group men.

Prostate cancer will respond to treatment with some cytotoxic agents but these are generally used only in patients whose cancer no longer responds to hormones. Hormones are usually more reliable, more effective and less toxic than cytotoxic agents in treating prostate cancer. Studies are now being made, especially in Germany, to determine whether better results can be expected from using regional cytotoxic chemotherapy before surgery in treating patients with locally advanced prostate cancers or whether regional chemotherapy used before radiotherapy might make the operation unnecessary in some patients. In the past most clinicians found responses to cytotoxic chemotherapy to be disappointing no matter how it was given but an anti-cancer agent called *Mitoxantrone* gave encouraging responses, especially with relief of symptoms but no convincing evidence of improved survival. A newer anti-cancer agent called *Docetaxel (Taxotare)* given at 3 weekly intervals is now giving even better symptomatic relief with some improvement in long-term survival for those men with hormone refractory prostate cancer.

16.3.6   Treatment of Bone Metastases

If bone scans show "hot spots" of metastatic prostate cancer in bones that are painless, a decision must be made as to whether or not treatment is needed. For an elderly man with small painless lesions it may be better not to treat actively but to keep under observation in case they change. If a large bone metastasis is seen, especially in a weight-bearing bone that could easily fracture, local radiotherapy might be advisable.

In most men with bone metastases who are not already having treatment, a program of hormone treatment is usually recommended.

For men having bone pain that has not been well controlled by standard treatment with hormones and/or local radiotherapy and/or standard pain-relief measures, treatment with *bisphosphonates* or *strontium-89* will often give good pain relief. There is also evidence that these treatments might sometimes help prevent further bone metastases from developing (Sects. 8.6.2 and 12.11) (Fig. 16.2).

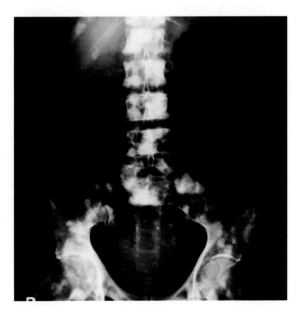

Fig. 16.2. Widespread metastatic prostate carcinoma in bones of pelvis, vertebrae and ribs

16

Why is there controversy about most appropriate management of men
with prostate cancer?

CASE REPORT

Prostate cancer

Karl is a 76-year-old businessman who, at the age of 69, when he had a
routine health check, was found to have a PSA of 6.1 ng/mL. At the time
he had been well and was a keen golfer. With a digito-rectal-examination
(DRE) his doctor felt a slightly enlarged prostate but no other abnormality.
Concerned about the raised PSA, the family doctor arranged a consultation with a specialist urologist.

The urologist did not feel anything abnormal except that as well as
being slightly enlarged the prostate gland was a little harder than normal.
No lumps were felt. The urologist arranged ultrasound studies of the prostate. No lumps were seen but three biopsies were taken from each side of
the prostate gland. The biopsies were all negative for cancer.

One year later the tests were all repeated. The PSA had risen to 8.3 and
ultrasound revealed a small nodular area in the right lobe of the prostate
gland. Biopsy of this showed a small collection of low-grade malignant
cells (Gleason 1) in one of the three right lobe specimens.

The urologist explained to Karl that the few positive cells might repre-
sent low-grade "latent" cancer that may or may not progress into a serious
cancer problem during his lifetime. The urologist explained that any surgical or other "curative" procedure would risk complications (especially
erectile dysfunction with impotence and possibly some incontinence) and
may not change his life expectancy. After discussion between Karl and
the urologist it was decided to repeat all tests in 4 months.

(continued)

(continued)

In 4 months the PSA had risen to 9.3 and biopsies showed positive cancer cells in two specimens with a slightly higher-grade in one specimen (Gleason 4).

Karl was otherwise still fit and well with an otherwise good life expectancy. In view of the apparent progress of the disease, which still appeared to be contained within the prostate gland and therefore was eminently resectable, Karl and his wife decided that they would accept the option of radical prostatectomy with all the risks rather than further "wait and see".

The operation was performed without a major problem and the surgeon tried to preserve the erectile nerve on the left side. There was no evidence of lymph-node involvement. Six weeks after discharge Karl's urinary function was good, except for occasional stress incontinence, but he was unable to achieve an erection in spite of his urge to have intercourse.

The options of management of erectile dysfunction were discussed between Karl, his wife, the family doctor and the urologist. For some months the tablet Viagra was used but not always with reliable success so that penile injection of prostaglandins has since been used with reliable success.

Karl is now alive and well 6 years postoperatively and plays golf regularly. Since operation his PSA has been less than 0.1. Apart from needing help to achieve an erection, and occasionally a little stress incontinence of urine, he has no significant health problem.

Comment

Karl has heard that improvements in radiotherapy and especially brachytherapy with radioactive implants into the prostate gland, if available, may have been a preferred treatment option with equally good long-term results and fewer side-effects, especially with erectile dysfunction. The urologist explained that this may be so with presently available radiotherapy facilities but when he was first treated there was no proof that his long-term cure would be the same. As more cases of early, limited prostate cancer have been treated by brachytherapy it does appear that in suitable patients long-term results can match results of surgery with the advantage of less fewer side-effects.

Cancers of Bladder and Kidneys

17

17.1   Bladder Cancer

Many years ago bladder cancer was found to be increased in industrial workers who were exposed to aniline dyes and certain other chemical compounds. It has since been found to be more common in smokers and in people who abuse the use of analgesics. Cancer may also develop in a papilloma, a small benign fern-like or cauliflower-like tumour of the bladder. Some patients have several small papillomas in the lining of the bladder wall and any one of these can change to become a cancer if not treated. In some countries, including Egypt and some other North African countries, infestation with the fluke parasite, Schistosoma or Bilharzia, is common. If these flukes infest the bladder they can cause inflammation and erosions of the mucosa and penetrate into the bladder wall. In those countries this is a well-recognised cause of bladder cancer.

Most bladder cancers develop in the transitional cells that line the bladder cavity. They are about twice as common in males as in females and in both sexes are more common in developed than developing countries. They most commonly present in men between 50 and 70 years. The most common symptom of bladder cancer is blood in the urine (haematuria). The blood may be intermittent at first but becomes more constant as the tumour grows and invades the bladder wall. At a later stage there may be discomfort in passing urine (dysuria) and symptoms of bladder infection (cystitis) such as frequency, burning and pain when passing urine. Sometimes a ureter may become obstructed by the growth and pain may be felt in the loin due to backpressure on the kidney.

F. O. Stephens and K. R. Aigner, *Basics of Oncology,*
DOI: 10.1007/978-3-540-92925-3_17, © Springer-Verlag Berlin Heidelberg 2009

After losing blood in the urine for some time, anaemia may develop and symptoms of anaemia (pallor, tiredness, palpitations, etc.) may be noticed.

17.1.1   Investigations

The urine is examined for blood and may also be centrifuged and examined for cancer cells. Excretory urograms, (IVP X-rays as described in Sect. 7.4) may show a *filling defect* or lump in the bladder. They may also show evidence of obstruction to a ureter if present.

CT scans may reveal a lump in the bladder wall but the ultimate investigation is with a cystoscope. The cystoscope (described in Sect. 7.4) is passed into the bladder through the urethra usually under general anaesthesia, and the inside of the bladder is examined. A section of any suspected cancer together with a small piece of adjacent bladder wall is taken as a biopsy for microscopic examination.

17.1.2   Types of Bladder Cancer (Pathology)

There are various degrees of bladder tumours ranging from a single benign cauliflower-like papilloma to an invasive ulcerated thickened cancer. Between these extremes there may be several papillomata, one or more of which may show signs of early malignancy, or there may be a malignant lump or malignant ulcer in the bladder wall. Superficial non-penetrating bladder cancers tend to remain confined to the bladder-wall for a long time before they spread but more penetrating bladder cancers often metastasise at an early stage. After a time, bladder cancers may involve the whole thickness of the bladder-wall and even invade the rectum or other organs nearby. Penetrating cancers often spread to nearby lymph nodes but they do not commonly metastasise more widely.

There are various degrees of bladder tumours ranging from a single benign cauliflower-like papilloma to an invasive ulcerated thickened cancer.

17.1.3   Treatment

Small papillomata of the bladder are usually treated by burning them off with an electro-cautery. The electro-cautery instrument is used through a cystoscope. The patient is cystoscoped regularly thereafter in case the tumour recurs.

For larger papillomas or early invasive cancers, treatment by radiotherapy or surgical excision or a combination of both radiotherapy and surgical excision may offer good prospects of cure.

Early non-invasive bladder cancer will often respond to Bacillus Camille Guerin (BCG) irrigation. BCG is a harmless bacterium that seems to stimulate an immune healing response. This treatment is repeated at intervals as necessary to control the cancer. However if the cancer becomes invasive surgical resection or radiotherapy will be needed.

For more advanced cancers, surgery to remove the whole of the bladder (cystectomy), may be necessary. A new type of bladder is then usually surgically constructed from a part of the bowel.

When cure by surgery is impossible, palliative radiotherapy may give relief.

Chemotherapy has a limited place in the treatment of bladder cancer, although studies are being carried out in the hope of improving prospects of cure or worthwhile palliation with the use of newer agents and newer techniques of giving chemotherapy. Systemic chemotherapy is used with some benefit in treating bladder cancer if it does become widespread or metastatic.

17.2   Kidney Cancers

Kidney cancers are not common but there are three well recognised types. The Wilm's tumour (nephroblastoma) occurs in infants or young children. In adults kidney cancers are either adenocarcinoma (sometimes called hypernephroma or Grawitz tumour), or carcinoma of renal pelvis (usually squamous or transitional cell type).

17.2.1   Wilm's Tumour (Nephroblastoma)

The Wilm's tumour usually is found in children of less than 4 years. It can even be present at birth. Whilst in most cases only one kidney is affected, occasionally there is a cancer in both kidneys.

This cancer is most commonly found as a lump in the loin of an infant. It may present by causing the child to be in poor general health with a fever, anaemia, or sometimes blood is seen in the urine. It may spread to nearby lymph nodes or into the large veins. From these veins cancer cells may be carried by the blood to the lungs where metastases may develop.

The Wilm's tumour usually is found in children of less than 4 years. It can even be present at birth.

17.2.2   Adenocarcinoma (Hypernephroma or Grawitz Tumour)

This is the most common type of kidney cancer and is usually seen in adults of middle age or older. It is about twice as common in men than women and is more common in smokers of either sex. The first symptom is usually passing blood in the urine, most often painlessly. (Passing blood in the urine with severe pain in the loin is more likely to be caused by a kidney stone.) There may be a fever or a lump may be felt in the loin or sometimes there is local pain. This cancer may spread into nearby lymph nodes but commonly grows into the large renal vein and may spread by the bloodstream into the lungs, liver or bones. Occasionally the first evidence of this cancer is the presence of metastases in a lung or in one or more bones.

The first symptom is usually passing blood in the urine, most often painlessly.

17.2.3   Carcinoma of the Renal Pelvis Or Ureter (Transitional Cell Carcinoma)

This cancer is rather like cancer of the bladder and behaves in a similar way. The first sign of this cancer is also usually blood in the urine. Smoking and analgesic abuse are commonly associated with development of these cancers. They also sometimes develop as a reaction from a stone present in the kidney for a long time.

17.2.4   Investigations

X-rays of the abdomen may show an enlarged kidney. Excretory urograms (intra-venous pyelograms or IVP), CT scans, ultrasound, and arteriography (as described in Sect. 7.3) are all useful investigations to help diagnose a tumour in a kidney and to help determine whether a kidney lump is solid and likely to be cancer, or a fluid-filled cyst and probably benign.

Other investigations include examination of the urine for blood or malignant cells and X-rays of lungs for evidence of metastatic cancer, or bone scans or X-rays to show evidence of metastases if there are any swelling or painful areas in bones.

17.2.5   Treatment

Cancer of a kidney is best treated by an operation to remove the kidney (nephrectomy). For Wilm's tumour (nephroblastoma) in children, results are much better if radiotherapy and chemotherapy are used in combination with nephrectomy.

For adenocarcinoma nephrectomy is the only likely cure for a patient. Radiotherapy and chemotherapy may be used as palliative treatment in advanced cases but results other than by complete surgical removal have been disappointing. Sometimes these cancers will show a temporary response to male or female hormones and some studies have reported responses in patients with metastases treated with the immunological agents interferon or interleukin 2. Adenocarcinoma of a kidney is one cancer that sometimes spreads to a lung as one single metastatic lump, resembling a "cannon ball", and this can sometimes be cured by an operation removing the part of the lung containing the lump.

For cancer of the renal pelvis, the best results are achieved if the kidney is removed together with the whole of the ureter and a small part of the bladder because seedlings of this cancer sometimes grow in the ureter between the kidney and the bladder.

CASE REPORT

Wilms' tumour

Andrew is a 4-year-old boy who was brought to the Emergency Room of the Children's Hospital after his parents noticed he was passing heavily blood-stained urine. On examination in the Emergency Room, he looked well, with normal male genitalia, and no evidence of penile ulceration or excoriation. A firm non-tender mass was palpable below the liver on the right side of his abdomen. His blood pressure was 140/90. A specimen of urine was frankly blood-stained.

An abdominal ultrasound revealed a right-sided renal mass consistent with a right-sided renal tumour. Examination of the inferior vena cava by ultrasound revealed a patent vessel with no evidence of tumour thrombus in the cava. CT scan of chest, abdomen and pelvis revealed no evidence of metastatic disease and no other abnormalities.

A needle biopsy of the renal tumour was performed under general anaesthesia guided by image intensification in the Medical Imaging department. Histopathology confirmed a Wilms' tumour (nephroblastoma), with the histology being of the usual ("favourable") type. No evidence of anaplasia was seen. A central venous catheter was inserted in the operating theatre under a separate general anaesthetic. A low dose of an oral anti-hypertensive agent was administered for a few weeks after diagnosis to control the hypertension.

Andrew received 7 weeks of outpatient chemotherapy (using vincristine, and actinomycin-D and doxorubicin). This was associated with intermittent fever, episodes of abdominal discomfort, and constipation, and mild inflammation of the oral mucous membranes and temporary mild bone marrow depression following each of two pulses of actinomycin-D and doxorubicin. The renal mass was noted to be somewhat smaller by the seventh week.

Eight weeks after diagnosis, Andrew underwent a right radical nephrectomy, from which he recovered uneventfully. Histopathologic examination of the excised kidney indicated a significant degree of tumour cell destruction from the initial chemotherapy and no visible spread of the tumour beyond the renal capsule. He is currently continuing adjuvant chemotherapy (with vincristine, actinomycin-D and doxorubicin), which will be continued for 12 months. Blood pressure fell to normal levels immediately after the nephrectomy.

(continued)

17

(continued)

Andrew has an excellent prognosis. The definitive surgery is typically delayed a few weeks after diagnosis to allow shrinkage of the tumour to occur with the initial induction chemotherapy, to lessen the likelihood of intraoperative haemorrhage, facilitate early ligation of the renal vein, and improve the safety of the procedure.

Around 90% of children with localised Wilms' tumour with the usual histology will be cured permanently using this combination of induction chemotherapy, surgery and adjuvant chemotherapy.

Comment

Survival historically with surgery alone was no better than 20%. Radiation therapy to the renal fossa and rear of abdomen is reserved for those patients where regional spread has occurred at diagnosis, and where localised residual disease is considered likely after nephrectomy. Preservation of unaffected kidney tissue in the diseased organ may be attempted in patients whose tumour is confined to one or other poles of the affected kidney.

Cancers of the Brain and Nervous System

18

18.1 Brain Cancers

Although most brain cancers occur in people over the age of 45, with a peak incidence between 60 and 70 years, in fact the brain is also one of the more common sites for primary cancer in children and young adults. Brain cancers are more common in developed than developing countries (see Appendix), but the reason for this is not known.

There are two groups of cells in the brain that may form tumours. The glial cells (true brain cells) from which most of the malignant tumours develop, and the non-glial cells or supporting cells (such as cells of the meninges or cells of the nerve sheaths) from which develop the majority of benign tumours.

Cancers that arise from true brain cells or glial cells are called *gliomas*. There are a number of different types of gliomas ranging from the more slowly growing types called *astrocytoma* or *oligodendroglioma* to more rapidly and highly malignant types called *medulloblastoma* (usually in children) or *glioblastoma multiforme* (more often in adults). These different types of glioma tend to occur in different parts of the brain in children and adults. They also have other differences for example medulloblastomas are usually highly radiosensitive and are sometimes cured by radiotherapy but other types are less radiosensitive (if at all).

There are no known causes of cerebral tumours. The commonly held belief that electromagnetic fields, (including the use of mobile telephones), may play

F. O. Stephens and K. R. Aigner, *Basics of Oncology,*
DOI: 10.1007/978-3-540-92925-3_18, © Springer-Verlag Berlin Heidelberg 2009

a part has not as yet been substantiated with statistical evidence. However the possibility remains and anecdotal evidence justifies further study.

18.1.1   Clinical Features (Symptoms and Signs)

Brain cancers tend to cause two types of clinical features:

(a)   General features due to generalised pressure on the brain
(b)   Focal or local features due to pressure or interference by the tumour on parts of the brain or nerves near the tumour.

18.1.1.1   General Features

The common general features of cancer in the brain are due to pressure and swelling on the brain as a whole. This causes headache, nausea, vomiting and disturbances of vision due to swelling of the optic nerve at the back of the eye (seen as papilloedema). The most significant single feature is persistent headache. Other features may be listlessness, tiredness and mood or personality change. The sufferer may progressively withdraw from social contacts and gradually become confused and stuporous and may lapse into coma. In young children the increased pressure may cause the head to enlarge and *hydrocephalus* (so-called "water on the brain") may develop.

Fitting alone is rarely caused by cancer in children.   It should be noted that in children, convulsions or fitting are most often caused by a fever or other less serious problem. Fitting alone is rarely caused by cancer in children. In an adult, however, with no previous history of epilepsy, injury or fitting from another known cause, the sudden onset of a fitting attack may be the first sign of a brain tumour.

18.1.1.2   Focal Features

Focal features are due to interference of function of a local region of the brain. These features will depend upon the site of the tumour. In one place it may be interference with speech, in another it may be loss of movement of an arm or leg, or elsewhere or loss of sensation in a part of the body. Tumours elsewhere might cause local twitching or focal fitting with different sensations such as olfactory or visual hallucinations like the flickering of lights. There may be disorders of balance, or clumsy movement or interference with a cranial nerve such as the optic nerves for vision, the nerves that move the eyeball or the facial nerves that move the muscles of the side of the face. In the frontal lobes, the earliest features might be mood or personality change.

18.1.2   Pathology Types

Astrocytomas can range from relatively low-grade to anaplastic high-grade cancers called glioblastoma multiforme. Low-grade astrocytomas develop more slowly with more prolonged symptoms and a longer life-expectancy but the majority of primary brain cancers, especially in adults, are glioblastoma multiforme with a more rapid onset of headache and other symptoms.

Medulloblastomas are malignant tumours in the cerebellum and are the most common brain cancers in children causing headaches and problems of balance and loss of co-ordination, possibly with fitting.

18.1.3   Investigations

CT scans and MRI scans have revolutionised investigations for brain tumours. Before these scans were invented, cerebral angiography (arteriography after injecting a radio-opaque iodine compound into one of the internal carotid arteries), radio-isotope scans, and air encephalograms (described in Sect. 7.3) were used almost routinely together with a number of other investigations such as the electroencephalogram (EEG), which records brainwave activity. Nowadays, however, the CT scan or the MRI scan, usually supplies most of the information of other investigations and even more precisely. Angiography may still give added information particularly concerning the vascularity of a tumour. Surgeons often use angiograms to plan operations. The surgeons then know exactly where the tumour is in relation to nearby blood vessels. The angiograms also indicate which vessels are supplying blood to the tumour.

18.1.4   Treatment

Whilst the majority of benign cerebral tumours, like meningiomas, can be cured by surgical removal, malignant tumours, other than radiosensitive medulloblastomas, are not often curable. For this reason, it is vital to determine – often at operation – whether a tumour in the brain is benign or malignant. If malignant, it is also important to determine the type of malignancy because the outlook for some is better than others and some, such as medulloblastomas, may be curable.

Whilst the majority are not curable, most patients with brain cancer can be given considerable relief of symptoms by a number of means. First, corticosteroids can be used to reduce swelling and so reduce pressure on the brain, which will relieve headaches and other pressure symptoms. Then surgical operation can be carried out to remove at least most of the cancer, giving further and more prolonged relief of symptoms. Following surgery, radiotherapy alone will usually further improve the immediate outlook but not in the long term.

18

Recent studies have shown that post-operative chemotherapy with radiotherapy has given added benefit and some apparent cures have been reported, particularly in the case of medulloblastomas but also in some cases of other cerebral malignancies.

CASE REPORT

Glioblastoma multiforme

Elsie is a 60-year-old retired teacher who does not smoke and seldom drinks alcohol. She had enjoyed good health. She is right-handed.

Elsie gave a very short history. About 7 days before consulting her doctor she had experienced a visual disturbance, which lasted for less than 2 h. She was reading but could not interpret the words.

For 3 days she had had some unusual visual sensations. On one occasion she thought she saw something in the peripheral right visual field, like a street sign, but there was no such sign. In speech there were some errors of word selection. She knew what she wanted to say but sometimes the wrong word "came out". For example on one occasion she told someone that she had three wolves at home when she was meaning to say three dogs.

On examination there were no abnormalities on visual field testing. The fundi and optic discs were normal. The lower cranial nerves were intact. No abnormality was found on neurological examination of the limbs.

A CT scan of the brain demonstrated a spherical lesion 1.5 cm in diameter in the inferior and medial aspect of the left temporal lobe with swelling and oedema around it.

The differential diagnosis of such lesions includes a primary brain tumour or a solitary metastasis. Blood tumour markers were negative for the most common undiagnosed cancers likely to metastasise to brain in a woman of her age, breast cancer and bowel cancer (CA 15-3 and CEA both normal).

A mammogram and breast ultrasound showed no abnormality. A CT scan of the chest, abdomen and pelvis was clear. A PET scan of the brain was consistent with a high-grade tumour.

Anticonvulsants and corticosteroids were commenced.

A neurosurgical operation was done. The tumour was biopsied, and frozen sections indicated a high-grade glioma, glioblastoma multiforme, (a malignant primary brain tumour). Most of the tumour was then removed. She woke with no new deficits. After recovering from the surgery a course of radiotherapy was commenced but her outlook must be very guarded.

CASE REPORT

A large benign cerebral tumour (meningioma)

Gur is a 47-year-old successful businessman who had smoked for many years. He drank little alcohol, and was being treated for hypertension. His brother had been treated for a cerebral meningioma some years before.

For some months Gur had been aware of cognitive problems, with insidious onset and progression. He misplaced things continuously. This had been noticed by his family and golf partners. His handwriting had altered greatly.

Normal tasks required great effort. Although very experienced he dithered and dawdled in running his business, and in organising the purchase of a new house.

He often woke up at night because of a throbbing pain in the head. He had lost some weight recently but was not aware of a change in appetite. He was aware that he had become quite moody. He was left-handed and his wife would chasten him because of a tendency to carry things around in his left hand unknowingly. He took the flag out appropriately at one of the holes when his golf-playing partner was putting, but then continued to carry the flag in his left hand while attempting to shape up for his next stroke.

On examination he was slow in responding. His writing was shaky and difficult. When asked to undress for physical examination he undressed in a very odd fashion. He was holding his wallet in his left hand. He did not put the wallet down. For the whole period while he took off his shoes and socks the wallet stayed where it was and he removed his shoes and socks one-handed with his right hand. Neither arm swung when he walked. There was an increase in left upper limb tone, the limb appeared stiff but power was normal. Coordination was slightly less in the left upper limb but sensory examination was normal. Stance and heel-toe walking was good. The reflexes were brisker for the left biceps, knee and ankle jerks and the left plantar response was equivocal.

A CT scan indicated an unusual tumour with a large cystic component. An urgent MRI scan showed a very significant tumour in the right medial frontal lobe, abutting the sagittal sinus and probably arising from the falx, uniformly enhancing with contrast. Around the tumour and cyst there was some brain oedema.

Dexamethasone (a corticosteroid) was given to relieve the cerebral pressure and oedema and anticonvulsants were commenced.

At operation a giant meningioma (a usually benign tumour of the meninges) was diagnosed. Even though it was so large and odd, the histology was benign. The tumour was entirely removed, and his cognitive functions improved rapidly over the next 3 months.

He is now back to normal and has a good prognosis.

18

CASE REPORT

Malignant astrocytoma

Mr P is a 59-year-old barrister who at the age of 56 years first noticed that he was beginning to feel "old and tired". During a stormy court case he had occasionally lost the word he was trying to express. He concluded that he had been working too hard and arranged to take a holiday in a month's time.

Unfortunately before his holiday period he began to have headaches that he felt "all through" his head. Sometimes the headaches were more pronounced in the left temporal region just above his ear. He took some proprietary headache tablets with only limited relief. One morning the right side of his face began to spasm in a most alarming fashion. He was unable to speak and a few minutes later the spasm moved into his right shoulder and arm.

Terrified of this symptom (as most people are with their first seizure) he sat on the edge of his bed until he was able to call his wife who drove him to the nearest Hospital Emergency Department.

On examination he was found to be a middle-aged man who had a partial weakness of the right side of his face and right arm and shoulder although he appeared otherwise fit. His tendon reflexes were much increased on the right side and papilloedema (swelling of the optic nerve) could be seen when his eye was examined with an ophthalmoscope. MRI studies showed a moderate sized tumour within the brain in the left temporo-parietal region.

Mr P was referred to a neurosurgeon who informed him that this was almost certainly a malignant brain tumour but that he would not recommend surgery because it would not be possible to remove the tumour without damaging the part of his brain controlling speech and movement of the right side of his body. He advised, and carried out, a needle biopsy of the tumour to establish its exact nature.

Biopsy showed it to be a high grade malignant astrocytoma.

Mr P was advised that his tumour might respond to combined therapy using a new agent called temozolomide and radiotherapy. After consultation with a neuro-oncologist and radiotherapist he was treated with this drug and radiotherapy synchronously.

Over the next 12 months MRI studies showed that the tumour gradually regressed. Three years later, at the age of 59, Mr P has returned to his practice as previously. He remains well but continues to have 6-monthly courses of temozolomide and 6 monthly MRI studies.

(continued)

(continued)

Comment

In the past results of treatment of aggressive brain cancers, especially in adults, have been so negative that it is very encouraging to see results of the combined treatment as given to Mr P. Whilst several similar results have now been reported it is too early in this clinical study to speculate what percentage of patients so treated will have similar responses or for how long such responses will be maintained. This is an example of the cutting edge of clinical studies in cancer treatment. Such studies are practiced in all areas of cancer treatment, especially where there is no established successful alternative.

EXERCISE

Drawing on case reports in this and other chapters of this book, construct a case report of a typical patient presenting with and being investigated and managed for a medulloblastoma.

18.2 Secondary Cancers in the Brain

The brain is sometimes the site of a metastatic cancer. Cancers of lung, breast and melanomas are the most common primary cancers that metastasise to brain but occasionally the brain may harbour secondary cancer from almost any other primary site or from leukaemia.

Cure by any means is unlikely for metastatic cerebral tumours but considerable, although temporary, relief is often gained by surgical removal, radiotherapy or even sometimes chemotherapy. A combination of these treatment modalities is often more effective.

18.3   Nerve Cell Cancers

18.3.1   Neuroblastoma

Neuroblastoma is a malignancy of primitive nerve cells. After acute lymphoblastic leukaemia and brain tumours, it is the most common malignancy of childhood, about 10% of childhood cancers. About 80% of cases occur in infants less than 4 years.

Neuroblastomas can occur anywhere in the sympathetic nervous system from the neck to pelvis and including the adrenal glands.

18.3.2   Presentation

The child is usually failing to thrive, often irritable and may have lost bladder or bowel control.

There may be an abdominal mass but symptoms and signs will depend upon which site in the sympathetic nervous system the tumour started and which tissues are involved in tumour invasion (e.g. the neural canals), or metastases (bone, subcutaneous tissue or liver are common).

Occasionally, especially in infants less than 1 year, the tumour may resolve spontaneously but treatment usually requires a combination of surgery, chemotherapy and radiation therapy, sometimes to a degree requiring bone-marrow transplantation to restore blood-forming tissues. Local tumours are often controlled by treatment but widespread metastases are rarely controlled.

18.4   Retinoblastoma

A retinoblastoma is an uncommon childhood cancer in the eye of infants and children up to 4 years. In about 25% of patients it is bilateral and in almost half of the cases there is a genetic factor with a family history of a similar tumour, and invariably both eyes are enucleated to prevent the development of cancer.

Retinoblastoma is an anaplastic malignancy of the retina. It can spread from the eye to involve brain and meninges, and cause premature death in infancy.

18.4.1   Presentation

The first sign is often a white reflex through the child's pupil (leukocoria) noticed by the parents. a squint may have developed in the eye.

Treatment often involves cryosurgery, radiotherapy and chemotherapy (both induction and adjuvant chemotherapy), with or without enucleation of the eye.

If diagnosed early (before local spread or metastases) a high incidence of cure is achieved. Neurosarcomas are discussed in Chap. 20.1.5

The Leukaemias and Lymphomas

19

19.1 The Leukaemias

Leukaemia is a cancer of blood-forming cells. Leukaemias are classified into two broad groups according to the type of blood-forming cell that has become malignant. These are called lymphatic leukaemia and myeloid (or non-lymphatic) leukaemia.

In lymphatic leukaemia the cells that have become malignant are the bone marrow cells that normally make lymphocytes. Lymph nodes and lymphoid tissue are usually involved and some nodes become enlarged. In myeloid leukaemia the cells that have become malignant are cells in the bone marrow that normally make the other types of white blood cells (that is myeloid cells that make polymorphs and other white cell types). The spleen usually becomes involved and enlarged.

Leukaemias may be acute or chronic according to whether the disease would tend to run a rapid and rapidly fatal course (acute leukaemia) or whether the disease would progress more slowly (chronic leukaemia).

Thus there are four main types of leukaemia:

- Acute lymphocytic (lymphatic) leukaemia (ALL)
- Acute myeloid (non-lymphatic or granulocytic) leukaemia (AML or ANLL.)

F. O. Stephens and K. R. Aigner, *Basics of Oncology,*
DOI: 10.1007/978-3-540-92925-3_19, © Springer-Verlag Berlin Heidelberg 2009

- Chronic lymphocytic leukaemia (CLL)
- Chronic myeloid (non-lymphocytic or granulocytic) leukaemia (CML or CNLL or CGL)

It is important to distinguish between the major types of leukaemia because they tend to run different courses and respond differently to different treatments.

19.1.1   Incidence and Prevalence of Leukaemias

Leukaemias occur throughout the world but the incidence varies in different countries and in different races. All types of leukaemia are slightly more common in males. The Scandinavian countries and Israel have the highest incidence and the lowest reported incidence is in Chile and Japan but in general they are more common in developed countries (see Appendix). In the USA the highest incidence is in Jews and the lowest is in African Americans.

Acute leukaemia accounts for about half of all cancers in children
The overall incidence of ALL and AML is about equal but there is a distinct age difference. Acute leukaemia accounts for about half of all cancers in children and acute lymphocytic leukaemia is the most common of all cancers in young children, with a peak incidence of between 2 and 4 years. The incidence of AML is low in children but increases with age.

The causes of leukaemia are unknown although some predisposing factors are recognised. Leukaemias, especially myeloid leukaemias, have been linked with ionising radiation. There is also evidence that exposure of a foetus to X-rays during its mother's pregnancy is associated with a slightly increased risk of leukaemia developing later in childhood. However, there is no evidence that normal use of diagnostic X-rays in adults is associated with leukaemia. Myelofibrosis (myeloplastic disease) is a disorder of bone marrow cell proliferation that sometimes presents in adults as anaemia of no obvious cause and commonly degenerates into an acute leukaemia.

Excessive exposure to some chemical agents such as benzene is associated with a slightly increased risk of leukaemia. AML will occasionally develop in patients who have had some other form of cancer including Hodgkin lymphoma, or cancer of the ovary, that has been treated with chemotherapy.

Use of anti-cancer cytotoxic drugs for other cancers, and especially their pronged use with radiotherapy, also slightly increases the risk of later development of leukaemia.

Familial leukaemia is rare although some families with multiple cases of leukaemia have been reported. In general, siblings of a child with leukaemia have only a slightly higher risk of developing leukaemia although if one identical twin develops acute leukaemia the other twin has about a 20% chance of developing the disease.

People with Down's Syndrome have a twenty times greater risk of developing acute leukaemia than other people. Women who become mothers at an advanced age not only have an increased risk of producing children with Down's syndrome but otherwise normal children born of older age group mothers have a slightly greater risk of developing acute leukaemia.

Genetic mutations and complex gene rearrangements are of basic importance in the pathogenesis of leukaemias and lymphomas. There is presently a great deal of study of these chromosome changes. Studies indicate that the chromosomal and genetic changes not only show different patterns in different forms of leukaemias but genetic patterns may also indicate likely responses to different treatments and an indication of likely progress.

There were increased numbers of people with leukaemias after the atomic bomb explosions at Hiroshima and Nagasaki and after the Chernobyl atomic energy plant disaster in Russia, CML was the most prevalent.

Viruses are known to cause leukaemia in some animal species but only one type of leukaemia in humans has been linked to a virus. Adult T-cell leukaemia/lymphoma, prevalent in the Carribbean, Japan and New Guinea, is probably caused by a Human virus designated "T-cell leukaemia virus" (HTLV-1). The Epstein-Barr virus has been implicated in Burkitt's Lymphoma/leukaemia.

19.2 The Acute Leukaemias

19.2.1 Clinical Presentation

19.2.1.1 Acute Lymphatic (Lymphoblastic) Leukaemia (ALL)

This is the most common form of leukaemia in children with an age peak of about 5 years. Symptoms are caused by replacement of normal blood-forming cells of bone marrow by malignant leukaemic cells and infiltration (invasion) of other tissues such as spleen, lymph nodes, tonsils and sometimes liver, kidneys, lungs and brain.

Fever, weakness, anorexia (loss of appetite), pallor, and infection are common. Infection is especially common in the region of the tonsils or anus and the lungs may also become infected causing pneumonia. There may be pain in bones or joints.

Lymph nodes, tonsils and spleen are commonly enlarged. Sometimes the liver and kidneys are enlarged.

Platelets may be deficient and there may be petechial spots or bruising or signs of bleeding from any site especially from the gums, the digestive tract or anus. Bleeding in the brain or from the lungs may also occur. Thrombosis (clots) may also develop in veins.

Meningitis due to leukaemic cell spread into the meninges frequently occurs in patients with ALL unless prevented by radiotherapy or chemotherapy.

19.2.1.2   Acute Myeloid Leukaemia

AML more commonly affects adults. Anaemia, bleeding or bruising and infection are the likely presenting features. But as with ALL, general ill health with fever, lassitude, loss of appetite and involvement of other tissues or organs with septicaemic infection is likely.

19.2.2   Investigations

The diagnosis of leukaemia can be made only after careful examination of blood and bone marrow. Blood is taken by a needle from a vein in the arm and bone marrow is usually taken with a small instrument that is used to puncture a bone of the pelvis (the iliac crest). Bone puncture is painful so it is done under local or even general anaesthesia. A pathologist then examines the blood and bone marrow for leukaemic cells and for other features of leukaemia. These may include anaemia (with a reduction in numbers of red blood cells), reduction in number of normal white blood cells, and reduction in the number of platelets. About one third of patients with acute leukaemia will have an elevated white blood count, one third will have a low white blood count and in one third the white cell count is about normal.

Patients with AML are usually found to have abnormalities of chromosomes. There may also be changes in blood chemistry, including increased uric acid, that may be associated with features of gout.

Cytogenetic studies on bone marrow are now part of a full investigation of leukaemia patients. These studies identify specific molecular genetic syndromes and help in selecting the best therapy. They also give a good indication of the likely prognosis.

19.2.3   Treatment

Encouraging progress has been made in recent years in the treatment of the acute leukaemias.

Encouraging progress has been made in recent years in the treatment of the acute leukaemias.

The best opportunity to achieve the maximum cure of leukaemia is when the disease is first diagnosed. Cells that remain after the first treatment tend to develop resistance to drugs. It is therefore important that patients with acute leukaemia should immediately be referred to a readily available specialist clinic so that the most effective treatment can be given under expert supervision without delay.

Chemotherapy using cytotoxic drugs and cortisone forms the basis of modern treatment. Combinations of effective cytotoxic drugs have produced best results.

With the best current treatment methods, more than 90% of children and about 80% of adults with ALL now achieve complete remission (that is, the disease apparently disappears and the patient feels and looks well again).

Because after a time most ALL patients will develop the disease in the meninges, the lining around the brain, and because anti-cancer drugs do not pass in high concentration into the nervous system, injections of cytotoxic drugs are given into the meningeal space around the brain and the brain is also treated by radiotherapy. In the case of AML, nervous system involvement does not occur so often but this treatment is also given immediately there is any sign that there may be brain or central nervous system involvement.

With AML, good results of chemotherapy have not been as reliable as with ALL. Recently, in attempts to further improve results, bone marrow transplantation has been used effectively, especially in younger people (aged under 50). In marrow transplantation the leukaemic cells are destroyed by big doses of chemotherapy and radiotherapy (total body irradiation). This is a dangerous procedure and is carried out only in highly expert units within specialised hospitals. The patient is then given an infusion of bone marrow taken from a matched donor (that is, a donor with similar body cells unlikely to cause a rejection reaction). The best donor is often a sibling or other family member. Bone marrow transplantation involves a number of risks and should therefore be carried out only by appropriately trained experts, in specially equipped hospitals. Results have been most encouraging in this otherwise fatal illness. An alternative source of haemopoietic stem cells for transplantation is to use peripheral blood stem cells or umbilical cord stem cells Blood stem cells are collected from the blood after stimulation by colony stimulating factors (like G-CSF). Although controversial from an ethical and moral point of view embryonal stem cells may have the ability to respond in the bone marrow in a similar way to bone marrow derived cells.

In recent years, treatment with immunotherapy has been further investigated. Although major success has not as yet been achieved there have been interesting results that give hope for better treatments in the future.

Transplantation of *matched unrelated bone marrow* (bone marrow from a matched donor person not related to the patient) is used to elicit graft vs. leukaemia effect. The immunological effect of the graft might be as important or even more important than chemotherapy. In recent years *mini-allogeneic transplants* have been used (allogeneic stem cells are used without myelo-ablative chemotherapy). Studies are proceeding to determine whether such interventions might be safer and equally effective.

During the acute illness there may be special problems of anaemia, lowered resistance to infection, bleeding or even clotting. These may require blood transfusion or platelet transfusion and antibiotics or other treatment for infection. Aspirin should be strictly avoided because it interferes with blood clotting.

CASE REPORT

Acute lymphoblastic leukaemia

Elizabeth is a 5-year-old girl whose mother took her to their family doctor with a 4-week history of increasing lethargy, loss of appetite, pallor, and low grade intermittent fevers. The doctor noted that Elizabeth was pale, had a pulse rate of 140 per minute with a systolic flow heart murmur. She had scattered petechiae (little red spots) on the lower limbs, and a moderately enlarged but non-tender liver. Blood count revealed low haemoglobin (56 g/L), a raised white cell count (9×10^9/L), differential predominately blasts cells, and a low platelet count (15×10^9/L).

Elizabeth was admitted immediately to the Children's Hospital, where compatible platelets and packed red blood cells were administered to correct the thrombocytopenia and anaemia. Under general anaesthesia, a bone marrow aspirate was performed, confirming the diagnosis of ALL. A lumbar puncture contained no white cells (suggesting that cerebral involvement was unlikely). An indwelling central venous catheter was inserted.

Elizabeth commenced chemotherapy treatment (a national childhood ALL protocol, was used. This is an international program based on a very effective German protocol) in which a steroid (prednisolone) is given first. Her peripheral blast, white cell, count fell (to less than 0.1×10^9/L) after the first week of oral prednisolone. She continued induction therapy (receiving intra-venous vincristine, daunorubicin, and asparaginase), in addition to the oral prednisolone. A repeat bone marrow aspirate at the completion of the first 5 weeks of therapy indicated haematologic remission with no detectable blast cells (primitive white cells). Chemotherapy continued on an outpatient basis, followed by four doses of high-dose methotrexate intravenously over 8 weeks, and a final extended phase (using mercaptopurine daily and methotrexate weekly) for a total of 2 years of therapy. Minimum residual disease (MRD) assays performed on marrow obtained at the completion of both the first (induction) phase and completion of the second (consolidation) phase were both negative for disease.

Comment

Elizabeth has as good an outlook as is possible to have for childhood ALL. Her gender, age at diagnosis, and peripheral white cell count at diagnosis are all long-recognised indicators of a favourable prognosis. The favourable response to prednisolone as a single agent is a highly reliable indicator of responsiveness established by German studies in the late 1980s as a key determinant of required intensity of therapy. The negative MRD assays at day 33 and day 72 are, in 2005, the most advanced and sensitive indicators of an optimal response to therapy. Elizabeth has a better than 90% chance of being cured.

19.3   Chronic Lymphocytic (Lymphatic) Leukaemia

CLL tends to occur in older people with an average age of about 60 years and is usually a very slowly progressive disease. In this disease there is an overproduction of mature and relatively normal looking lymphocytes resulting in increased numbers of lymphocytes in the blood.

19.3.1   Clinical Presentation

The most obvious feature is lymph-node enlargement. Enlarged lymph nodes may be felt as lumps in the sides of the neck, in the axillae or groins. Enlarged lymph nodes in the abdomen are more difficult to feel but enlarged lymph nodes in the chest may be detected in a chest X-ray. The spleen and sometimes the liver may also be enlarged. The normal bone marrow may be replaced by malignant lymphocytes and the patient may become anaemic and deficient in platelets. This may lead to bleeding and clotting problems. Due to the replacement of normal white cells by abnormal white cells the patient has decreased ability to combat infection and may also have immunologic abnormalities.

19.3.2   Investigations

Blood count, bone marrow biopsy and tests of immune function will establish the diagnosis.

19.3.3   Treatment

CLL may be present for years without causing troublesome symptoms. Many patients may not need treatment for months or years. The median age is about 60 years and there is an increased family incidence. There is no evidence that chronic lymphatic leukaemia can be cured by early treatment, so treatment is usually reserved for episodes of the disease that are causing the patient to feel ill or causing other problems. Eventually fatigue, malaise, weight loss, bleeding and symptoms of anaemia will develop. In its early stages treatment of symptoms only may be all that is needed but eventually more aggressive treatment may be necessary.

Treatment should be initiated for CLL only when anaemia, thrombocytopenia or other disease-related symptoms appear.

Large and conspicuous lymph nodes and a large spleen can be reduced by radiotherapy. If the patient's general health is poor, treatment with anti-cancer cytotoxic drugs, often with cortisone, will usually cause reduction of enlarged lymph nodes and spleen, improve the bone marrow and make the patient feel better. Two cytotoxic anti-cancer drugs are commonly used – these are *chlorambucil* and *cyclophosphamide*. Both are given by mouth. More recently the development of new *purine analogues (fludarabine phosphatee or Fludara, 2CdA and Pentostatin)* is rapidly changing the treatment of this disease. Many experts advise that fludarabine phosphate should now be the initial treatment of choice. There is also interest in the development of monoclonal antibodies to CD20 and CD52 (Rituxan and Campath-1H respectively). These agents are now undergoing trials in association with cytotoxic chemotherapy. Rapid changes and advanced trials are proceeding into treatments of these leukaemias.

Unlike CML, CLL only very rarely changes into an acute type of leukaemia but in about 10% of cases it will change into a high-grade B-cell lymphoma-like disease as described in the following pages. This is known as *Richter's transformation.*

19.4 Chronic Myeloid Leukaemia (CML)

CML can occur at any age but the median age of people affected is about 50 years. Males are affected more often than females. There is an association with a specific chromosomal abnormality called the "Philadelphia" chromosome, which produces an enzyme called tyrosine kinase that is involved in the cellular changes of CML. Although there is no known specific cause in most cases, it was found that in Japan there was an increase in both acute and CML 5–8 years after the atomic bomb explosions.

In CML there is a marked increase in the number of white cells in the blood. This is associated with a big increase in the number of cells in bone marrow. There may also be a considerable increase in the numbers of blood platelets. Bone marrow occupation by non red-cell precursors leads to gradual but progressive anaemia.

19.4.1 Clinical Presentation

One of the more common symptoms is a pain in the left upper abdomen due to an enlarged spleen. Usually the spleen is felt easily in patients with this disease (a normal spleen cannot be felt with examining fingers). There may also be features of anaemia, tiredness, weight loss or fever. Sometimes, abnormal bruising, bleeding or clotting problems may be the first evidence of the disease.

19.4.2 Investigations

Blood count and bone marrow biopsy will usually establish the diagnosis. As for the other forms of leukaemia and the lymphomas, genetic arrangements and genetic mutations are not only associated with CML but may indicate likely patterns of progress of the disease, most appropriate treatments and likely outcomes.

19.4.3   Treatment

There are two phases of CML. The chronic phase is the least dangerous and with modern treatment may last for many months or years before the dangerous acute phase takes over.

During the chronic phase, the disease can usually be kept under good control with cytotoxic chemotherapy. The drug most commonly used with good effect has been *hydroxyurea*, although other drugs are now found to give equally good or possibly better disease control. With these treatments the blood count may return to normal and the spleen may be reduced considerably in size.

The immunological agent *"interferon"* is proving to be effective in producing remission but because in most cases it does not eliminate the "Philadelphia chromosome", it is unlikely to cure the disease. Interferon alpha with hydroxyurea significantly prolong survival (by about 20 months) of patients with chronic-phase CML compared to previously standard treatment with *busulfan*. For patients who do not tolerate interferon, hydroxyurea alone has also been shown to give better results than busulfan.

For younger patients in good health, allogenic bone marrow transplantation (BMT) appears to be a preferred option. Bone marrow transplantation is more likely to be successful in the chronic phase than in the acute phase. If the spleen remains large and causes pain or other problems due to its large size and over-activity it may sometimes be necessary to have the spleen removed by a surgeon.

Sooner or later, a more acute and more dangerous episode of this disease will develop resembling acute leukaemia. This phase of the disease is more difficult to control. Sometimes other cytotoxic chemotherapy with cortisone might give control for a period. Studies are also being made to control this acute phase of the disease with intensive radiotherapy and bone marrow transplantation. Although a number of problems still need to be overcome, results have been encouraging especially in younger people.

The most exciting new addition to the treatment of CML is the tyrosine-kinase inhibitor STI 571 *(Glivec or Gleevec)* which is a newly discovered agent. STI 571 inhibits intracellular tyrosine kinase. Tyrosine kinase is targeted because it is a growth promoting enzyme involved in the cellular changes of CML.

Recent studies have shown a remarkable high response rate. STI 571 counteracts tyrosine kinase. Further studies are needed but responses to date appear to be dramatic. In a third of cases there is a complete cytogenic remission with apparent elimination of the Philadelphia chromosome. Studies are now being conducted on the possible potential of *tyrosine kinase inhibitors* being effective in treating other cancers.

The most exciting new addition to the treatment of CML is the tyrosine-kinase inhibitor STI 571 *(Glivec or Gleevec).*

19

Consider why recent results of treatment of CML has caused such intense interest in possible new treatments of other cancers.

. . . .
. . . .
. . . .
. . . .
. . . .

19.4.4   Hairy Cell Leukaemia

This uncommon form of chronic leukaemia is so named because of the unusual features of its cells, which appear to have fine hair-like projections from the surface. It is of special interest because it is a leukaemia that usually responds well to immunological treatment with interferon (see Sect. 8.4.2). Treatment with interferon and purine analogues *(2CdA and Pentostatin)*, has been very effective. Previous treatment by splenectomy as first-line treatment is no longer indicated.

CASE REPORT

Acute myeloid leukaemia

Brett is a 34-year-old swimming instructor at a private school. He had noticed that over the last few weeks his energy levels were not as good as usual and in the last week a few little "blood spots" had appeared on his lower legs round the ankles. He hadn't taken much notice of this until he had a bad nose-bleed which he could not stop, so he went to the Emergency Department of his local hospital clutching a handkerchief around his bleeding nose.

The Emergency doctor noticed that he was pale and that he had the blood spots about his ankles. After he had packed his nose the doctor ordered some blood tests.

Within an hour the laboratory had phoned to say that the blood test was very abnormal and that Brett was very anaemic with a haemoglobin level of 60 g/L, a low platelet count, and a very high white cell count.

(continued)

(continued)

It became clear that Brett had had a serious bleeding episode and that this was probably caused by the low platelet count. Brett was admitted to the hospital for a blood and platelet transfusion, and a specialist haematologist was consulted. The specialist advised Brett of the abnormal blood result and recommended a bone marrow biopsy. (The bone marrow acts like a factory for blood cell production.)

The bone marrow test confirmed a diagnosis of AML. This was based on the appearance of the leukaemic cells in the bone marrow but also on some special tests that determine the genetic make-up of the cells and what chemicals are present on their surface.

Naturally Brett was very upset to hear the diagnosis as was his wife and family of two young children. After the transfusions the bleeding stopped and Brett felt much better. The haematologist explained that he would require anti-leukaemia treatment with powerful cytotoxic drugs and that this would mean hospitalization for probably 4–6 weeks. While the leukaemia drugs are usually given for about 7 days the drugs are very powerful and cause the blood counts to become very low so that blood and platelet transfusions are very commonly needed during and after the treatment until the bone marrow and blood recovers. In addition intravenous antibiotics may be needed to protect against infection.

After storing some sperm samples in case his fertility was affected, Brett agreed to start treatment and appears to be doing well after the first 2 weeks. Although it is still early days, plans are underway to test his two brothers to see if they could donate stem cells for a stem cell transplant after the initial chemotherapy. This determination can be done by simple blood tests.

CASE REPORT

Chronic myeloid leukaemia

Richard is a 48-year-old publisher with an English publishing group. He has enjoyed good health except for a soccer related knee injury when he was 17.

He presented to his general practitioner with left upper quadrant abdominal pain and a feeling of early satiety after eating meals. He looked reasonably well but on examination his GP had found an enlarged spleen, 8 cm below the left costal margin. The spleen was not tender to palpation and the liver edge was not palpable.

(continued)

(continued)

His GP arranged for some routine blood tests and was telephoned later that day by the local pathologist to indicate that the white cell count was grossly elevated at 112×10^9/L. The haemoglobin level was slightly reduced at 127 g/L and the platelet count was slightly elevated at 521×10^9/L.

Richard was referred to a haematologist who, other than the spleno-megaly, found little else of note. Review of the blood film confirmed the grossly elevated white cell count, which showed a spectrum of myeloid cells, ranging from a few myeloblasts through promyelocytes, myelocytes, metamyelocytes and mature neutrophils.

A bone marrow examination was arranged and showed a hypercellular marrow with active proliferation of myeloid cells. A cytogenetic (chromo-some) analysis of these bone marrow cells revealed the presence of the Philadelphia chromosome in 100% of the cells examined, confirming the diagnosis of CML.

[The Philadelphia chromosome is a small chromosome derived by the reciprocal translocation of genetic material (DNA) between chromosomes 9 and 22 leading to the juxtaposition of DNA and the creation of a so-called new "fusion gene" that can lead to the production of new protein. In this particular case the new protein, which has tyrosine kinase activity, is called BCR-ABL protein because of its origins from the genetic material on chromosome 22 (bcr) and chromosome 9 (abl).]

In Richard's case, a sample of his blood and bone marrow cells were sent to a specialized laboratory to analyse the cells for the presence and quantification of the bcr-abl gene transcripts, by the polymerase chain reaction (PCR), to allow for future disease monitoring.

The nature of the disease was explained to Richard and he was com-menced on a new oral drug Imatinib, (400 mg/day), a specific tyrosine kinase inhibitor which has specificity for the *bcr-abl* gene transcripts. Imatinib is also known by its proprietary names Gleevec or Glivec.

Richard's blood counts quickly reverted to normal within 2 months, his spleen became impalpable and at 6 months from starting Imatinib, the Philadelphia chromosome had disappeared from his blood and marrow, although the bcr-abl gene transcripts could still be detected by PCR.

Comment

Although, at the time of writing, this drug, imatinib, has only been avail-able for treating CML for a few years there is good reason to believe that it will herald a new era in the treatment of this disease and it also has potential in treating other cancers, especially gastro-intestinal stromal cancers.

19.5 The Lymphomas

The lymphomas are a group of cancers of the body tissues that constitute the body defence system known as the reticuloendothelial (immune system). The majority of lymphomas arise from lymph nodes but they may arise from B and T cells in extra nodal sites such as in lymphoid tissue elsewhere for example the tonsils, spleen, stomach or bowel lining, liver, lung, kidneys or skin.

There are two main types of lymphoma called Hodgkin lymphoma (or Hodgkin disease, HD) and the so-called Non-Hodgkin lymphomas (NHL). NHLs are the more common. They tend to affect a rather older age group than Hodgkin lymphoma. Both types are more common in developed countries (see Appendix).

About 15% of cases of lymphoma are Hodgkin lymphoma, which predominantly originates in lymph nodes. NHLs are predominantly of the "B" cell type. "B" cells are especially concerned with humoral immunity i.e. the circulating immune system, including manufacture of immune antibodies.

The NHLs may also develop in lymph nodes but they develop almost as commonly in lymphoid tissue in other organs.

Lymphoma is predominantly a disease of adults and other than common skin cancers in the US it is the fifth most common cancer in men (after prostate, lung, colo-rectal, and bladder). In women other than skin cancers, it is also the fifth most common (after breast, lung, colo-rectal and uterus). The average age is about 32 years for Hodgkin lymphoma and somewhat older, about 42 years, for NHL.

The lymphomas are a group of cancers of the body tissues that constitute the body defence system known as the reticulo-endothelial (immune system).

19.5.1 Causes of Lymphoma

The causes of most lymphomas are not known. Viruses are known to cause lymphomas in some animals but, with one exception, have not been found to be a significant factor in lymphoma in humans. A lymphoma called *Burkitt's lymphoma* which is uncommon in most countries but is more common in children in tropical Africa and New Guinea, has been found to be associated with infection by the *Epstein-Barr* virus. This same virus causes glandular fever and in Western societies people who have had glandular fever have a slightly increased risk of developing a lymphoma later in life. On the other hand, doctors and nurses who specialise in caring for people with lymphoma have not been found to have any increased risk of developing the disease.

It is well recognised that people with a deficiency of their immune systems, do have an increased risk of developing a lymphoma. This is especially seen in AIDS patients but also in people who have had an organ transplant and are given drugs to suppress the rejection of the transplanted organ. In Western countries between 3 and 4% of patients with AIDS develop lymphomas. This represents more than

100 times the incidence in the general population. It is uncertain whether this is a direct effect of the HIV virus or a general deregulation of the immune system.

There is also a slightly increased tendency to develop lymphomas in some families but this may be due to an hereditary tendency towards immune deficiency in these families or possibly there is an, as yet unknown, environmental factor.

19.6   Hodgkin Lymphoma

19.6.1   Presentation

Hodgkin lymphoma is more common in upper socio-economic groups and especially in males (about 2:1 ratio males/females). The most common presentation, especially in young people, is of enlarged lymph nodes usually in one side of the neck. The nodes are rubbery and movable and usually feel distinctly different to the hard, enlarged nodes that may result from metastatic spread from other cancers.

Sometimes, other symptoms are a general feeling of ill health, lassitude, fever, weight loss and/or night sweats. An unusual feature sometimes complained of, is pain in swollen lymph nodes after drinking alcohol.

The disease usually progresses from the site of origin (most commonly the lymph nodes in the neck) to other lymph nodes nearby – then to lymph nodes in the chest or abdomen – to the spleen – and eventually to the liver and bone narrow. The earlier the disease is detected before it has spread widely, the greater the likelihood of cure by modern treatment (Fig. 19.1).

19.6.2   Investigations

In order to decide what is the best treatment it is important to find out as accurately as possible exactly which lymph nodes and organs are involved. A thorough examination of the patient is needed including all lymph node areas, spleen, liver and chest. X-rays are taken of the lungs, especially, to look for enlarged lymph nodes between the lungs (mediastintal lymph nodes).

To establish a diagnosis the most obvious and easily removed lymph node is removed surgically and to have it examined microscopically. In fact any lymph node of diameter greater than 1 or 1.5 cm that remains enlarged for more than about a month without an obvious cause, may need to be removed and examined in case it is an early indication of a serious disease like Hodgkin disease. The pathology microscopic hallmark of Hodgkin disease is a large multinucleated cell, called the *Dorothy Reed-Sternberg* cell.

If a positive diagnosis of Hodgkin disease is established, a number of other tests should be done, including a blood count, because anaemia may develop.

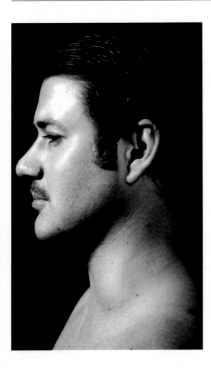

Fig. 19.1. Photograph of a 20-year-old man with enlarged rubbery lymph nodes in his neck. This was his first evidence of a Hodgkin lymphoma

Other features of Hodgkin disease may also be found in immuno-histochemical studies. CT scans and ultrasound help in discovering if there are any enlarged abdominal lymph nodes as well as any enlargement of the liver or spleen. Gallium isotope scans (see Sect. 7.3.8) may now be used to show abnormal or enlarged lymph nodes.

A liver biopsy and bone narrow biopsy may indicate spread of the disease to these tissues. Likewise, studies of kidney function or a kidney biopsy may indicate involvement of the kidneys.

19.6.3 Staging and the Staging Laparotomy

Some patients who had Hodgkin lymphoma a few years ago (then called Hodgkin disease) will remember that an operation was done by a surgeon to find out what organs and tissues in the abdomen were involved. This operation is rarely needed nowadays because of the accuracy of CT scans, ultrasound, isotope scans, gallium scans and by lymphoscintigram studies. These may even be replaced one day by PET scans which have shown promising results in studies but are very expensive and are not available in most places. In any case, it is still uncertain whether PET scans will add anything to the combined information from the other tests.

19.6.4   Treatment

Treatment of Hodgkin lymphoma is either by radiotherapy or chemotherapy or both. In experienced hands well-delivered treatment can now improve greatly the outlook for this once lethal illness. It is now possible to cure most patients, especially those who do not have extensive disease.

In general, limited areas of disease are best treated by radiotherapy (a modern linear accelerator is the most appropriate equipment) but the exact doses, techniques of delivery and fields of irradiation must be expertly arranged.

For widespread disease (in which tissue other than lymph nodes and spleen are involved), treatment is usually with chemotherapy, using appropriate combinations of cytotoxic drugs. Present-day lymphoma specialists are now able to achieve very good results and keep toxic side effects (see Sect. 8.3.4) to a minimum. For advanced cases chemotherapy and radiotherapy may both be required in an integrated treatment program.

CASE REPORT

Hodgkin lymphoma

Julie is a 22-year-old law student coming up to her final exams. She was under a lot of stress and studying hard. She was often up late at night and was also having difficulty sleeping. Like a lot of girls in this situation she was probably not eating regular meals and noticed that she was losing weight. She had woken up a couple of times in the last week with bad sweats and on the last occasion she had been drenched with sweat, so much so that she had to change her pyjamas. She also noticed a swelling in the area above her left clavicle although there had been no pain, but she was persuaded by her flatmate to go to her local family doctor.

The doctor saw Julie and confirmed that there was a swelling above her left clavicle but could not find any other abnormal findings. She arranged for some blood tests and a chest X-ray. When the results came back she arranged for Julie to attend for follow up consultation.

The blood tests showed that Julie was mildly anaemic with a haemoglobin level of 98 g/L, and her kidneys and liver function tests were normal. Her chest X-ray showed a mass of lymph nodes between her lungs. After discussing the results, Julie was referred to a surgeon who arranged a biopsy of the mass above the clavicle. Within 2 days the result confirmed that the biopsy had shown Hodgkin lymphoma.

(continued)

(continued)

The surgeon explained that this was a type of cancer of the lymph nodes and referred Julie to a specialist as, with appropriate treatment, this type of cancer can often be cured. Julie saw a specialist within a few days. The specialist explained that it was important to "stage" the disease, i.e. find out where else the disease might be. Julie had a CT scan (to assess if there were any other enlarged lymph nodes or other organs), a PET scan to assess if there were any areas of increased metabolic activity and a bone marrow biopsy to see if the disease had spread to the bone marrow. After these tests, Julie was said to have Stage IIB Hodgkin lymphoma. This meant that she had disease in two sites (the neck and chest) (II), and she had night sweats (B symptoms).

Julie has now started a course of cytotoxic chemotherapy called ABVD, (after the initials of the drugs used). She has treatment every 2 weeks at the hospital's out-patient cytotoxic unit, and after two courses she noticed that her sweats had disappeared. She has deferred her final exams until after her chemotherapy is finished and spoke to a gynaecologist about her fertility before starting treatment. At Julie's age and with this type of chemotherapy the gynaecologist felt that there was a good chance that her fertility should be retained.

Comment

Julie has a very good chance that her disease will be eradicated by the treatment but will require further blood tests and scans to be sure.

19.7   Non-Hodgkin Lymphomas

NHL is not just one disease. It is a range of diseases of the reticuloendothelial system grouped together and called the NHLs. The particular type of lymphoma depends upon the predominant type of malignant cell in the tissue in which it arose. One uncommon form of NHL is a "T" (tissue) cell lymphoma that predominantly involves skin. It is called *mycosis fungoides* (Fig. 19.2).

NHL is not just one disease. It is a range of diseases of the reticuloendothelial system.

19.7.1   Presentation

Like Hodgkin lymphoma, this group of diseases begins in reticulo-endothelial tissues (the "immune" body defence system) and may first be noticed in lymph nodes. However, the first indication of NHLs may be enlargements of the spleen, tonsils or lymph nodes, or lumps in other organs such as stomach,

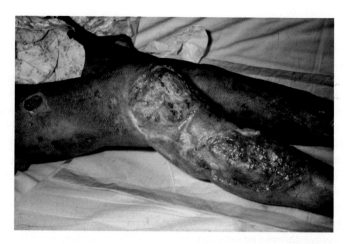

Fig. 19.2. Photograph showing advanced mycosis fungoides (a rare form of lymphoma that predominantly develops in skin). This patient was a 63-year-old woman

bowel, lung, bone or skin. NHL is more common than Hodgkin lymphoma in older age groups. The gender ratio is about 2:1 males/females. The incidence increased over the last two decades of the twentieth century and is still increasing. About 3–4% of Aids patients will develop NHL. Treatment is somewhat controversial and complex. It depends on the tissues involved and the stage of the disease. For early disease, radiotherapy is used while for more advanced disease, chemotherapy using an alkylating agent. High-dose chemotherapy with rescue may be indicated for very advanced disease.

The purine analogues (as mentioned early under treatments for chronic lymphocytic anaemia, CLL) and monoclonal antibody therapy (Rituxan and Campath 1H) have become important in treating some lymphomas (Fig. 19.2).

19.7.2   Investigations

Diagnosis is usually made by surgical removal of an enlarged lymph node or biopsy of a lump in another tissue with microscopic examination and also by immuno-histochemical features in blood, especially LDH (lactodehydrogenase).

The disease tends to involve a number of tissues other than lymph nodes and the best form of treatment will depend upon the predominant type of malignant cell rather than the organs or tissues involved. However, similar investigations as for Hodgkin disease are usually required including full blood count, chest X-ray, CT scan, bone marrow biopsies and liver biopsy. PET scans may be of additional diagnostic help when these become more readily available. Surgery to determine the stage of the cancer is now rarely needed.

19.7.3 Treatment

Just as for Hodgkin lymphoma, treatment of the NHLs is by radiotherapy, chemotherapy or both. However, depending on the type of lymphoma, different plans of radiotherapy or different programs of chemotherapy are used. With this information lymphoma therapy teams can arrange the most appropriate treatment plan.

In general, radiotherapy is best used for localised disease. Because NHL are likely to involve more than one site treatment by general body chemotherapy (systemic chemotherapy) is usually required. Sometimes, in some types of lymphoma, the use of a single anti-cancer cytotoxic agent will achieve good results but, in general, best results are achieved when a combination of two or more cytotoxic drugs is used.

Over recent years, results of treatment of most NHLs have improved significantly with modern treatment regimens. This is especially so in some specific types of lymphoma. For some patients, especially younger ones, very high dose toxic treatment followed by a bone marrow transplant may be used for advanced disease. Results to date have been encouraging especially in young people.

CASE REPORT

Non-Hodgkin lymphoma

Arthur is a 67-year-old farmer who was still working on his farm but for a few weeks he had noticed that his energy had not been as good as usual. He had lost his appetite and he had noticed his clothing, particularly his trousers, had become a bit looser than normal. One day while taking a shower he noticed a swelling in his left groin. The swelling was not painful and he wondered if it was a hernia. He mentioned this to his wife who suggested he get things checked by the local doctor.

Next day the doctor confirmed that Arthur had a swelling in his groin but it was firm and was not reducible and did not feel like a hernia. There was also a vague sensation of a mass in the abdomen. His doctor referred him to a surgeon at the local hospital who agreed that the mass in the groin was worrying and recommended a biopsy to see what the problem was. Within a week Arthur was in the Day-surgery area having a biopsy and it showed that the mass was a collection of enlarged lymph nodes affected by NHL.

(continued)

19

(continued)

The surgeon explained that this is a type of cancer of the lymph nodes and that in broad terms these types of cancer can be divided into two main types depending on microscopic findings. The more common type is called NHL and the less common type is Hodgkin lymphoma. It is important to differentiate, as the treatments for the two diseases are different.

Even within these two broad categories there are many different sub-types which the pathologist can identify and aid treatment strategies.

In Arthur's case the diagnosis was diffuse large cell lymphoma, which is one of the common types of NHL. Arthur was seen by a specialist who arranged some blood tests and staging procedures (CT scan, PET Scan, Bone marrow biopsy) to identify where else the disease was present. In addition, as Arthur had been on treatment for blood pressure, a gated heart pool scan was arranged to ensure his heart would tolerate treatment. The scans showed that Arthur did indeed have a mass of lymph nodes in his abdomen (about 4×3 cm in diameter) and an enlarged lymph node (2 cm) in his left axilla. Arthur was thus classified as Stage III (having lymph nodes enlarged above and below the diaphragm). The bone marrow test was clear.

After these tests were completed, Arthur was started on a program of intravenous chemotherapy called R-CHOP (after the initials of the drugs used). This contains a new product (R) called a monoclonal antibody (Rituximab) in addition to standard chemotherapeutic agents and has been shown to be of benefit in patients with diffuse large-cell lymphoma. The monoclonal antibody directs the chemotherapy directly to the target tumour cells. This treatment is given as an outpatient every 3 weeks.

Comment

In Arthur's case the specialist indicated that the treatment had a reasonable chance of success and that the aim of treatment was to eradicate the disease. If this could be done the chances of being alive in 5 years was about 30–40%.

A major improvement in treatment outcome has been the development of a genetically engineered antibody directed against the lymphoma cells. This is produced using biotechnology industrial processes using mouse cells to produce a humanized antibody. The antibody is named *Mabthera (Ritiximab)* and is used in combination with chemotherapy. The results of treatment for some of the early stage lymphomas can be excellent with a high cure rate, particularly for the so-called diffuse large B cell lymphomas.

19.8 Multiple Myeloma

This tumour occurs in bone but is not truly a tumour of bone. It is in fact a malignant tumour of plasma cells in bone (plasmocytoma). Plasma cells are cells responsible for making antibodies or immunoglobulin molecules, they are a type of blood forming cell in bone. Plasmocytoma shows in X-rays as a "hole" or "holes" in one or more bones. Usually there are many lesions in a number of bones although occasionally a single "hole" only is present. A single lesion is called a solitary plasmocytoma.

Multiple myeloma most often affects adults over 40 or 50 years and is more common in "developed" countries. It causes local pain and swelling and sometimes fractures in affected bones. Back pain is sometimes associated with collapse of a vertebral body.

19.8.1 Investigations

X-rays may show typical "punched out" areas in bones. A blood count is taken because patients usually have anaemia. Other changes in the blood proteins may confirm the diagnosis. The lesions and pain are often in vertebrae or near the ends of long bones so that pain is often felt in the back or limbs. There may be hypercalcaemia and kidney failure and sometimes, unexplained fevers or infections.

The urine is also examined for a particular type of protein (Bence-Jones protein) which, if present, is diagnostic for multiple myeloma.

19.8.2 Treatment

Because this tumour is usually widespread, it cannot be eradicated by surgery. Treatment by chemotherapy with local radiotherapy of painful lumps offers the best relief of symptoms and sometimes long-term control. As yet there is no known cure but interferon has been found to increase duration of chemotherapy and has induced remissions and *thalidomide* (and especially the thalidomide analogue *lenalomide*) has demonstrated efficacy, probably because of its *anti-angiogenic* effects. (That is it prevents the tumour developing new capillaries on which all tumours depend for nourishment and further growth.) Treatment of anaemia may require blood transfusion. Bisphosphonates are used to reduce pain and help stabilise diseased areas of bone.

Autologous stem cell transplantation using blood-derived stem cells has been shown to be beneficial in patients fit enough to undergo the procedure. Combinations of *lenalomide* with high dose chemotherapy and stem cell transplantation is now regarded as most appropriate treatment for most patients, especially for patients under 65 years.

Soft-Tissue Sarcomas

20

In this chapter you will learn about:

> *Fibrosarcoma*

> *Liposarcoma*

> *Rhabdomyosarcoma*

> *Leiomyosarcoma*

> *Neurosarcoma*

> *Malignant fibrous histiosarcoma (MFH)*

> *Angiosarcoma*

> *Synovial sarcoma (synoviosarcoma or malignant synovioma)*

A sarcoma is a cancer of connective tissue such as muscle, bone, cartilage, fat, nerves, fascia, tendons, and blood and lymph vessels. Hence sarcomas can develop in any part of the body although they are not as common as carcinomas that develop from epithelial tissues such as skin and other lining cells and glands. This is probably because there is not such a constant turnover of cells in connective tissues as in epithelial tissues.

Sarcomas are classified into two groups, soft-tissue sarcomas and hard sarcomas of bone or cartilage (osteosarcomas and chondrosarcomas). There are no known causes.

The soft tissues are those connective tissues that surround the bones of the body and include muscles, fat, fascia, nerves, tendons, blood vessels and lymphatic vessels. The majority of soft-tissue tumours are not malignant – it is only when they are malignant that the term sarcoma applies. Thus most tumours of fatty tissue are lipomas – it is only when one of these is malignant that it is called a liposarcoma. Similarly, most tumours of fibrous tissue are benign and are called fibromas, and most tumours of nerves are benign and are called neuromas. Most tumours of blood or lymph vessels are benign and are called angiomas, either haemangiomas composed of primitive blood vessels, or lymphangiomas composed of primitive lymphatic vessels (Fig. 20.1).

Soft-tissue sarcomas are classified according to the type of tissue from which they arise and the type of tissue they most resemble.

F. O. Stephens and K. R. Aigner, *Basics of Oncology,*
DOI: 10.1007/978-3-540-92925-3_20, © Springer-Verlag Berlin Heidelberg 2009

20

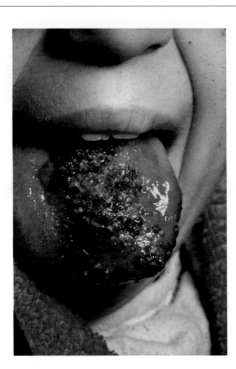

Fig. 20.1. Photograph of a large benign haemangioma of tongue in a young woman

The following is a list of tissues from which soft-tissue sarcomas develop:

Fibrous tissue – fibrosarcoma
Fatty tissue – liposarcoma
Nerve tissue – neurosarcoma
Histiocytes (protective cells – malignant fibrous histiocytoma (MFH)
Synovial membrane lining a joint or tendon sheath – synovial sarcoma (synovioma)
Blood vessels – haemangiosarcoma
Lymphatic vessels – lymphangiosarcoma
Muscle – myosarcoma

Myosarcomas may be further classified as rhabdomyosarcoma and leiomyosarcoma. A rhabdomyosarcoma is a malignant tumour of a voluntary muscle (that is, one of the muscles of the body over which we have control in moving arms, legs, abdomen, back, head and neck or the muscles used in breathing). A leiomyosarcoma is a malignant tumour of involuntary muscle, that is, one of the muscles over which we have no conscious control such as the muscle in the wall of the stomach or bowel, or the muscles in the wall of the uterus or the wall of large blood vessels.

Soft-tissue sarcomas make up only about 2% of malignant tumours. They can occur in people of all ages from birth to old age and are relatively more common in children and young adults than are most carcinomas. Unless radically excised sarcomas have a tendency to recur locally. Whilst most cancers tend to metastasise via the lymph vessels, to lymph nodes first, most sarcomas have a greater tendency to metastasise via blood vessels to lungs rather than to lymph nodes.

20.1 Classification: Pathological Types

20.1.1 Fibrosarcoma

These tumours develop in fascia or fibrous tissue that covers and surrounds muscles, nerves and other tissues and is distributed widely throughout the body. Thus a fibrosarcoma may develop almost anywhere in the body especially in a limb or in the tissues of the trunk. One very fibrous and slowly growing type of fibrosarcoma, called a *desmoid tumour*, has a tendency to grow into nearby tissues and to recur locally after surgical excision but rarely metastasises to other organs. Other more cellular and less fibrous types have a greater tendency to metastasise.

20.1.2 Liposarcoma

These tumours develop from fatty tissue and may arise in any tissue or organ where fat is present. They tend to vary from a low-grade malignancy likely to recur locally after excision but unlikely to metastasise, to a high-grade malignancy in which both local recurrence and metastatic spread to lungs is common. As a rule the deeper they are (sometimes they are deep in muscle tissue) and the larger they have become, the more likely they are to be a higher grade of malignancy (Fig. 20.2).

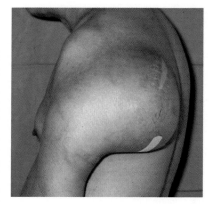

Fig. 20.2. A large liposarcoma of shoulder region in a 73-year-old man

20.1.3   Rhabdomyosarcoma

This tumour presents most commonly in infants and young children as a swelling in voluntary muscle, especially in muscles of the head and neck, genitourinary tract, thorax and limbs. It is the sarcoma most likely to metastasise to lymph nodes although it does metastasise to lungs (Fig. 20.3).

20.1.4   Leiomyosarcoma

This tumour may occur at any site where there is smooth muscle, including the wall of the stomach or bowel or the uterus or the wall of large blood vessels.

20.1.5   Neurosarcoma

This tumour may develop on any nerve. Sometimes it is purely a tumour of nerve cells, and sometimes it is a mixture of fibrous tissue and nerve tissue and it may then be called a neurofibrosarcoma.

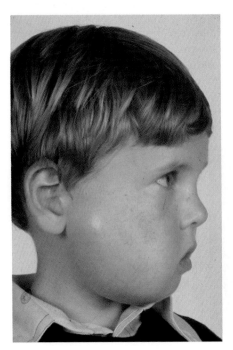

Fig. 20.3. The swelling in the jaw in this 4-year-old boy proved to be a rhabdomyosarcoma

20.1.6 Malignant Fibrous Histiocytoma (MFH)

These tumours most commonly develop in muscles, fascia or fatty tissues in limbs. They are firm rounded tumours rather like liposarcomas or fibrosarcomas. If deep in muscle, they may become quite large before they are noticed as they cause few if any symptoms until a lump is felt (Fig. 20.4).

20.1.7 Angiosarcoma

These tumours may develop from endothelial cells of blood vessels or lymph vessels. They develop as enlarging vascular masses (clumps containing partly formed blood vessels). They are softish tumours and may contain either blood or lymphatic fluid and thus may be called haemangiosarcoma or lymphangiosarcoma.

Angiosarcoma is a poor prognosis neoplasm because of the high propensity of blood-born metastases.

20.1.8 Synovial Sarcoma (Synoviosarcoma or Malignant Synovioma)

This tumour of synovial membrane is often a highly aggressive malignant tumour and occurs most commonly in limbs near joints or in association with the sheaths around tendons.

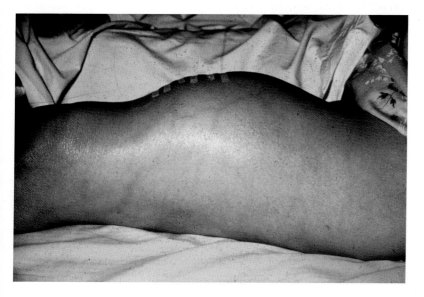

Fig. 20.4. A large malignant fibrous histiocytoma caused this swelling in the thigh of a 77-year-old woman

20

20.1.9   Presentation

Sarcomas
occasionally
develop from
previously
benign
tumours of a
similar type.
More often,
however,
these tumours
arise as a local
swelling from
no apparent
pre-existing
abnormality.

Sarcomas occasionally develop from previously benign tumours of a similar type. For example, a previously benign lipoma may begin to enlarge, showing evidence of malignant change to become a liposarcoma. More often, however, these tumours arise as a local swelling from no apparent pre-existing abnormality. Usually, though not always, the lump is painless. Occasionally the swelling develops at a site of recent injury and the possibility of a sarcoma developing as a result of injury cannot altogether be dismissed. It is more likely, however, that in most cases the injury drew attention to a lump that was already present.

Rarely the first evidence of a soft-tissue sarcoma is found on a chest X-ray showing lung metastases.

20.1.10   Investigations

Like all health problems the first requirement is to take a history of the presentation of the problem from the patient's point of view. In the case of a sarcoma it will usually include a history of the lump and how and when it was first noticed; the presence, or absence of pain or other possible associated symptoms and if, when and how rapidly it started to enlarge or otherwise change; then the general health of the patient and any relevant previous or family history. The lump is measured, the local draining lymph nodes and other lymph nodes are examined and a chest X-ray and full blood count are performed. CT scans or MRI scans, ultrasound and angiography (as discussed in Chap. 7) may also give more information about the tumour (Fig. 20.5). MRI scans are now used preferentially in most centres. Microscopic examination of a biopsy specimen of the lump will establish the diagnosis.

More recently,
induction, or
neo-adjuvant,
chemo-therapy
has been
used before
operation to
reduce the
size, extent
and viability
of large or
aggressive
primary
sarcomas
before surgery.

Whether further information of value can be learned from PET scans is presently being investigated.

20.1.11   Treatment

The standard treatment of soft-tissue sarcomas is excision at a surgical operation. Because the risk of local recurrence of sarcoma is high, the surgeon must remove a great deal of apparently normal tissue around the tumour to be as sure possible that all of the malignant cells have been removed. For large sarcomas in a limb, sometimes amputation of the limb may offer the best chance of surgical cure. Because of the high risk of local recurrence amputation was the preferred choice of treatment for most large sarcomas in limbs and even moderate sized sarcomas, until the mid or late 1970s until it became appreciated that whilst these tumours are usually not particularly sensitive to radiotherapy, sometimes radiotherapy before or after local surgery could achieve better results than surgery alone.

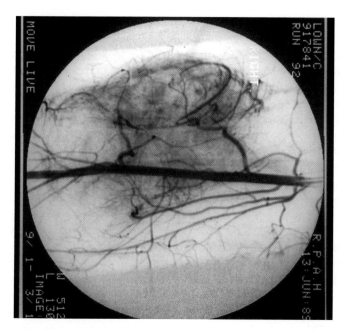

Fig. 20.5. Angiogram showing vascularity of a large synoviosarcoma in the popliteal fossa of a 43-year-old woman

Many of these tumours respond to cytotoxic chemotherapy. Early medical experience with chemotherapy to treat metastatic sarcoma, especially in the lungs, achieved some regression, with improved length of survival for some patients, but dramatic improvement in results was rare. More recently, induction, (or neoadjuvant), chemotherapy has been used before operation to reduce the size, extent and viability of large or aggressive primary sarcomas before surgery. This chemotherapy (see Sect. 8.3.4.9), will be more concentrated if given by regional infusion into a supplying artery and good results have been reported when this procedure is followed by surgery.

Another form of combined therapy proving to be effective in many cases is concomitant chemotherapy and radiotherapy. In experienced hands this is proving very effective in treating a number of locally advanced cancers, however it is potentially considerably more toxic to local tissues than serial use (i.e regional chemotherapy followed by surgery).

Combined treatments with chemotherapy and surgery with or without radio-therapy have often avoided the need for amputation and should now be considered by experts experienced in these techniques before a decision to amputate is made. Liposarcomas and malignant fibrous histiocytomas are the most common of the soft-tissue sarcomas and even when very large they usually respond well to chemotherapy, especially when given directly to the tumour site by regional infusion before surgery. This will often reduce them to smaller, less aggressive and locally resectable tumours, making follow-up surgical resection possible and successful in most cases without the need for amputation.

Another effective technique being studied in treatment of large or aggressive sarcomas in limbs is by closed circuit infusion with chemotherapy and TNF (tumour necrosis factor) (Sect. 8.4.2.4). Good results that avoid amputation have also been reported.

With some sarcomas, the risk of metastatic spread to lungs is considerable and there may be virtue in also giving a post-operative course of systemic adjuvant chemotherapy (Sect. 8.3.4.5) to reduce this risk. Studies are being carried out to determine whether routine use of adjuvant treatment is worthwhile for patients with aggressive sarcoma.

Sometimes after successful treatment of a soft-tissue sarcoma one solitary metastatic deposit will be seen in a follow-up chest X-ray. This may have the appearance of a small round "cannon-ball" and is referred to as a "cannon ball metastasis". Occasionally such a lesion can be resected and if it truly is a solitary metastasis the patient may be cured.

Angiosarcoma being of and in blood or lymph vessels metastasises early and although surgery, radiotherapy and chemotherapy are the mainstays of treatment, because of the poor outlook, biotherapy treatments are now being closely investigated.

CASE REPORT

Rhabdomyosarcoma

John is a 3-year-old Turkish boy whose mother took him to their family doctor after noticing a swelling of the muscles in the posterior aspect of his left leg. The family doctor found a firm, non-tender, slightly mobile, mass, that was attached to the muscles below and behind the left knee. Physical examination was otherwise unremarkable, and plain X-ray of the lower legs detected no abnormality. An MRI scan of the legs detected a localised lesion in the left soleus muscle measuring 5.6 cm (superior to inferior) by 2 cm (anterior to posterior) by 4 cm (left to right). The mass had a slightly increased density compared to muscle. Multiple septations (lobules) were identified within the mass. No fat-like component or haemorrhage was identified. The appearances were reported as being suggestive of a sarcoma or fibrosarcoma in the left soleus muscle. John was admitted urgently to the Children's Hospital. A biopsy of the lesion performed under general anaesthesia revealed rhabdomyosarcoma

(continued)

(continued)

(of the aggressive alveolar type). Staging investigations, including a CT scan of chest, abdomen and pelvis, bone scan, gallium scan, bone marrow aspirate, and PET scan, detected no distant metastases. However a discrete PET-enhancing scan suggested a lesion in the left popliteal fossa, remote to and above the primary tumour, consistent with an infiltrated regional lymph node. A central venous catheter was inserted under the same anaesthetic for the biopsy. Cardiac, liver function, and glomerular filtration tests were all normal.

John commenced intensive systemic chemotherapy (using a combination of vincristine, actinomycin-D, doxorubicin, and cyclophosphamide, given in pulses every 3–4 weeks for three courses. G-CSF, a bone-marrow cell stimulating factor, was administered subcutaneously daily between courses to hasten bone marrow recovery. Each chemotherapy course caused severe mucositis, severe bone marrow depression, fever and presumed sepsis requiring broad-spectrum IV antibiotics, and anaemia and thrombocytopenia, requiring transfusion support. John remained hospitalised for the first 2 months of therapy to receive either planned chemotherapy or supportive care while recovering.

Progress MRI and PET scans performed 2 months after the initial scans revealed some reduction in size of the primary tumour, and persistence of the regional abnormal lymph node.

John is currently recovering from the third course of chemotherapy and is under consideration for a surgical procedure, which would remove the muscles from the rear compartment of his left leg along with the regional lymph node. This is considered an effective method of gaining control of the visible component of the disease, with an acceptable level of consequent orthopaedic disability. The alternative is radiation therapy to the left lower leg, which would cause sufficiently severe long-term effects to require probable late amputation of the lower leg. Adjuvant chemotherapy is to be continued following a stem-cell harvest, collected to permit a high dose marrow-ablating chemotherapy treatment with stem-cell rescue to be given to complete planned chemotherapy around 9 months from diagnosis.

Comment

Sadly this boy has a poor prognosis despite the intensity of treatment given. The alveolar subtype of histology documented in the primary tumour and the detectable regional node involvement at the time of diagnosis are poor prognosis features.

EXERCISE

Drawing on case reports in this chapter and other chapters of this book,
construct a case report of a typical adult patient presenting with and being
investigated and managed for a very big (10-cm diameter) sarcoma of thigh
that proved to be a liposarcoma. What alternative plans of management
might be considered?

Malignant Tumours of Bone and Cartilage

21

In this chapter you will learn about:

> *Osteosarcoma*
> *Osteoclastoma (central giant cell tumour of bone)*
> *Ewing's tumour*
> *Chondrosarcoma*

21.1   Osteosarcoma

A malignant tumour of bone-forming cells is called an osteosarcoma. This is a highly malignant cancer and tends to affect children and young adults, with the highest incidence between 10 and 25 years. The cause of osteosarcoma in young people is not known although it does occur most often in the growing parts of bone near the bone ends while the patient is still growing and developing.

A rare and virtually incurable osteosarcoma sometimes develops in old people but in these people the sarcoma has almost always occurred in a bone with a long-standing bone disease called *osteitis deformans or Paget's disease of bone.*

21.1.1   Presentation

Osteosarcoma in young people usually first develops as a painful lump near the end of a long bone. There may be an obvious swelling occasionally with overlying redness and sometimes a fever. The swelling may be tender and may at first look like an acute infection in bone. This sarcoma tends to metastasise to lungs early in its course so that best results are achieved if it is diagnosed and treated very early.

Osteosarcoma in young people usually first develops as a painful lump near the end of a long bone.

F. O. Stephens and K. R. Aigner, *Basics of Oncology,*
DOI: 10.1007/978-3-540-92925-3_21, © Springer-Verlag Berlin Heidelberg 2009

21.1.2 Investigations

Bone X-rays showing a diseased area with "sunray" appearance is typical of osteosarcoma. There is evidence of bone destruction and irregular new bone formation in the same area of bone. More precise information can be learned from CT studies or MRI studies. PET scans if available may give even more information about the tumour. However, the ultimate deciding test is a biopsy in which a small piece of the tumour is taken for microscopic examination. Chest X-rays will also be taken to look for evidence of spread to the lungs although there is commonly micro-metastatic spread to the lungs before becoming visible in chest X-rays.

21.1.3 Treatment

In the pre-chemotherapy days, osteosarcoma could rarely be cured. Treatment was by early amputation of an affected limb, sometimes in combination with radio-therapy, but death usually resulted due to development of lung metastases.

The outlook has been greatly improved with modern chemotherapy given before and after surgery (Sect. 8.3.4.8).

The outlook has been greatly improved with modern chemotherapy given before and after surgery. At first, amputation was commonly used to eradicate the primary sarcoma and the chemotherapy was used to eradicate any small microscopic metastases in the lungs before they could grow into larger incurable metastases. From almost no cures previously the cure rate was improved to about 50% but in virtually all cured patients a limb was amputated.

The use of chemotherapy has now been taken even further. Rather than amputation of the limb induction chemotherapy is given first. The chemotherapy will affect the primary sarcoma in the bone making it smaller and less aggressive. At the same time the circulating chemotherapy helps eradicate any micro-metastatic deposits of sarcoma in lungs or elsewhere. In some specialised treatment centres the primary cancer can be exposed to an even greater concentration of chemo-therapy if given by intra-arterial infusion. Having passed through the limb, the chemotherapy then flows into the general circulation as systemic chemotherapy and affects micro-metastatic deposits in lung or elsewhere. Although attractive as a potentially more effective method of exposing the primary cancer to more con-centrated chemotherapy, the technique requires close nursing attention and expert management and as yet studies have not been carried out to determine whether the advantage gained justifies the more complex and more expensive technique.

Reports of cures without amputation in 80% of cases in which intra-arterial chemotherapy was given first as induction treatment have now been matched by reports of equally successful results with treatment by *intense high-dose chemotherapy* given systemically pre-operatively. In both cases post-operative systemic "adjuvant" chemotherapy is given to deal with any residual cancer cells wherever they might be, most likely in the lungs.

After reduction of the size and aggressiveness of the primary tumour, either by systemic or regional chemotherapy, the section of bone containing the residual primary sarcoma must be excised and replaced by a metal or plastic prosthesis to reconstruct the bone. An experienced orthopaedic surgeon is needed to carry out this operation. If there is any remaining doubt about any malignant cells still being present, radiotherapy might also be given after the surgery (Fig. 21.1).

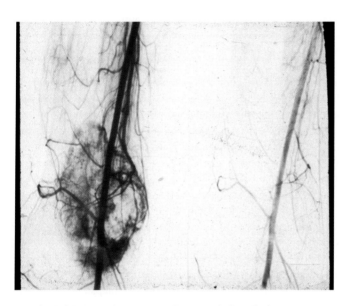

Fig. 21.1. On the *left* is an angiogram showing vascularity of a large osteosarcoma of lower femur of a 22-year-old man. On the *right* is a repeat angiogram of the same leg showing the response to chemotherapy. In this case the pre-operative "induction" chemotherapy was give by infusion into the femoral artery. The lower femur still with residual but much reduced sarcoma was then resected and the bone reconstructed with a metal prosthesis. The patient was then given adjuvant chemotherapy by intravenous infusions at monthly intervals for 6 months. When last seen 8 years later he was well and walking well with no evidence of residual sarcoma

EXERCISE

What investigations are helpful in diagnosing the presence, size, blood supply and extent of sarcomas?

. . . .

. . . .

. . . .

. . . .

. . . .

21

Osteosarcoma

Mohammed was a 12-year-old boy who had complained of pain in the right knee region. The pain had been first noticed 5 weeks previously and had been gradually increasing, causing him to limp. For 2 weeks his mother noticed swelling just below the knee. The swelling had been slowly increasing. His mother also said that Mohammed had appeared feverish.

His family doctor arranged X-rays of his knee. The X-rays showed an area of mixed destruction and increased calcification in the upper end of the tibia with slightly raised periosteum. There were small spicules of bone protruding at right angles from the lesion in the bone.

Mohammed was referred to an orthopaedic specialist who arranged an MRI scan of the knee and a chest X-ray.

No abnormality was seen in the chest X-rays but the presence of a destructive lesion consistent with osteosarcoma was confirmed in the MRI.

A core biopsy of the lesion, CT scans of lungs and radio-isotope bone scans were arranged. The biopsy confirmed the presence of osteosarcoma. No lesion was seen in the lung CTs and other than the lesion in the upper tibia no other bone lesion was detected.

Mohammed was treated with three cycles of chemotherapy (cisplatin and adriamycin were used by systemic infusion).

The pain and swelling decreased and after completion of chemotherapy the lesion had regressed significantly but blood counts showed reduced white cells requiring antibiotic cover.

Four weeks later when the blood count had returned to normal the lower femur and upper tibia were excised and a joint prosthesis inserted.

Histopathology confirmed almost total destruction of the sarcoma.

Four cycles of post operative adjuvant chemotherapy was administered using the same chemotherapeutic agents.

Five years later Mohammed remains well with no evidence of disease.

21.1.4   Intra-Operative Irradiation

A recent study in treatment of osteosarcoma is for the surgeon to excise the section of bone containing the tumour, and have that section heavily irradiated (with a certain tumouricidal irradiation dose) and re-implanted into its original site. The irradiated bone forms as a strut around which new tumour-free bone develops so acting as a graft. Encouraging results are being reported.

Consider why amputation of a limb for advanced soft tissue sarcoma
or osteosarcoma is now a relatively rare event.

21.2   Osteoclastoma (Central Giant Cell Tumour of Bone)

This tumour occurs most commonly in the ends of long bones of middle-aged
adults, most often around the knee joint. It is a tumour of low-grade malignancy
in that it does not often metastasise to other organs or tissues but does tend to
develop locally, and commonly recurs locally after attempts at removal. Sometimes recurrent osteoclastomas develop malignant changes.

21.2.1   Presentation

The first evidence of this tumour is usually swelling near a joint, such as the
knee joint, often with pain. It may be first noticed due to a fracture of the
weakened bone.

21.2.2   Investigations

X-rays, CT or MRI will usually show a typical cystic appearance of this tumour.
A pathologist will establish the diagnosis after microscopic examination of a
biopsy specimen.

21.2.3   Treatment

If possible, the tumour is removed surgically. If inadequately removed, radiotherapy may be given post-operatively.

  Recurrent osteoclastoma tends to be more malignant and treatment by amputation may then be required.

Recurrent
osteoclastoma
tends to be more
malignant and
treatment by
amputation may
be required.

21

21.3   Ewing's Tumour

This is an uncommon highly malignant tumour that occurs most often in the shafts of long bones of children and adolescents from 5 to 15 years. Although it occurs in bones, it is not truly a tumour of bone cells but is a tumour of undifferentiated connective tissue or neurogenic tissue in bone.

21.3.1   Presentation

Pain, swelling, fever and anaemia are common features of Ewing's tumour, so much so that a diagnosis of infection (osteomyelitis) may be thought to be present. Sometimes lesions are present in more than one bone. Metastases to lungs or other bones are common.

21.3.2   Investigations

An increased erythrocyte sedimentation rate (ESR), increased white cell count and a degree of anaemia are usual features. X-rays of the bone typically show a laminated "onion peel" appearance due to periosteal reaction. Further information may be gained from CT or MRI studies or from isotope scans. Biopsy and microscopic examination will establish the diagnosis.

This is a tumour where, if available, PET scans may be especially helpful to detect any focus of tumour in bones at other sites and to evaluate response to chemotherapy and radiotherapy.

21.3.3   Treatment

In the past, standard treatment was by surgery (usually amputation), but was generally unsuccessful. Fortunately Ewing's tumour is radiosensitive and chemosensitive.

With modern treatment using induction chemotherapy, radiotherapy and possibly local surgical excision of the affected piece of bone, and further post irradiation or post-operative adjuvant chemotherapy, significantly better results are now being achieved. Recently myelo-ablative chemotherapy followed by autologous bone marrow transplantion for poor prognosis patients has given good results.

From being a malignancy considered almost universally incurable a few years ago most of these patients are now cured.

21.4 Chondrosarcoma

21.4.1 Presentation

Chondrosarcoma is a malignant tumour of cartilage and most often affects middle-aged adults. It varies from low-grade (the majority) to high-grade malignancy. This tumour may develop on any bone, especially at the ends of long bones or in bones of the pelvis, shoulder or ribs. It usually presents as a slowly growing painful lump on a bone, often near a large joint.

21.4.2 Investigations

X-rays will often show typical appearance of a chondrosarcoma: a cartilage-like swelling. Biopsy will establish the diagnosis. CT or MRI studies will help show the exact position, nature and extent of the tumour.

21.4.3 Treatment

If possible, radical surgical excision of the tumour with adjacent bone is carried out. This may require amputation of a limb.

These sarcomas are not sensitive to standard radiotherapy or chemotherapy but, because they are slowly growing and usually do not metastasise until late in the disease most can be cured as long as the primary tumour can be widely excised before the sarcoma is very advanced.

Encouraging responses with high percentage of apparent cures of chondrosarcomas in inaccessible surgical sites, especially the base of skull, are now reported from Boston , USA and other clinics with proton-beam radiotherapy facilities.

Metastatic (Secondary) Cancer

22

In this chapter you will learn about:

› *The most likely sites of metastatic spread from primary cancers*

A metastatic (secondary) cancer is the term used to describe a cancer that is growing in an organ or tissue some distance away from the tissue or organ in which it originated. The most important differences between benign tumours and malignant tumours are that benign tumours tend to be slowly growing and remain localised to the tissue in which they arose. Malignant tumours tend to grow more rapidly, grow into surrounding structures and spread and establish secondary growths in tissues or organs away from their primary site of development. To spread to distant sites, malignant cells usually grow into blood vessels or lymph vessels. Individual cells or clumps of cells break off and are carried by the bloodstream or the lymphatic vessels to a distant organ or tissue or to lymph nodes where they may grow as secondary or metastatic tumours. It is somewhat akin to the spreading cancer cells acting like "seeds" and being transported along blood or lymph vessels to a new "soil" where they may take root and grow. Malignant cells may also sometimes spread along nerve sheaths, or, across body cavities such as the abdominal cavity or a pleural cavity.

The most common site for metastatic spread of carcinomas as opposed to sarcomas, is via lymph vessels into lymph nodes. First, they grow in lymph nodes near the original cancer and then spread into lymph nodes further away (Fig. 22.1). The next most common sites of spread are by the bloodstream to the lungs or liver.

Other common sites of metastatic spread are to bones, the brain, under the skin, or to the ovaries. No tissue is exempt from developing a metastasis, including the adrenal glands and the kidneys. However, some organs and tissues tend to have a relatively low incidence of metastatic growth of most cancers for no obvious reason. These include the spleen and muscles.

F. O. Stephens and K. R. Aigner, *Basics of Oncology,*
DOI: 10.1007/978-3-540-92925-3_22, © Springer-Verlag Berlin Heidelberg 2009

22

What primary sites are likely to have resulted in metastatic involvement of cervical (neck) lymph nodes?

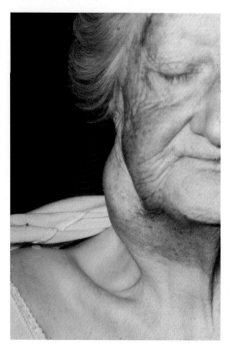

Fig. 22.1. This elderly woman had metastatic cancer in enlarged, hard cervical lymph nodes from a squamous cancer under the right side of her tongue. She had not been aware of any trouble in her mouth

The likelihood of a tumour metastasising to a particular site depends to a considerable degree on the type of tumour and its place of origin.   The likelihood of a tumour metastasising to a particular site depends to a considerable degree on the type of tumour and its place of origin. Stomach, pancreas and bowel cancers, for example, tend to spread first to abdominal lymph nodes and by portal vein to the liver. Breast cancer tends to spread first to nearby lymph nodes and later to the lungs, liver and bone. Prostate cancer tends to spread local lymph nodes and to bone. Skin cancer and cancers in the mouth and throat tend to spread to nearby lymph nodes with the exception of basal cell cancer which rarely spreads anywhere other than into surrounding tissues. Lung cancers, on the other hand, tend to spread early not only to lymph nodes but to almost any other organ or tissue in the body including bone and brain. Like lung cancer melanoma tends to spread not only to lymph nodes, lung, liver, lung, bowel and brain but also to the spleen.

Sarcomas are more likely to first spread via the bloodstream to the lungs rather than to lymph nodes. The most likely sites of cancer metastases are given in Table 22.1.

Table 22.1 Most likely sites of cancer metastases

Primary	Common sites for metastases	Chap.
BCC of skin	Very rarely metastasises	10
SCC of skin	Regional lymph nodes; the next group of lymph nodes; lungs very late in disease spread	10
Melanoma	Regional lymph nodes; next group of lymph nodes; lung; liver; brain; remote lymph nodes; small intestine; subcutaneous tissues; spleen; bone; adrenal glands	10
Lung	Mediastinal lymph nodes; remote lymph nodes; bone; brain; liver; subcutaneous tissue; adrenal glands	11
Breast	Axillary lymph nodes; supraclavicular lymph nodes; chest lymph nodes; lung; liver; subcutaneous tissues; brain	12
Oesophagus	Adjacent mediastinal lymph nodes; other intra-thoracic lymph nodes; supraclavicular lymph nodes sometimes liver and sub-diaphragm lymph nodes	13
Stomach	Peri-gastric lymph nodes; para-gastric lymph nodes; coeliac lymph nodes; small omentum lymph nodes; supra clavicular lymph nodes; (usually left side); liver; omentum; peritoneum; ovary	13
Liver	Other sites in liver, lungs, regional lymph nodes, rarely to bone	13
Gall bladder and bile duct	Small omentum lymph nodes; liver; peritoneum	13
Pancreas	Adjacent lymph nodes; coeliac lymph nodes; small omentum; liver; peritoneum; lungs	13
Small intestine	Mesenteric lymph nodes; para-aortic lymph nodes; liver	13
Colon and rectum	Para-colic lymph nodes; next group of lymph nodes; para-aortic lymph nodes; liver; peritoneum	13
Anus – upper anal canal Lower anal canal	Pelvic lymph nodes; para-aortic lymph nodes; liver; inguinal lymph nodes	13
Lips	Submental and submandibular lymph nodes; cervical lymph nodes; parotid lymph nodes	14
Tongue, floor of mouth, buccal mucosa	Submental lymph nodes; submandibular lymph nodes; cervical lymph nodes; supra clavicular lymph nodes	14
Posterior tongue, tonsillar region and pharynx	Tonsillar lymph node; cervical lymph nodes; supra-clavicular lymph nodes; lung	14

(continued)

Table 22.1 (continued)

Primary	Common sites for metastases	Chap.
Salivary glands	Adjacent lymph nodes; cervical lymph nodes; supra-clavicular lymph nodes	14
Thyroid gland follicular cancers	Adjacent lymph nodes; more distant lymph nodes; also bones; lungs; liver	14
Uterus	Adjacent lymph nodes; pelvic lymph nodes; ovaries; peritoneum	15
Ovaries	Adjacent lymph nodes; pelvic lymph nodes; the other ovary; fallopian tubes; abdominal lymph nodes; small intestine; peritoneum; liver	15
Vagina	Adjacent lymph nodes; pelvic lymph nodes; inguinal lymph nodes	15
Vulva	Inguinal lymph nodes; more distant lymph nodes	15
Penis	Inguinal lymph nodes; more distant lymph nodes	16
Testis	Para-aortic lymph nodes; more distant lymph nodes; lungs	16
Prostate	Adjacent lymph nodes; pelvic lymph nodes; bone; lung; liver	16
Bladder	Adjacent lymph nodes; pelvic lymph nodes; peritoneum	17
Kidney renal pelvis	Hilar lymph nodes; para-aortic lymph nodes; lung (sometimes a solitary metastasis); also ureter	17
Brain	Rarely metastasises before causing death from primary tumour	18
Leukaemia and lymphomas	These are systemic diseases	19
Soft tissue sarcomas	Predominantly lung (sometimes a solitary metastasis)	20
Osteosarcoma	Lung (multiple and early)	21
Osteoclastama	Rarely metastasises unless it degenerates then to lungs	21
Ewings tumour	Lung; bone	21
Chondrosarcoma	Lung, other bones but rarely metastasises until large, painful and degenerate	21

This table provides a summary of most primary tumours, their most likely sites of cancer metastatic spread and reference to the relevant chapters in this book where further details of each type of cancer is discussed

List the more common primary sites of secondary cancers in:

1. Lung

2. Liver

3. Bone

4. Brain

5. Spleen

6. Left supra-clavicular lymph nodes

Part IV
Making Progress

Techniques and Evidence of Progress

23

In this chapter you will learn about:

> *Evidence-based medicine*
> *Clinical trials*

23.1   Evidence-Based Medicine

It would be good to think that doctors would always know just what was the right thing to do about every health problem in different people under different circumstances but the reality is that this is not the case. The evidence is not always available for deciding just what is best for each individual patient.

Nowhere in the field of medical practice is the situation more uncertain than in some aspects of treating cancer.

The objective of all doctors has always been to get best evidence of most effective management. However, the advent of computerised information with a variety of approaches in statistical and mathematical analysis and randomised studies, made it appropriate to link new scientifically studied and mathematically confirmed clinical information under the group umbrella known as "*evidence-based medicine*". This label distinguishes such evidence from information based on a "one-off" experience, a collection of anecdotes, traditionally accepted beliefs, medical folklore, wishful thinking or grandmothers' tales.

Nowadays most acceptable evidence is based on randomised trials.

Nowhere in the field of medical practice is the situation more uncertain than in some aspects of treating cancer.

23.1.1   Randomised Trials

In a randomised trial all patients referred to a specialised clinic with a problem that needs to be studied to discover best method of care are invited to take part. There are strict ethical standards that must be observed in conducting randomised trials. Approval must be obtained, not only from the patients involved, but from independent ethics committees.

F. O. Stephens and K. R. Aigner, *Basics of Oncology*,
DOI: 10.1007/978-3-540-92925-3_23, © Springer-Verlag Berlin Heidelberg 2009

The nature of the trial is fully explained to patients considered appropriate for the study and if they agree they are allocated randomly to one of two "test groups" over which the researchers have no control. In some special studies there may be more than two test groups. The researchers have no control over which patients are allocated to each group. Patients in one of the two groups are treated by the best known available standard treatment and patients in the other group are treated by the new technique under study that is believed may be a better method of treatment. Ideally results are recorded "blind" that is by a third party who does not know what treatment each patient was given. Results of the two groups are compared, usually by an appropriate form of statistical analysis, to discover which was the better form of treatment. Such studies are known as randomised controlled studies and are stopped as soon as there is enough evidence that one method is better than the other. The better method is then usually recommended for all patients.

Although this is not the only way of finding convincing "evidence" of best practice, it is usually regarded as the most persuasive.

23.1.2   Other Historic Methods of Gathering Evidence

Much evidence accumulated over many years of medical practice has not been evaluated scientifically or statistically proven to give best clinical information.

In the past, doctors had to make decisions and introduce practices and concepts based on best available evidence but this was usually gathered from historical evidence or evidence learned by "trial and error". Trial and error is based on the principle of trying not to repeat mistakes, or making least mistakes. This often masquerades as experience, but one way or another, inevitably by making some mistakes, new information was produced and progress was made.

Often traditional or historically accepted practices just "grew" and became accepted without close analysis or criticism

Often traditional or historically accepted practices just "grew" and became accepted without close analysis or criticism. The dominant medical or surgical teacher may have been skilled in practice but unskilled in critical analysis. Each practitioner's own personal experience was often taken as convincing evidence without proper analysis or fair comparison with other evidence or under different circumstances. This type of a teacher's belief, or of personal experience in a limited practice, is often referred to as "anecdotal evidence". Although anecdotal evidence may well be true, there is no proof that the outcome will be consistent when used by different practitioners, in different circumstances, and for different patients.

However there are some notable exceptions to the value of a "one off" experience.

Edward Jenner was so convinced that "immunisation" with the mild disease cowpox would give protection against the deadly and virulent small pox disease, that he tested his belief on himself. He injected himself with cowpox and had a mild reaction. He later injected himself with small pox and did not get the disease. His belief was based on "anecdotal" observations and historic evidence.

There was no scientifically proven information or randomised trial yet vital medical progress was made. In fact Jenner's discovery of 1796 has still not been proven by randomised trials.

Alexander Fleming, working in London in 1928, noticed a mould growing on a culture stopped the growth of bacteria. Later, in 1940, an Australian, Dr Howard Florey, also working in Britain, showed that an extract of Fleming's mould, called penicillin, could be used effectively and safely in people to kill bacteria causing infection in humans. So penicillin was discovered and the era of present-day antibiotic treatment of bacterial infections began. Success of treatment of pneumonia and other infections with penicillin was so obvious that no randomised trial was ever initiated.

The approach of Edward Jenner, in using himself as a test case, is still occasionally used in testing strongly held beliefs in other areas of medicine.

In 1983 Dr Robin Warren and Dr Barry Marshal in Australia reported in *Lancet* their finding of a bacterium called the *Helicobacter pylori* was present in the gastric mucosa of patients with gastric ulcers. They believed that rather than being a coincidental finding it would be found to be a cause of gastric ulcers. To prove that this bacterium actually was a cause of gastric ulcers rather than an incidental finding Dr Marshal and a friend swallowed cultures of the bacterium. Both contracted gastritis with vomiting and abdominal pain and underwent gastroscopic examination. Biopsies showed the organism in the inflamed gastric mucosa. This confirmed the association between *H. pylori* and gastritis and subsequent epidemiological studies confirmed that without treatment, ulcers could develop in the inflamed gastric mucosa.

Another report of this type of approach was published in *The Medical Journal of Australia* in 1997 in relation to prostate cancer. A doctor was diagnosed by biopsies as having prostate cancer. Because he believed that there was good evidence that plant phytoestrogens could influence the growth of prostate cancer, (as do human oestrogens), he gave himself 7 days of treatment with a moderate dose of phytoestrogens before undergoing radical prostatectomy. After the radical prostatectomy, the pathologist was asked to examine the prostate cancer cells and compare their appearance with the appearance of the cancer cells taken in the biopsies prior to any treatment.

The pathologist found clear evidence of *apoptosis* (inbuilt cell death) in the cancer after the treatment without any evidence of apoptosis in the biopsy specimens taken 3 weeks earlier. This of course was a "one off" study as were the studies of Edward Jenner and Barry Marshal. Although it did not prove anything as convincingly as would a scientifically controlled "randomised study", it certainly indicated that further study would be justified.

An attempt to more scientifically determine the most likely outcome of different medical practices or treatments has now evolved, especially over the last two or three decades of the twentieth century. Led by medical scientists with a statistical frame of mind and epidemiologists' aptitude, *"randomised trials"* have now become the doctor's basic "measuring stick" of new information and the foundation upon which "new" and "old" practices are now compared and judged.

This is a great leap forward in ability to make acceptable medical progress more efficient. Where possible, progress in medical practice is best made in scientifically tested studies where the evidence can be tested and comparisons made and measured against existing best practices.

However, it should not be forgotten that much of our present knowledge, "know how" and effective practice is based on a broad range of skills in gathering evidence and it is still true that not all relevant information can be measured or converted into a computerised model. There is still need for solutions based on logic and close and personal relationships between practitioners and their patients. These relationships and evidence gained must not be lost in the momentum for mathematically based science. Such factors as warmth of relationship and personal understanding of priorities in social, domestic spiritual and other circumstances between practitioners and their patients cannot be measured but are important in decision making. Because they cannot be measured does not mean that they should be ignored or discarded. They do make a difference to outcome as far as people are concerned and patients are special people.

Historical evidence, clinical experience, patient belief systems, personal and social priorities and needs and other considerations still must play an important part in clinical decision making. The patient must always be a person first, a person with a health problem, not primarily a health problem to be solved. The relationship between the doctor and patient must be personal and sacrosanct, based on many unmeasurable and intangible aspects of human emotion as well as knowledge, and applied to the immediate health needs as worked out between patient and doctor, not as dictated by "scientific data" alone.

Scientific limitations, variations and uncertainties are very evident in determining best treatment for women with breast cancer and men with prostate cancer. Outcomes of investigation and treatment are still unpredictable. Patients' priorities are often quite different. What will be the right decision for one patient will not necessarily be right for another patient. Individual judgement and understanding must play important roles but these are difficult to measure scientifically.

Some years ago from randomised controlled studies in women with breast cancer it was learned that the standard operation of radical mastectomy with removal of underlying muscles and all adjacent lymph nodes from the axilla did not result in any more cures than a "modified" radical operation. In the modified operation, no muscle was removed. From further randomised trials it is now known that for women with a relatively small cancer in the breast, cure is just as likely by a "breast saving operation". In a "breast saving operation" only that part of the breast containing the cancer is removed together with any likely involved axillary lymph nodes. This is followed by radiotherapy to the remaining breast tissue. Yet some women who have a breast cancer are not comfortable unless the whole breast is removed and they should be entitled to make this decision for themselves if that is their wish. To these women the saving of the breast would be more worry to them than the loss of the breast.

To other women, and especially to most younger women, the breast is emotionally very important to them. If the whole breast must be removed they would choose to have an artificially reconstructed breast operation immediately rather than be left for a period without a breast. Until recently most surgeons were reluctant to reconstruct an artificial breast for at least 2 years, by which time recurrence of the cancer in the breast region was unlikely. Randomised studies have now shown that this delay does not improve the outlook for the patient and in most cases she should be allowed to choose immediate reconstruction if she wishes. There are sometimes other variables in patients' wishes that may need to be considered such as whether or not to have adjuvant chemotherapy or hormone therapy, or radiotherapy or chemotherapy for widespread asymptomatic disease. Some women wish to have their other breast removed, especially if there is a high incidence of breast cancer in their families. The ultimate decision on these and other matters must be based on the patient's special and personal priorities and needs together with an understanding of the best evidence available of possible outcomes of different courses of action as explained by the doctor and treatment teams.

In the case of prostate cancer, a histological diagnosis of cancer does not mean that the cancer will progress during the patient's lifetime. In only about 1 in 4 patients is the prostate cancer potentially life threatening before he dies of other causes yet there is no certain way of determining which cancers must be treated as a life saving measure. Most men with prostate cancer are in the older age group and side effects of treatment aimed at cure are likely to be severe. Decisions must be made on best available evidence but modified by the patient's lifestyle needs and priorities.

There are so many variations in disease processes, environmental and social situations, human needs, beliefs, emotions, priorities and interpersonal relationships, as well as medical skills, facilities and practices that it is not always possible to subject even basic information to scientifically designed statistical analysis. The following truisms sums up the complexities involved.

Not all evidence can be justified by statistics and
Not all statistics can be justified as evidence

It is also important to keep in mind that:

The absence of evidence
is not the same as
Evidence of the absence.

"The absence of evidence" Is not the same as "Evidence of the absence."

In other words because there is no statistical evidence to prove that something is true does not, in itself, prove that it is untrue.

In those instances where anecdotal or historic evidence or information based on a logically proposed hypothesis is still the best available evidence, it must inevitably still play a part in medical thinking and gathering of knowledge.

Evidence based on a logical hypothesis, but not yet ready for a "randomised trial", can still be put to the test under a label of scientific study sometimes called "a pilot study". The idea and study proposed is usually put to a group of "peers" or well-informed colleagues for comment and approval before being "trialled" in a small group of well-informed, consenting and interested patients. If the initial "trial" is successful a further and larger group is studied. This allows new ideas to be tested and new evidence gained but under well-organised, closely observed and safe conditions.

An obvious example of important but uncomplicated information gathered without scientific analysis is that there has been no randomised study to prove that people who develop pneumonia will have a better outcome if they are treated with antibiotics than with the treatment that was standard in the pre-antibiotic era. Similarly anecdotal and historic evidence alone suggests that surgical removal of an acutely inflamed appendix is likely to achieve a better outcome than the treatment that was used in pre-anaesthetic days without the intervention of surgery. There has been no randomised trial to prove this.

In a more recent context the traditional and most effective known treatment for people with an advanced cancer (usually a sarcoma) in a limb that was too big for successful local surgical removal, was amputation. Anything less was known to result in a high risk of local cancer recurrence. Experience in some clinics now indicates that, rather than amputation, in most cases equally satisfactory results can be achieved by first "reducing" the cancer with chemotherapy, followed by local surgical removal of the remaining cancer (Chap. 8). This has never been proven in a strictly randomised controlled study and, in fact, in some clinics amputation is still regarded as the treatment of choice. Ideally it should be studied in a properly organised trial but who would be prepared to ask patients to enter a study in which the amputation of a limb depended on the luck of the draw? Even if such co-operative patients could be found would this not be a rather select group of people who would seem to be different to the rest of us?

23.2   Clinical Trials

With so many different ways of treating cancers in general it is important for major treatment teams to continue to discover which method or methods of treatment are most likely to achieve best results. This will depend on many variable factors such as the age and place of living and home circumstances of the patient, the type of cancer and its degree of advancement, the range of treatments available, any potential side effects of treatment and the acceptance by the patient of treatment options. In order to compare different treatments of different cancers in different patients and different circumstances it is important for studies to be continued in well-conducted clinical trials. In such trials, when it is not known which option of treatment is best for patients who have a particular problem, studies are conducted by experts who agree to compare treatment options.

If more than two treatment options are being studied, the trial is said to have "more than two arms". Such studies must be well considered and planned by teams of experts and well conducted in a closely supervised fashion. Usually such trials are best conducted in major teaching hospitals. This is the way much progress has been made and will continue to be made in improving treatment for patients with all types of cancer.

Patients should have the conditions of the trial fully described to them. They should know why the trial is needed, why they have been selected as good patients for the trial, what potential benefits may result, what are the potential problems, if any, and the advantages or disadvantages of taking part in the trial (especially any potential side effects). If patients are invited to take part in a clinical trial, it is because the specialists cannot be sure that one treatment to be used is better than another. However in taking part in a study to try to find the answer, patients will certainly be given closely supervised and highly skilled care. They must be reassured that their entry into the trial is completely voluntary and they can withdraw at any time but their participation should help the expert teams discover just which treatment achieves best results. This information will be important for the future care of patients perhaps including members of their own family or friends or even themselves.

Clinical trials of drugs under study are carried out in three phases:

Phase I is planned to determine the maximum well tolerated dose of a drug that can be safely given. Usually beginning with small doses in a small number of patients (usually two or three) and gradually increasing the dose in successive small groups of patients until a maximal well tolerated dose is apparent.

Phase II is planned to determine how effective the safe maximum dose determined is in treating a number of patients.

Phase III is a randomised trial of sufficient numbers of patients to compare results of treatment with the new agent under study compared to results of treatment by standard best practice.

23.2.1 Ethics Approval

In medical practice and research there are different types of clinical trials but all require informed consent from patients and approval of independent ethics committees. To achieve best information, especially when dealing with relatively uncommon health problems, it is often necessary to organise multi-centre studies. Multi-centre studies involve patients in a number of different hospitals or institutions under the care of a number of different practitioners. Such trials require strict ethical standards of data collection and privacy, approved by independent ethics committees as well as agreed methods of gathering, analysing and publishing results.

Future Directions

24

In this chapter you will learn about:

> *Prevention*
> *Improved cancer screening and diagnostic techniques*
> *MRS (magnetic resonance spectroscopy)*
> *Combined imaging using PET and CT or PET and MRI*
> *Magnetic resonance-guided focused ultrasound surgery*
> *Vaccines*
> *Improved treatment agents*
> *New agents*
> *Therapeutic viruses*
> *Targeted therapies*
> *Improvements in radiotherapy*
> *More effective integrated treatments with chemotherapy, radiotherapy and surgery*
> *Prevention of metastases*
> *Heat therapy*
> *Other physical treatments – cryosurgery, electrolysis*
> *Immunotherapy*
> *Stem cell research*
> *Genetic engineering and gene therapy*
> *Studies in cell mediated anticancer activity*
> *Molecular characterisation in future cancer treatment*
> *Learning from "alternative" and "naturopathic" practices*
> *Improved palliative care and supportive care*
> *Hope for the future*

The future for cancer sufferers is a mixture of hope and caution. Certainly there is much that can be done by application of present knowledge. There is also great expectation of future improvements in prevention, diagnosis and care. However, just as there will be great advances in management of cancer in the future, so too there will be new challenges. AIDS in Western countries is most prevalent in promiscuous male homosexuals and intravenous illicit drug users who share needles but in some parts of Africa and Asia it is widespread and increasing in

F. O. Stephens and K. R. Aigner, *Basics of Oncology,*
DOI: 10.1007/978-3-540-92925-3_24, © Springer-Verlag Berlin Heidelberg 2009

both sexes. Affected people have increased susceptibility to infections and to developing malignant tumours. As yet no cure is in sight.

People who have undergone organ transplantation and are dependent upon immune-suppressive drugs to prevent rejection of the transplanted organ, also have an increased risk of developing a cancer and the sexual revolution has exposed young women to an increased risk of developing cancer of the cervix. Lastly it is quite unknown what potential other modern drugs, especially the illicit drugs, might have in regard to increasing the risk of some cancers. It took many years before the dangers of tobacco smoking became manifest.

24.1   Prevention (See Chap. 3)

The most obvious measure in reducing the incidence of cancer is to avoid smoking. This has been known for years, but human nature being what it is, this precaution has been widely disregarded. While ever there are large profits to be made from the sale of tobacco products, there will be resistance to the introduction of more severe statutory measures aimed at reducing smoking. Tobacco smoking is related to a greater incidence of cancers of lung, mouth, throat, larynx, oesophagus, stomach, pancreas, large bowel, kidneys, bladder and even breast cancer.

Another useful active measure is to encourage fair-skinned people to take greater protection against exposure to the sun and ultraviolet irradiation and especially for young people to avoid sunburn.

More attention can be paid to removal of pre-malignant conditions such as hyperkeratoses, leukoplakia, stomach and bowel polyps and papillomas and to avoid and prevent such infections as hepatitis and AIDS.

Some changes in lifestyle should be encouraged, including a reduction of animal fats, and artificial additives and chemical preservatives and other contaminants in the diet. A greater intake of fibre, nuts, grains, fresh fruits and vegetables including legumes should also be encouraged as should moderation in the use of alcohol, although the possibility of some cancer protective value of a little red wine cannot be denied. There will continue to be advances based on epidemiological information such as a better understanding of protective qualities of high fibre diets and apparent protective qualities of diets high in other possible protective agents such as phytoestrogens and lycopene.

Slim, fit, active people have a lower risk of several cancers

General physical fitness with absence of obesity is desirable from every point of view. Slim, fit, active people have a lower risk of several cancers including lung, breast, colon and rectum, prostate and pancreas, as well as better ability to tolerate treatment programs.

Reduction of atmospheric pollutants, vigilant observation of protective industrial laws and protection against radioactive sources are also important preventive factors.

24.2   Improved Cancer-Screening and Diagnostic Techniques (See Chap. 7)

Another measure of increasing importance is regular screening of people at special risk for certain kinds of cancer so that any early lesion may be treated before an advanced cancer develops. This may be most appropriate to detect early breast cancer, cancer of the cervix, cancer of the stomach in some communities and large bowel cancer. Screening for prostate cancer can often give a valuable guide but is not universally practiced. It will be more widely accepted if a method can be developed for determining which prostate cancers are likely to become aggressive during the patient's otherwise expected lifetime.

A newer technique of *"digital mammography"* is showing promise of improving the accuracy of diagnostic screening of breast cancer in women younger than 50.

It is anticipated that improved, more accurate and simpler screening measures for increasing numbers of different cancer types will become available. These may include simple blood screening tests for cancer antibodies or other tumour markers to indicate the presence of early cancer at a more curable stage and before symptoms have developed.

Improved diagnostic measures will also allow more certain and more accurate diagnosis at an earlier stage. Already improvements in CT scanning and other organ imaging techniques have made considerable progress and further advances are assured. Magnetic resonance imaging (MRI) has added to these improved diagnostic and imaging methods and it is anticipated that positron emission tomography (PET) scanning might make an even greater impact than CT and MRI scanning within a few years (Chap. 7). PET gives information about activity, composition and survival of tumour cells as well as detection of metastatic cells at an earlier stage than has been possible in the past.

Fine-needle aspiration cytology, frozen section techniques and other improved pathology techniques have allowed major progress in establishing early detection and the nature of early tumours. Improvements in the ability to examine body cavities with the use of flexible fibre-scopes and endoscopes have allowed considerable progress in detecting and assessing early cancers in recent years. Such instruments and their application will undoubtedly continue to be improved.

Studies are being made in a number of laboratories to develop *tumour markers* that will detect cancers in their earliest stages. One such study with encouraging potential is a test for a molecule present when cells are abnormally dividing. Studies of bowel cancer are showing this molecule is a possible indicator of the presence of a bowel cancer in its preclinical stages. A future screening test for bowel cancer may result. Studies are also being made in relation to other cancers including breast, bladder, cervix, mouth and lung.

Studies are being made in a number of laboratories to develop tumour markers that will detect cancers in their earliest stages.

24.2.1   MRS (Magnetic Resonance Spectroscopy)

MRS is an application of MRI. It is evolving technology that has potential to diagnose many tumours and characterise their metastatic potential. It is a non-invasive diagnostic test that uses strong magnetic fields to measure and analyse the chemical composition of human tissues.

New laboratory testing methods will also give information as to which treatment methods and which anti-cancer agents are likely to be of greatest benefit in treating each individual cancer; for example a tumour cell scanning technique under study known as magnetic resonance scanning is investigating better methods of screening for and determining more specific anti-cancer chemotherapy for different cancers, and trying to match each individual cancer with the agent or combination of agents to which it is most sensitive.

Experience with MRS of primary breast cancers indicates that it may also have a valuable application in other cancers. For example it may be possible to predict the metastatic potential of melanoma by spectroscopic analysis of the primary tumour and to distinguish naevi from melanomas, thus better selecting patients for surgery.

24.2.2   Combined Imaging Using PET and CT or PET and MRI

Early imaging studies combining PET and CT or PET and MRI have shown prospects of demonstrating both functional and anatomical information of primary and metastatic cancers. Such combined imaging has considerable advantage in diagnosis and assessing response of cancers to treatment. Such techniques are sure to be further developed in the very near future.

24.2.3   Magnetic Resonance-Guided Focused Ultrasound Surgery

Magnetic resonance guided focused ultrasound surgery (MRgFUS) is a non-invasive technique that can coagulate tumours, both benign and malignant. It has been used in some clinical studies and has been shown for example to have potential as a non-invasive replacement for some open operative procedures such as lumpectomy of breast lumps. Undoubtedly it will become more widely used to remove other tumours in the future.

24.3   Vaccines

An effective vaccine traded as "Gardasil" (Merk) against the human papilloma virus has now been developed and successfully trailed for clinical use against cancer in humans. It is now used in several countries to vaccinate teenage girls.

Progress is also being reported in developing vaccines against breast, colo-rectal, ovarian and kidney cancers and melanomas.

24.4 Improved Treatment Agents

Improved treatment with more effective and more specific anti-cancer drugs is proceeding and there is constant progress in how best to use anti-cancer drugs in appropriate combinations and treatment schedules. New and more effective anti-cancer agents like the *Taxanes* (derived from a plant) are adding to the range of available anti-cancer drugs and many drugs are being made safer and more effective by increasing availability of agents that protect bone marrow and other body tissues.

Solving many of the problems of bone marrow transplantation has also allowed stronger and more effective anti-cancer treatment to be given with improved safety. It is anticipated that heavy-dose chemotherapy with life-saving bone marrow transplantation may be used effectively in treating patients with more types of widespread cancer. At present only limited numbers of tumour types, mostly lymphomas and leukaemias, can be effectively treated this way with relative safety.

A new class of agents, *Cox-2-inhibitors*, is being tested in both prevention and clinical trials. Epidemiological studies have shown that people who regularly take non-steroidal anti-inflammatory drugs, such as aspirin, for arthritis, have lower rates of colorectal polyps and colorectal cancers. These block certain enzymes (cyclogenase enzymes) that are produced in the body when there is inflammation and are also produced by precancerous tissues. Inhibition of Cox-2 enzymes may help treat and prevent cancer. Clinical trials of new Cox-2 inhibitors (one is called celecoxib), in cancer prevention and cancer treatment are under study.

24.5 Self Rescuing Concept (SRC)

S-1 is an active oral flourouracil anti-tumour drug, which is called a "self-rescuing" drug. The first of a new concept of combining an anti-cancer agent (5-FU) with a protective or self regulating agent to give dual actions that is enhancement of pharmacological actions of 5-FU and reduction of its adverse reactions. By making use of the biochemical and enzymological properties of 5-FU in combination with FT, which is gradually converted to 5-FU in the body, with a 5-FU's adverse reaction reducing substance.

It seems that the combined regimen of S-1 with other anti-cancer agents and with other therapeutic modalities will contribute to the routine medical practice of cancer treatment in the future.

S-1 based combination therapies with other promising drugs like cisplatin, irinotecan and taxanes, are expected to yield good results. Above all, S-1 plus CDDO therapy showed a high efficacy and is expected to become a standard therapy for advanced gastric cancer.

24.6   New Agents

A whole range of new anti-cancer agents is presently undergoing trials in cancer treatment and some are proving to be very effective. Some under study have been mentioned in this book in treating different cancers (Chaps 8 and 19). The most significant of these new agents are gemcitabine, vinorelbine, topoisomerase I inhibitors (topotecan, irinotecan), liposomal anthracyclines, new fluoroprimidines and tyrosine kinase inhibitors but as progress is made more agents will be added to this list and some older agents will no longer be used.

24.7   Therapeutic Viruses

A new approach in anti-cancer treatment is to find a virus that will specifically damage cancer cells without damaging normal cells. In some laboratories, genetically engineered anti-cancer viruses are being designed. Present laboratory studies in relation to breast cancer cells have been encouraging although the anti-cancer potency has been shown to become less effective with prolonged use. An adenovirus (OnyxO15) has been developed which specifically kills head and neck cancer cells with $p53$ mutations, though not as simply as originally thought. A variant of this has been licensed in China, though its approval and use remains controversial At the time of writing, safety and effectiveness in clinical studies has rarely yet been demonstrated.

24.8   Targeted Therapies

Recently, a new avenue of cancer chemotherapy began to show promise with the discovery of an antagonist to the enzyme involved in myeloid leukaemia, tyrosine kinase, STI571 (*Gleevec or Glivec*) The discovery of this agent has stimulated further research to discover more inhibitors of possible enzymes involved in production of other cancers (see Sect. 19.4). Future enzyme treatment of prostate cancer and certain gastro-intestinal cancers appears promising.

A great number of new targeted therapies are under consideration at the clinical level and the use of multi-target tyrosine kinase inhibitors is increasing for solid tumours. Focusing on EGFR-tyrosine inhibitors (gefitinib or erlotinib) some positive clinical results for lung cancer patients have been encouraging.

Other new studies of special interest in cancer treatment are those investigating the use of "angiostatic" and "angiotoxic" agents. These drugs have potential to eliminate cancers by destroying the new fragile blood vessels that cancers depend upon for their survival. One such agent under investigation is Thalidomide (see Sects. 8.5.2 and 19.8.2). Thalidomide taken by mothers to reduce morning sickness in early pregnancy some years ago, was responsible for many birth defects. The birth defects resulted from thalidomide damaging newly developing blood vessels in the foetus. It is precisely this damaging property to developing capillaries that may help destroy blood supply to developing cancers. Another new agent called "Avastin" damages tumour capillaries and when used with chemotherapy it magnifies the cancer destructive activities of the chemotherapy. Encouraging results have been reported in treating bowel cancer and studies in treating a range of other cancers are under investigation.

Lastly the search goes on for agents to promote apoptosis in cancer cells (see Chap. 1). There is some evidence that it may be possible to restore the self-destructive features of normal cells to at least some types of cancer cells, possibly by administration of some biological agents. One of the more interesting studies of this type is being made in relation to phytoestrogens or related compounds that seem to have ability to restore apoptosis properties to prostate cancer cells. Breast cancer cells are similarly under study.

24.9   Improvements in Radiotherapy

Radiotherapy is also being constantly improved with different types of radio-emission and different treatment schedules integrated with anti-cancer drugs or hormones for more effective treatment. Improved techniques of administration include more effective doses of radiation delivered to the tumour volume with reduced risk of damage to normal tissues. Because tissue sensitivity to radio-therapy, including that of cancer cells, is dose-dependent, techniques of delivering increased doses of irradiation more precisely to cancer tissue and sparing normal tissues are constantly under investigation. Such techniques will continue to improve local tumour control. The combination of external radiotherapy and brachytherapy in treatment of prostate cancer is one example (Sect. 16.3) and further advances continue to be made in treating this and other cancers. The combined synchronous use of radiotherapy with chemotherapy or sometimes more precisely with regional chemotherapy is another avenue being studied. A further study using reduced oxygenation with chemotherapy together with radiotherapy is showing encouraging results in the treatment of advanced head and neck cancers. Radiotherapy together with immunological agents is similarly under study. Further treatment progress can be anticipated from of these studies.

Implantation of radioactive "seeds" is now established treatment for some prostate cancers but encouraging results are now being studied using more effective "seeds", implanted more precisely into other types of cancer in different situations. Cancers in the liver for example are now under study and encouraging results have been reported.

Anticipated technical advances in radiotherapy include three-dimensional planning techniques, radio-surgery and ionising magnetic radiotherapy (IMRT) will increase the likelihood of delivering high doses to smaller well-delineated tumour regions.

Photon therapy with more specific use of X-rays, gamma rays, proton rays and neutron rays are under study for more specific therapy of some cancers.

24.9.1   Improvements in Focussing Radiotherapy

Treatment by radiotherapy is also being constantly improved with sophisticated computer planning technology coupled with CT, MRI and PET scans that accurately image tumour targets. The ability to combine radiotherapy with chemotherapy has improved treatment results. More effective use of chemotherapy and radiotherapy integrated with surgery can be anticipated as cancer specialists become better organized in multidisciplinary teams focusing on specific tumour types. The best example of this has been in the treatment of breast cancer. The combined effects of earlier diagnosis, less mutilating surgery combined with either adjuvant chemotherapy and or hormonal therapy has seen the death rate from this disease fall by over 20% in the last 15 years.

Newer forms of radiation therapy being tested in trials in a small number of world specialist centres include a *cyberknife, tomotherapy and proton beam therapy.*

A *cyberknife* is basically an advanced linear accelerator technique that rotates around the tumour region focusing the irradiation onto a limited central region. At the time of writing this equipment and technique is being especially studied in a small number of centres including Washington. Tomotherapy, now available in a number of US centres, is also a technique of focusing irradiation onto a central tumour with minimal irradiation of surrounding tissues. *Proton beam therapy* directs irradiation to a deep especially targeted tumour region. At the time of writing this equipment and technique is being especially studied in a small number of centres including Boston.

24.10   More Effective Use of Chemotherapy and Radiotherapy Integrated with Surgery

With a few possible exceptions such as organ replacement or the use of regional tissue perfusion techniques, it does not seem that surgical measures for cancer eradication will advance greatly over present techniques. However, there is need for an increasing role for better-organised and better-planned combined, integrated treatment schedules in which chemotherapy, radiotherapy, and surgical modalities are used more effectively in planned combined approaches from the outset to improve the treatment of advanced cancers. Further studies are seeking to refine surgically and radiologically placed intra-arterial catheter techniques to more selectively distribute anti-cancer agents in greater concentration to the region of a tumour. Together with PET imaging, it is anticipated that future treatments will be directed more selectively and more precisely to those parts of the body where it is needed.

24.11   Prevention of Metastases

Recent reports that bisphosphonates appear to help prevent bone destruction by secondary cancers have created much interest (Chap. 8). These substances seem to have ability to protect bone from osteoclast activity and they possibly also promote apoptosis in secondary cancer-forming cells in bone.

24.12   Heat Therapy

Heat is another treatment modality as yet not well exploited. Cancer cells have increased susceptibility to destruction by heat. The application of heat to selectively eradicate cancer cells, possibly in combination with anti-cancer drugs, may in the future produce improved treatment techniques for certain types of cancer (see Sect. 8.5.1).

24.13   Other Physical Treatments

New studies in progress include cryosurgery and electrolysis in cancer treatment. Some cancers in liver are being treated and some cancers in lung and other tissues are being investigated, but as yet, apart from very effective treatment of liver metastases by cryosurgery, no new major clinical application has been substantiated (see Chap. 8). Radio-frequency ablation therapy either alone or in combination with other treatments is being widely investigated for treatment of liver metastases, with a number of successes being reported.

Perhaps the greatest hopes for the future are in the fields of immunotherapy, genetic engineering molecular biology and Nanotechnology. (Nanomedicines and nanopharmaceuticals). This relates to small molecules 2–15 nm in size (similar to proteins) used for drug delivery or analysis.

24.14   Immunotherapy

Perhaps the
greatest hopes
for the future
are in the fields
of immuno-
therapy,
genetic
engineering
and molecular
biology.

Cancers are often thought to be due to a deficiency in the body's immune defence system. Whereas abnormal cells are usually recognised and eradicated by the immune defences, in cancer patients, the abnormal cells have continued to survive and multiply. There is a great deal of supportive evidence for this "immune surveillance theory", including the fact that, very occasionally, a really advanced and aggressive type of cancer will suddenly and spontaneously disappear without trace, for no apparent reason. This suggests that somehow the body's natural defence mechanisms have taken charge again and eradicated the abnormal cancer cells.

A great deal of work has been carried out in leading hospitals, cancer institutes and other institutions in search of greater knowledge about and better application of the immunological defence mechanisms. There is hope that specific immunological tumour markers will reveal evidence of more cancers very early, and before they can otherwise be detected clinically. Related research indicates that tumour antibodies may not only reveal early evidence of cancer but may be used in treatment either in a direct attack upon cancer cells or by carrying cytotoxic chemical agents specifically to the cancer cells. In time a more reliable means of stimulating the immune defence system to eradicate cancer cells may also emerge from these studies. Preparations of monoclonal antibodies are now available for some tumours, and treatments based on their use are under study. Studies with such products of the immune defence system as interferon and the interleukins (see Chap. 8) have not yet had the impact originally hoped for but more recent products, tumour necrosis factor (TNF) and Herceptin (a monoclonal antibody product) have immediate valuable clinical application, especially when used in combination with other anti-cancer agents (Chap. 12).

24.15   Stem-Cell Research

Stem cells are undifferentiated "immortal" cells capable of differentiating into any type of cell and tissue. They have been extracted from bone marrow of adults, they are present in umbilical cord blood or may be taken from very early human embryos at the stage of little more than a fertilised ovum. They are used in research in attempts to replace or to change special body tissues or to restore normal tissues where needed. They are thus used to develop tissues needed to solve many health problems such as diabetes, cystic fibrosis and spinal cord injuries as well as tissues involved with cancer. Taking stem cells from embryos for research purposes is the subject of much ethical and moral controversy.

24.16 Studies in Cell-Mediated Anti-Cancer Activity

Further basic studies of dendritic cells are leading to a greater understanding of cell-mediated anti-cancer activity.

Dendritic cells that develop from stem cells in bone marrow give rise to immature dendritic cells in myeloid or lymphoid pathways and they develop into mature dendritic cells under inflammatory microenvironments. They therefore consist of heterogenous (different types) of myeloid or lymphoid cells at different stages of maturity. They are widely distributed in both lymphoid and non-lymphoid tissues.

Mature dendritic cells are major antigen-presenting cells capable of activating T cells to different cell-mediated immune responses.

Immature dendritic cells play a crucial role in inducing tolerance by induction of naïve T cells into accepting (anergic) regulatory cells.

In addition dendritic cells recognise various pathogens and can produce cytokines that activate other immune cells. Thus dendritic cells are crucial for a link between innate and adaptive immunity.

There is thus an increasing interest in development of immunotherapy with dendritic cells in cancer treatment as well as other immunopathogenic diseases.

24.17 Genetic Engineering and Gene Therapy

New techniques of molecular DNA biology offer a different approach in combating cancer. It may soon be possible to change the arrangement of genes in cells and thus change the nature of actually or potentially malignant cells into cells without the properties of malignant growth.

Present studies include replacement of abnormal genes with normal genes, transfer of a gene that can induce tumour cells to die or that can enhance the environment to generate a systemic immune response against the tumour. The former strategy includes suicide gene therapies, tumour suppressor gene therapy and oncolytic virus therapy. The latter adopts immunogene therapy. Other possible gene therapies under study include therapies to control cell cycle or apoptosis and therapies to promote antiangiogenesis.

24.18 Developments in Antibody Treatment

Developments in genetic engineering have promoted further activity in the use of monoclonal antibody therapy in three major pathways.

(a) Monoclonal toxicity ("killer" or cytotoxic antibodies) against the specific cancer cells.
(b) Antibodies to focus delivery of radiation specifically to the cancer cells.
(c) Antibodies to carry chemotherapeutic anti-cancer agents specifically to the cancer cells.

24.19   Molecular Characterisation in Future Cancer Treatment

In addition to histological typing, molecular typing of cancer will increasingly be necessary. For example, the Philadelphia chromosome (Ph), the hallmark of chronic myeloid leukaemia, is formed by the reciprocal translocation of genetic material between two chromosomes, designated chromosome 9 and chromosome 22. This gives rise to the juxtaposition of DNA from chromosome 9, at the site of the another gene, the ableson gene (*abl*), to sit beside DNA at the so-called breakpoint cluster region (*bcr*) on chromosome 22, giving rise to a gene caused by fusion of the two genes, called BCR-ABL This new gene will then produce new and different RNA and new protein that has tyrosine kinase activity. This is thought to be important in the pathogenesis of this type of leukaemia. This new RNA can be detected using molecular techniques involving the polymerase chain reaction (PCR).

The enzyme STI-571 (Gleevec), active in treatment of chronic myeloid leukaemia and some gastrointestinal stromal tumours, is the first clinical application of such molecular biochemistry in treatment of cancer (see Sect. 19.4).

This kind of knowledge at a molecular level has now been put into therapeutic practice with the design of molecules which can block the tyrosine kinase activity associated with this new protein, leading to disease control and perhaps even cure.

This is just one example of the way in which molecular knowledge can give rise to new and exciting ways to diagnose, monitor and even treat cancer in the future.

Similarly, mutation and polymorphism in the *p53* gene, microsatellite-instability, and up-regulation of enzymes such as thymidylate kinase, influence tumour sensitivity to chemotherapy. In future, identification of molecular changes in tumour cell DNA, RNA and proteins will influence estimation of prognosis and decisions about management.

24.20   Gene Expression Profiling for Prediction of Response to Chemotherapy

Numerous genes are involved in the development and progression of each cancer. The expression of these genes is controlled by complex regulatory interaction networks. The tumour characteristics of each tumour will be an end result of these genetic inter-reactions.

Recent studies of the DNA micro-array provides a potential opportunity to assess detailed characterisation of tumour cells indicating clinical behaviour and drug responsiveness. Thus individualised therapy with molecular targeted drugs should become more widely available in the near future.

24.21   Molecular Heterogeneity

Clinical trials in the twentieth century were based on the assumption that there was a uniformity of cancer cells and different agents affected different cancers more-or-less randomly. Further understanding and acknowledgment of hetero-geneity of cancer cells is vital for the development of individualised therapy in malignancies. The twenty-first century will be the Era of pharmacogenomics-based medicine obtained from personal genomic information. Already it has been developed and started personalised (tailored) treatment based on the expression of the specific gene or change in drug metabolic enzyme as a biomarker.

24.22   Learning from Alternative and Naturopathic Practices

Finally the possibility that more will be learned from alternative medicine and naturopathic practices as well as traditional practices from ancient and "unsophisticated" communities must not be ignored. A number of important medications and treatments have been developed from plants and practices of other eras, cultures and civilizations. However care must be taken to properly analyse such practices and not allow wishful thinking, emotion or "fashion" to cloud scientific and clinical judgement (see Sect. 8.6.8).

24.23   Improved Palliative Care and Supportive Care

For those people with advanced cancer who are in great discomfort or pain, methods of relieving suffering with understanding counsel and comfort are now better understood and better practised. Such measures are more readily available and palliative care has become a specialty in its own right. These specialists can now offer very much needed support in patients' physical, nutritional and emotional care so that there is little need for patients to suffer greatly from pain or other distressing symptoms of cancer. Palliative care now extends beyond immediate hospital needs into domestic, social and long-term needs of patients and their loved ones and communities (see Sects. 8.6.3 and 8.6.7).

Specialist "supportive care" teams are becoming more established to care for those cancer patients with treatment complications or patients with a good

long-term prognosis but needing active treatment other than traditional palliative care.

24.24   Hope for the Future

Oncology is an exciting but continuously evolving study with constant progress
in understanding, prevention, investigation and management. This includes a
constant search for better treatment agents and treatment methods. There is now
an increasing plethora of names of chemotherapeutic, hormonal, immunological,
and anti-enzyme anti-cancer agents and gene therapy. Some are of historic interest, some are presently in clinical use, some are under study in clinical trials
and some are still confined to laboratory investigation. Students are advised that
agents and protocols for use of agents are constantly changing. Newer agents and
newer techniques inevitably replace older ones. With constant progress in cancer
research and treatment schedules some names, doses and treatment programs
of today will become outdated. What we have learned today may have to be
changed or added to tomorrow. We must never stop being students.

The Western medical model of health care and education is complex. Some
of its main areas of speciality include medicine, surgery, pathology, radiotherapy
and palliation with further specialisations within each of these. In a medical
system of such complexity it is not possible, nor indeed necessary, for individual
practitioners, researchers or teachers to keep abreast of all areas of progress.
However it is the responsibility of all of us, both those caring directly for patients
and those teaching future doctors and health professionals, to seek the optimum
treatment for our patients and we can do this by either working in or keeping in
contact with collaborative teams that provide the range of skills to offer best care
to our patients.

The probability or possibility of cure or prevention is now available for
increasing numbers of patients with cancer and for some currently considered
incurable, new prospects of cure may be around the corner.

Further Reading

Traditional detailed teaching of cancer for students includes study of each cancer under sub-headings including *introduction, incidence, causes, symptoms, signs, pathology, clinical investigations, prevention, treatment, complications, prognosis, follow-up or long-term care and record-keeping.* Details of treatment included could be *surgical procedures, radiotherapy indications and techniques and medical management involving drugs, hormones or other agents used, their indications, doses, treatment schedules as well as special nursing, dietary, social and community care requirements and facilities.* To cover all known information about each cancer recorded in one book this way would not be possible and would require many volumes and indeed before it could be published much would already be outdated.

In this book a limited number of drugs and techniques only can be mentioned to help establish principles of cancer-care and understanding. Some likely future directions are also suggested but practitioners will need to be constantly updated as years pass.

Many books and multitudes of papers are available for further reading on different aspects of cancer, according to more specific needs or at a more advanced level.

Some we recommend are:

Aigner KR, "Regional chemotherapy". Regional Cancer Treatment, Editorial Review 2000; 55–66.

Aigner KR, Santinami M, "Regional chemotherapy for pelvic, rectal and urologic tumours". Regional Cancer Treatment 1994; 7: 1.

Allen-Mersh TG, Earlam S, Fordy C et al., "Quality of life and survival with continuous hepatic artery floxuridine infusion for colorectal liver metastases". Lancet 1994; 344: 1255–1260.

Andersson I, "Mammographic screening under age 50: A review". Breast 2000; 9: 125–129.

Bishop JF, "Cancer Facts". Harwood Academic, Singapore, 1999.

Bismuth H, Adam R, "Resection of non-resectable liver metastases from colorectal cancer after oxaliplatin chemotherapy". Seminars in Oncology 1996; 224: 509–522.

Bonadonna GN, Hortobagyi GN, Gianni AM, "Textbook of breast cancer". Dunitz, London, 1997.

Brennan MF, "Management of extremity soft tissue sarcoma". European Journal Surgical Oncology 1989; 158: 71–77.

Buthiau D, Khayat, "Virtual endoscopy". Springer, New York, 1999.

Buthiou D, Khayat D, "CT and MRI in oncology". Springer, New York, 1998.

Casper ES, Gaynor JJ, Harrison LB, et al. "Preoperative and postoperative adjuvant combination chemotherapy for adults with high-grade soft tissue sarcoma". Cancer 1994; 73: 1644–1651.

Chow WH, Johansen C, Gridley G, et al. "Gallstones, cholecystectomy and risk of cancers of the liver biliary tract and pancreas". British Journal of Cancer 1999; 79: 640–644.

Coates A, Rumpke P, Systemic chemotherapy – new strategies. In: "Malignant Melanoma", Lejeune, Chaudhiri, DasGupta (eds.). McGraw-Hill, New York, 1994: 287–294.

Cox K, "Doctor and patient – exploring clinical thinking", University of NSW Press, Sydney, 1999.

Cristofanilli M, Charnsangavej C, Hortobagyi GN, "Angiogenesis modulation in cancer research – novel clinical approaches". Nature Reviews 2002; 1: 415–426.

Dart DA, Picksley SM, Cooper PA, Double JA, Bibby MC, "The role of p53 in chemotherapeutic responses to cisplatin, doxorubicin and 5-flurouracil treatment" International Journal of Oncology 2004; 24: 115–125.

Dawson AE, Mulford DK, Taylor AS, et al. "Breast carcinoma detection in women age 35 years and younger: Mammography and diagnosis by fine needle aspiration cytology". Cancer 1998; 84: 163–168.

DeVita V, Jr., Hellman S (eds.), "Principles and practice of oncology, 6th edn." Lippincott Williams and Wilkins, Philadelphia, PA, 2001.

Dowell SP, McGoogan E, Picksley SM, et al. "Expression of p21, WAF1/CIP1,MDM2 and p53 in vivo: Analysis of cytological specimens". Cytopathology 1996; 7: 340–351.

Early Breast Cancer Trialists' Collaborative Group, "Tamoxifen for early breast cancer. An overview of the randomised trials". Lancet 1998; 351: 1451–1467.

Eckardt A, "Intra-arterial chemotherapy in head and neck cancer". Einhorn-Presse, Reinbek, 1999.

Eggermont AM, Schraffordt Koops H, Leinard D, et al. "Isolated limb perfusion with high dose tumour necrosis factor in combination with interferon-gamma and melphalan for non-resectable extremity soft tissue sarcomas: a multicentre trial". Journal of Clinical Oncology 1996; 14: 2653–2655.

Elting Linda S, Shih Ya-Chen Tina, "The economic burden of supportive care of cancer patients". Supportive Cancer Care 2004; 12: 219–226.

Fisher B, Constantino J, Redmond C, et al. "Lumpectomy compared with lumpectomy and radiation therapy for the treatment of intraductal breast cancer" New England Journal of Medicine 1993; 328: 1591–1596.

Fossa SD, Droz JP, Stoter G, et al. "Cisplatin, vincristine and ifosphamide combination chemotherapy of metastatic seminoma: Results of EORCT trial 30874". British Journal of Cancer 1995; 71: 619–624.

Girard P, Decroux M, Baldeyrou P, et al, "Surgery for lung metastases from colorectal cancer." Journal of Clinical Oncololgy 1996; 14: 2047–2053.

Greenberg PAC, Hortobagyi GN, Smith TL, et al. "Long-term follow-up of patients with complete remission following combination chemotherapy for metastatic breast cancer". Journal of Clinical Oncololgy 1996; 14(8): 2197–2205.

Griffiths K, Adlercreutz H, Boyle P, et al. "Nutrition and cancer". Isis Medical Media, Saxon Beck, Oxford, UK, 1996.

Harker G, "Evaluation of intra-arterial versus intravenous cisplatin infusion on sheep epidermal cancer cell model". Regional Cancer Treatment 1993(Suppl 1): 26.

Harnett P, "Oncology: A case based manuel, 1st edn." Oxford University Press, New York, 1999.

Hortobagyi GN, Khayat D, "Progress in anti-cancer chemotherapy, Vol III". Springer, New York, 1999.

Hortobagyi GN, "Drug therapy : Treatment of breast cancer", New England Journal of Medicine 1998; 339(14):974–984.

Hortobagyi GN, "Long-term results of combined modality therapy for metastases. The University of Texas M. D. Cancer Center Experience". Journal of Clinical Oncology 2001; 19(3): 628–633.

Hortobagyi GN, Buzdar AU, Frye D, et al. Primary chemotherapy for breast cancer: Response to pre-operative chemotherapy as a prognostic factor. In "Cancer Treatment an Update", Banzet, Holland, Khayat, Weil (eds.). Springer, Paris, 1994: 106–109.

Ivan Damjanov, "Anderson's Pathology, 10th edn". Mosby, St Louis, 1996.

Kemeny Nancy, Huang Y, Cohen AM, et al. "Hepatic arterial infusion of chemotherapy after resection of hepatic metastases from colo-rectal cancer". New England Journal of Medicine 1999; 341: 2039–2048.

Khayat D, Waxman J, Antoine EC, "Cancer chemotherapy treatment protocols". Blackwell Science, London, 1998.

Khayat D, "The many causes of quality of life deficits in cancer patients". International Journal of Pharmaceutical Medicine 2000; 14: 70–73.

Klein ES, Berkenstadt H, Koller M, Paoa MZ, Ben Ari GY, Lieberman N, Klein ES, He W, Shmizu S, Asculai S, Falk RE, Ben-Ari GY. "Hyaluronic acid on experimental tumor uptake of 5-flourouracil". Regional Cancer Treatment 1994; 7: 163–164.

Kune GA, "Causes of colorectal cancer". Kluwer, Boston, 1996.

Lai D, Fulham M, Stephen M, et al. "The role of whole-positron emission tomography with [18F] fluorodeoxyglucose in identifying operable colorectal cancer metastases to the liver" Archives of Surgery 1996; 131: 703–707.

LeJeune, Chaudhuri, DasGupta, "New strategies in malignant melanoma". McGraw-Hill, New York, 1994.

Lickiss J Norelle, Principles of palliative care. In "Cancer facts", James Bishop (ed.). Harwood Academic, NJ, 1999.

Link KH, Aigner KR, Pillasch J, et al. "Individual chemo-sensitivity testing for regional chemotherapy in a prospective correlative and a prospective decision aiding test". Regional Cancer Treatment 1993; 6: 113–120.

Lord RVN, Frommer DJ, Inder S, et al. "Prevalence of *Helicobacter pylori* infection in 160 patients with Barrett's oesophagus or Barrett's adenocarcinoma". The Australian and New Zealand Journal of Surgery 2000; 70: 26–33.

Marks R, Hill D, "Melanoma control" UICC, Geneva, 1992.

Menzies SW, Crotty KA, Ingvar C, McCarthy WH, "An atlas of surface microscopy of pigmented skin lesions". McGraw-Hill, Sydney, 1996.

Morris DL, Kearsley DL, Williams CJ, "Cancer: A comprehensive clinical guide, 1st edn." Harwood Academic, Amsterdam, 1998.

Morris DL, Ross WB, Igbal J, et al. "Cryoablation of hepatic malignancy. An evaluation of tumour marker data and survival in 110 patients". GI Cancer 1996; 1: 247–251.

Ngan SY, Burmeister BH, Fisher R, et al. "A phase II trial of preoperative radiotherapy with protracted infusion 5-FU for resectable adenocarcinoma of rectum: A multicentre trial for the Trans-Tasman Radiation Oncology Group". International Journal of Radiation Oncology Biology Physics 2000; 48(3): 119–120.

Nishio M, Kawakara K, Tamaki T, "Application of PET-CT for diagnosis of cancer". Japanese Journal of Cancer and Chemotherapy 2005; 32(8): 1091–1095.

Parsonnet J, "Helicobecter pylori and gastric cancer". Gastroenterology Clinics of North America 1993; 22: 89–104.

Perel A, "Hemodynamic effects of aortic stop flow and total abdominal ischemic perfusion". Regional Cancer Treatment 1994; 7: 82–85.

Peterson DE, Elias EG, Sonis ST, "Head and neck management of the cancer patient". Kluwer, Boston, 1986.

Picksley SM, Lane DP, "p53 and Rb their cellular roles". Current Opinion in Cell Biology 1994; 6: 853–858.

Picksley SM, Dart DA, Mansoor MS, Loadman PM, "Current advances in the inhibition of the autoregulatory interaction between the p53 tumour suppressor and MDM2 protein". Expert Opinion on Therapeutics Patents 2001; 11: 1825–1835.

Pizzo PA, Poplack DG (eds.),"Principles and practice of pediatric oncology, 3rd edn." Lippincott-Raven, Philadelphia, 1997.

Pollock RE, "Manual of clinical oncology, 7th edn." Wiley Liss, New York, 1999.

Rose BR, Thompson CH, Tattersall MH, et al. "Squamous carcinoma of the head and neck: Molecular mechanisms and potential biomarkers". The Australian and New Zealand Journal of Surgery 2000; 70: 601–606.

Souhami R, Tobias J, "Cancer and its management, 5th edn." Blackwell, Oxford, 2005.

Spence RAJ, "Oncology, 1st edn." Oxford University Press, New York, 2001.

Stephens FO, "The cancer prevention manual". Oxford University Press, Oxford, England, 2002.

Stephens FO, "All about prostate cancer". Oxford University Press, Melbourne, 2000.

Stephens FO, "All about breast cancer". Oxford University Press, Melbourne 2001.

Stephens FO, "Induction chemotherapy: The place and techniques of using chemotherapy to downgrade aggressive or advanced localised cancers to make them potentially more curable by surgery and/or radiotherapy". European Journal of Surgical Oncology 2001; 27: 627–688.

Stephens FO, "The rising incidence of breast cancer in women and prostate cancer in men. Dietary influence. A possible preventative role for nature's sex hormone modifiers, the phytoestrogens". Oncology Reports 1999; 6: 865–870.

Stephens FO, "The case for a name change from neoadjuvant chemotherapy to induction chemotherapy". Cancer 1989; 63: 1245–1246.

Sugarbaker PH, "Management of gastric cancer". Kluwer, Boston, 1991.

Sugarbaker PH, Malawer MM (eds.), "Musculoskeletal surgery for cancer". Thieme Medical, New York, 1992.

Taguchi T, Nakamura H, "Arterial infusion chemotherapy". Japan Journal of Cancer and Chemotherapy Pub. Inc., 1994.

Tanock, Peckhan, "Oxford textbook of oncology". Oxford University Press, Oxford, 2001.

Thomas L, Delannes M, Matel P, "Intra-operative interstitial brachytherapy in the management of soft tissue sarcomas: Prelimary results of a feasibility Phase II study". Radiotherapy and Oncology 1994; 33: 99–105.

Thompson JC, Waugh RRC, Saw RPM, Kam P, "Isolated limb infusion (ILI) with melphalan for recurrent limb melanoma". Regional Cancer Treatment 1993(Suppl 1): 51–52.

Toner G, Stockler MR, Boyer MJ, Jones M, et al. "Comparison of two standard chemotherapy regimens for good prognosis germ cell tumours: A randomised trial". Lancet 2001; 357: 739–745.

Veronesi U, Paganelli G, Galimberti V, et al. "Sentinel node biopsy to avoid axillary dissection in breast cancer with clinically negative lymph nodes". Lancet 1997; 349: 1864–1867.

Veronisi U, Saccozzi R, DelVecchio M, et al. "Comparing radical mastectomy with quadrantectomy, axillary dissection and radiotherapy in patients with small cancers of the breast". New England Journal of Medicine 1981; 305: 6–11.

Voute PA, Kaiifa C, Barrett A (eds.), "Cancer in children: Clinical management, 4th edn." Oxford University Press, Oxford, 1998.

Wanebo H (ed.), "Surgery for gastrointestinal cancer: A multidisciplenary approach", Lippincott Williams and Wilkins, Philadelphia, PA, 2001.

Whiting JL, Hallissey MT, Fielding JWL, Dunn J, "Screening for gastric cancer by Helicobacter pylori serology: A retrospective study". British Journal of Surgery 1998; 85: 408–411.

www.cancerhelp.org.uk

Yu W, Whang I, Averbach A, Chang D, Sugarbaker PH, "Prospective randomized trial of early post-operative intra-peritoneal chemotherapy as an adjuvant to resectable gastric cancer". Annals of Surgery 1998; 223(3): 347–357.

Zhao-You Tang, "Results of treatment of primary liver cancer in China". Regional Cancer Treatment 1992; 5:136–139.

Glossary

Acute	Having a sudden onset.
Adenoma	A benign (not malignant) tumour in which the cells are derived from glands or from glandular epithelium (such as the lining of the stomach).
Adenocarcinoma	A cancer of glandular cells.
Adjuvant Chemotherapy	Chemotherapy given after operative surgery to help ensure complete eradication of all cancer cells.
Allele	One of two or more alternative forms of a gene.
Anaemia	A blood condition with a reduction in the amount of haemoglobin carried in the blood.
Anaplasia	More extreme abnormality of cells. Cancer cells are described as being anaplastic when they have lost the special features of the cells from which they developed. Anaplastic cells tend to grow and invade more aggressively. They more readily invade surrounding tissues and more readily spread to other places to form metastases.
Angiogram	An X-ray of blood vessels (see arteriogram).
Anorexia	A feeling of not wanting to eat (lack of hunger) or early satiety.
Antibody	A type of protein produced by the immune system that recognises invading organisms or other substances as foreign. The antibody attaches itself to the foreign or invading substance in an attempt to destroy it.
Apoptosis	An inbuilt ability of cells to undergo self-destruction after they have served their function; part of the ageing process of death and replacement and turnover of ageing cells during normal life. Cancer cells seem to have lost this inbuilt self-limiting life process.
Arteriogram	A radiograph (X-ray photograph) of an artery taken after injection of an iodine-based radio-opaque substance into an artery.
Aspiration	Act of sucking up or sucking out.

Ascites	Accumulation of abnormal amounts of fluid in the abdominal cavity.
Astrocytoma	A malignant tumour of connective tissue cells in the brain.
Atrophic	Wasted; degenerate; having lost special qualities.
Atrophy	Wasting away; losing special qualities (verb or noun).
Axilla	Armpit.
Bacteria	Germs. Microscopic organisms usually consisting of one cell only that normally occur in skin, mouth and the alimentary tract of humans and all animal species. Some bacteria are toxic and some tend to invade body organs or tissues causing damage and illness.
Barium Enema or Baryum Enema (French)	Similar to a barium (baryum) meal except that the radiopaque/contrast material is introduced via a tube through the anus to allow X-ray films and X-ray screening of the rectum and large bowel.
Barium Meal or (Baryum French) Meal	A test that involves swallowing a liquid containing the radio-opaque element – barium. This allows radiographs (X-rays) to be taken to show the size and shape of organs such as the stomach or duodenum.
Barium Swallow (Baryum Swollow)	Similar to a barium meal except that while the material is being swallowed, the shape and outline of the oesophagus can be studied.
Basal	The lowest part of a structure forming its base. The basal layer of the skin consists of the deep cells from which the upper or more superficial cells grow.
BCC	Basal cell carcinoma. A slowly growing skin cancer that has grown from the basal (deep) layer of skin cells.
BCG	Bacillus Calmette-Guerin. A bacterial preparation originally used as an active immunising agent against tuberculosis. It consists of harmless living organisms that promote a similar body defence action to that of tuberculosis bacteria. It is also used in the bladder as an immune stimulating agent against benign papillomata and non-invasive carcinoma.
Benign	Not malignant; favourable for recovery; unlikely to be dangerous. A benign tumour is one that remains localised and does not invade or destroy the tissue in which it originates and does not spread to distant sites in the body.

Benign Mammary Dysplasia	A condition of the breasts that is likely to cause cysts and other benign lumps in the breasts. This condition is probably more widely known as fibro-cystic disease, but other names are fibro-adenosis-cystica, hormonal mastopathy or "chronic mastitis". Cells in dysplastic tissues are not themselves malignant or pre-malignant but when a cancer develops in a breast with lumpy dysplastic changes it may be more difficult to identify. They do have a small but significantly greater potential for malignant change.
Biopsy	The removal of a small sample of tissue for microscopic examination.
Block Dissection	Total surgical excision of a whole group of lymph nodes in one piece of tissue.
Brachytherapy	A method of applying radiotherapy by placement of tiny radioactive pellets (seeds) or wires or needles directly into a tumour to destroy it.
Buccal Mucosa	The lining of the cheek in the mouth.
Calcitonin	A hormone produced by certain cells (C cells) in the thyroid gland. Calcitonin lowers the level of calcium and phosphates in the blood.
Cancer	A malignant growth of cells. A continuous, purposeless, unwanted and uncontrolled growth of cells that actually or potentially has power to invade and damage surrounding tissues and of metastasising to distant tissues or organs.
Cachexia	The wasting condition often associated with terminal cancer due to abnormal metabolism of glucose.
Capsule	The fibrous or membranous sac-like covering that encloses a tissue or organ.
Carcinogen	A substance that causes cancer.
Carcinoma	Cancer. More specifically a cancer of epithelial lining cells or of glandular cells.
Cervix Uteri	The neck of the uterus; the entrance of the womb.
Chemotherapy	Treatment with chemical agents or drugs.
Chronic	Persisting for a long time; having a long or protracted course.
Chronic Atrophic Gastritis	A gradual and persistent degeneration of the lining of the stomach.
Colostomy	An opening made surgically between the large bowel (colon) and the abdominal wall to allow evacuation of faeces when the lower bowel is blocked.
Congenital	Present from the time of birth.

Corynebacterium parvum	A harmless bacterium sometimes A bacterium used to stimulate an immune reaction defence reactions.
Cryotherapy	The use of cold or freezing as treatment.
Crohn's Disease	A chronic granular inflammatory condition that may affect the small intestine, the large intestine or both. It was first described by Dr Dalziel in Scotland and thoroughly studied and reported by Dr Crohn in America (see granulomatous colitis).
CT Scan	CAT scan or computerised axial tomography; a method of visualising body tissues by using computerised radiographic techniques. These give X-ray "pictures" of sections of body tissues.
Cytokines	Protein molecules released by cells when activated by an antigen. Cytokines are involved in cell-to-cell communication as enhancing mediators for immune responses through interaction with specific cell-surface receptors on white blood cells. Interleukins are cytokines produced by leukocytes. Interferons are cytokines produced by lymphocytes. Lymphokines and tumour necrosis factor (TNF) are also cytokines.
Cytotoxic	Having a toxic or harmful effect upon cells.
DNA	Deoxyribonucleic acid. The material from which the genes and chromosomes in body cells are made.
Dysplasia	An abnormal development of tissues. Dysplastic tissues are not in themselves malignant but have an increased potential for malignant change.
Endocrine Gland	A gland that secretes its product into the blood stream for wide distribution in the body. The thyroid, the pituitary and adrenal glands are examples.
Endoscope	An instrument used for visual examination of the interior of hollow organs or the interior of body cavities.
Epidemiology	The branch of medicine that deals with the distribution of diseases, their causes and the ways in which they appear and spread in different population groups and at different periods of time.
Epidemiological	To do with epidemiology.
Erythropoietin	A hormone secreted by certain cells in the kidneys to increase rate of red cell production.
ESR (erythrocyte sedimentation rate)	The rate at which red blood cells settle out of suspension in plasma. In general the ESR is raised in poor health conditions including cancer, inflammations, arthritic conditions etc.
Exocrine Gland	A gland that secretes its product through a duct into a body cavity. The parotid gland is an example.

Faeces	Waste material passed as a bowel motion. Stool, poo or shit (slang).
Familial Polyposis Coli	An inherited condition in which about half of the members of a family will develop polyps (small glandular tumours) in the wall of the large bowel. Eventually one or more of these will become malignant.
Fascia	A fibrous layer or covering.
Superficial Fascia	The fibro-fatty layer consisting mostly of fat under the skin.
Deep Fascia	The fibrous or membranous layer of tissue that covers muscles, nerves and blood vessels, or separates muscles or other tissues into different compartments.
Fibroma	A benign tumour composed of fibrous tissue and cells capable of forming fibrous tissue.
Floor of Mouth	The lower part of the mouth under the tongue.
Gastroscope	A long, thin, flexible instrument used for visual examination of the interior of the stomach.
Genome	The total genetic material of an organism, containing the genes in its chromosomes.
Germ Cells	Cells of embryonic tissue that have capacity to develop into spermatozoa or ova.
Gland	A tissue or organ that manufactures and secretes fluids and chemical substances necessary for maintenance of normal health and body function (e.g. a salivary gland secretes saliva, an adrenal gland secretes a number of hormones).
Glucan	A complex carbohydrate (type of sugar or starch) that constitutes much of the fibre in common vegetable and grain foodstuffs and has also been found to have immune stimulatory properties.
Goitre	Enlargement of the thyroid gland causing a swelling in the front part of the lower neck.
Granulomatous Colitis	A chronic inflammatory condition of the large bowel of no known cause (see Crohn's disease).
Hormone	A chemical substance produced by an endocrine gland and secreted directly into the bloodstream.
HRT	Hormone replacement therapy: Treatment with a low dose of hormones to reduce menopausal and post menopausal symptoms and other problems such as loss of calcium from bones.
Hutchinson's Freckle	A large freckle that develops slowly on the face or other sun exposed skin of elderly people. Sometimes it develops into a superficial melanoma.

Hyperkeratosis	A thickening of the flat protective surface layer of epithelium of skin or lip. The condition is usually characterised by the formation of crusts or flakes that drop off. There is a tendency for malignant changes to appear gradually and thus a skin cancer may develop.
Immunotherapy	The treatment of disease by giving immune substances or by stimulating the immune system of body defences.
Induration	Hardening or thickening of a tissue or a part of the body such as due to inflammation or infiltration with cancer.
Induction	The process of starting a change or starting something to happen. The first step in a process that will be developed.
Induction Chemotherapy	Induction chemotherapy is the use of chemotherapy to begin changes in a cancer as the first step in an integrated cancer treatment program. The cancer is usually made smaller and less aggressive by the use of induction chemotherapy, hopefully making it more curable by following treatment, usually surgery or radiotherapy or both.
Inflammation	A reaction of tissues due to injury.
Isoflavones	Members of a class of plant hormones (phytoestrogens) that are present in many plants but are especially plentiful in legumes like soybeans. The greatest known source is the red clover plant. The red clover is a legume that contains all the phytoestrogens known to be most active in human physiology.
Isotope	A different form of an element with the same chemical properties but different physical properties. Radioactive isotopes are unstable and slowly emit small amounts of irradiation and thus decay into other isotopes.
Kaposi's Sarcoma	A malignant tumour arising in blood vessels in the skin.
Kinase	An agent that can convert the inactive form of an enzyme (pro-enzyme) to the active form.
Langerhan's Cells	Cells of the immune system in skin.
Lesion	An abnormal area of tissue.
Leukocyte	A white cell. The "white" or colourless type of cell that circulates in the blood, has amoeboid movement, and is chiefly concerned with defending the body against invasion by foreign organisms.

Leukoplakia	A white patch. A condition distinguished by the presence of white thickened patches in mucous membranes, commonly in the mouth. There may be a tendency for malignant characteristics to appear gradually and thus for a cancer to develop.
Lipoma	A benign tumour composed of fat cells.
Lycopene	A recently studied anti-oxidant found in tomatoes and some other fruits that appears to have anti-cancer or cancer preventative properties. It is the red colouring component of tomatoes. Tissue culture and animal experiments suggest potential especially against prostate and breast cancer calls.
Lymphangiogram	A radiograph (X-ray photograph) of lymphatic vessels shown after injection of a radio-opaque substance (dye) into the lymphatic vessels.
Lymphocyte	One of the types of white cells that circulate in the blood and take part in immune reactions and the body's defence reactions. A mononuclear, non-granular leukocyte produced by lymph nodes and other lymphoid tissue.
Lymphoid	Resembling or pertaining to the tissue of the lymphatic system. Tissue that contains and produces lymphocytes.
Lymphoma	A malignant disease or cancer of lymphoid tissue.
Lymph Nodes	Small masses of lymphatic tissue contained in a bean shaped capsule measuring 1–25 mm. They are scattered along the course of lymph vessels and often grouped in clusters. They form an important part of the body's defence system. They function as factories for the development of lymphocytes and as filters for bacteria and foreign debris from tissue fluid. They are not glands but are sometimes referred to as lymph "glands".
Lymph Vessels or Lymphatics	Small vessels that drain tissue fluid into lymph nodes and inter-connect groups of lymph nodes. Eventually the larger lymph vessels drain this fluid into the blood stream.
Malaise	A general feeling of lassitude and ill-health; feeling unwell.
Malignant	Life threatening. A condition that in the natural course of events would become progressively worse resulting in death. A malignant growth or cancer is a growth of unwanted cells that tends to continue growing and invading, thus destroying surrounding tissues. It also tends to spread to other parts of the body causing eventual destruction of other tissues.

Malignant Fibrous Histiocytoma	A malignant tumour of histiocytes which are protective (immune) cells in soft tissues (muscles, fat etc.) or in bone.
Mediastinum	The central midline area within the chest and between the lungs. That part of the chest between the sternum (breast-bone) and the vertebrae (backbone), containing the heart, great blood vessels, trachea and oesophagus.
Medulloblastoma	An uncommon malignant brain tumour that usually develops from primitive brain cells in the cerebellar part of the brain, most commonly in children and young people.
Melanoma	A malignant tumour of pigment-producing cells most commonly arising in the skin, sometimes in the eye or occasionally elsewhere.
Menopause	The "change of life"; that time in the life of a woman when menstruation stops due to reduced activity of the ovaries and other glands. A number of other physical and emotional changes are likely to be associated.
Metaplasia	An abnormal change in a tissue, a cell or cell genes.
Metastasis	Metastatic cancer – a secondary growth of malignant cells that has spread from a primary cancer elsewhere.
Mitosis	A process of cell division in which a single cell including its nucleus and genes divide to form two identical cells.
Mitotic Figures	The numbers of dividing cells in a tissue
MRI	Magnetic resonance imaging; a special test based on certain laws of physics (electro-magnetic fields). The test allows very detailed pictures to be taken of cross sections of the trunk, head, neck or limbs. The resulting pictures are rather like those of CT scans.
Mucus	A protective slimy material secreted by certain glands and certain cells lining body cavities and hollow organs.
Mucous Membrane or Mucosa	The lining of most hollow organs and some body cavities, such as the mouth, stomach, bowel or vagina, all of which contain mucous glands and secrete protective mucus onto the surface.
Myelodysplasia	An abnormal change in bone marrow blood forming cells.
Naevus (or Nevus)	A localised collection of pigment-forming skin cells forming a circumscribed malformation, usually light or dark brown in colour, such as a mole or a birthmark.

Neoplasm	"New growth"; an abnormal growth of body cells. A neoplasm may be benign (innocent and usually harmless) with limited growth, or malignant (cancer) with continuing, unwanted and uncontrolled growth.
Neuroblastoma	A malignant tumour of primitive nerve-forming cells that usually arises in the autonomic nervous system.
Neuroma	A benign tumour composed of nerve cells.
Occult Blood	Hidden blood. Blood that cannot be seen with the naked eye but is found to be present on chemical testing.
Oesophagus	The gullet; the part of the digestive tract for passage of food from the mouth and pharynx above to the stomach below. It is a muscular tube lined with epithelium and extends from the neck, through the chest and into the abdomen
Oncology	The study of tumours and of patients suffering from tumours.
Osteomyelitis	Infection of bone. Acute osteomyelitis occurs when bacteria enter the bone via the bloodstream establishing a localised, painful swelling with fever and sometimes septicaemia. It most often occurs in children. Osteosarcoma in children can sometimes resemble acute osteomyelitis in its initial presentation.
Paget's Disease of Bone	A degenerative bone disease in which bones become thickened and disorganised.
Paget's Disease of the Nipple	A malignant condition of the nipple in which the nipple appears to develop a rash or "abrasion-like" appearance.
Palliative	Giving relief; relieving symptoms but not curing the condition.
Palliation	Relief.
Pancreas	A pale fleshy gland that lies across the back of the abdominal cavity behind the stomach. It is responsible for secreting digestive juices containing digestive enzymes into the digestive tract and for secretion of the hormone insulin into the bloodstream.
Papilloma	A benign wart like or fern like tumour derived from epithelium and projecting from an epithelial surface with a central core of small blood vessels.
PCR (Polymerase Chain Reaction).	Simple laboratory technique that involves repeat cycles of targeted replication of genes, to produce copies that can easily be analysed.

Petechiae	Small, often pinhead size, reddish or pink spots in the skin caused by minute haemorrhages. They are often associated with a deficiency of blood platelets but are sometimes associated with other conditions such as liver failure or some infections such as typhoid.
Petechial	Having to do with petechiae.
Pernicious Anaemia	A type of anaemia resulting from a failure of gastric mucosa (stomach lining) to produce a vital ingredient for making blood. This is called intrinsic factor.
PET Scan	Positron emission tomography scan. A special imaging technique that produces "pictures" of body tissues based on glucose metabolism in the cells of those tissues (cancer cells metabolise more glucose than do normal cells).
Philladelphia Chromosome	A chromosome detected in cells in patients with chronic myeloid leukaemia.
Phytoestrogens	Natural occurring oestrogen-like hormones present in all plants but in large quantities in certain leguminous plants such as soy beans. Thought to be at least partly responsible for the lower incidence of some diseases (especially breast and prostate) in people such as Asians living in Asia who have a high intake of legumes in their diets.
Platelets	Small disc-shaped particles in the blood that are essential for normal blood clotting.
Pleomorphic	Having a variety of appearances. Pleomorphic cells in a cancer are cells of different sizes shapes and other features in the cancer.
Pleura	The lining or membrane surrounding the lungs and surrounding the cavity in which the lungs move during respiration.
Polyposis Coli	A condition in which there are many polyps in the colon mucous membrane lining.
Polyp	A tumour projecting on a stalk from the mucous membrane lining the cavity of a hollow organ.
PMS	Post menopausal syndrome; symptoms of hot flushes, depression, vaginal dryness, bone wasting etc associated with menopausal changes.
PMT	Pre menstrual tension. Hormone produced emotional changes that often occur in women over a few days preceding menstruation.
Prosthesis	An artificial replacement for a missing body part.
Prosthetic	To do with a prosthesis.

PSA	Prostate specific antigen. The PSA test is a blood test to determine the amount of this special protein enzyme in the circulation. Prostate gland cells produce this enzyme and when the number of these cells is increased there is usually a raised level of PSA in the blood. High PSA levels can be an indication of the presence of prostate cancer although other non malignant conditions, especially prostate hyperplasia and prostatitis, can also cause the PSA level to be raised.
Radical	Extreme or very extensive. A radical mastectomy is removal of the whole breast together with lymph nodes in the axilla and other nearby tissues.
Radio-Opaque Material	A substance that does not allow penetration of X-rays. It thus shows as a white area on an X-ray film. It is commonly referred to as "dye".
Radiotherapy	Treatment with X-rays or gamma rays.
Reticulo-Endothelial System	Special defensive cells that form part of the immune system. These cells protect the body against foreign materials and invading organisms. The cells are predominantly found in bone marrow, spleen, liver and lymph nodes but are also found in other tissues such as skin and soft tissues and the wall of stomach and bowel.
Retinoblastoma	A rare malignant tumour of the eye retina that occurs in infants. Mono-lateral forms represent sporadic tumours, and bilateral forms are familial.
Sarcoma	A cancer that arises and develops in connective tissues such as muscle, fat, fascia or bone.
Science	The study of truth or fact; provable information.
Scientific Methods	Methods of determining what is truth as opposed to what might be unproven beliefs, theories, assumptions or concepts. The most accepted form of scientific method is to propose a hypothesis and then present it for scrutiny or testing. Different methods are used for testing hypotheses in different situations.
	In medicine the most commonly used method of scientific analysis is to propose a hypothesis and subject it to scrutiny by making statistical comparison with one other, or several other, concepts in the same field. The hypothesis is then further tested, by determining whether information gained will reliably give the same results when tested in different circumstances

Screening Test	A relatively simple, safe, inexpensive and easily performed test that can be carried out on large numbers of people to determine whether they are likely to have a cancer or other serious disease.
Sentinel Node	The lymph node into which tissue fluid first drains from a tissue via lymphatics.
Side Effect	An effect other than the effect wanted.
Sigmoidoscope	A sigmoidoscope may be a rigid, hollow metal tube or a long flexible tube containing multiple fibre-optic channels.
Sigmoidoscopy	Passage of a sigmoidoscope through the anus to allow visual examination of the inside of the lower bowel and biopsy of suspicious areas.
Squamous	Flat, like a scale or pavement. Squamous cells are flat scale-like cells that cover the skin, the mouth, throat, oesophagus, vagina and some other cavities.
Stem Cells	Cells that have the capacity to develop into all cells within the organ and repair or replace organ tissue; immortal, undifferentiated and uncommitted cells. Most commonly used in reference to stem cells in bone marrow.
STI 571	Code name for an agent that counteracts tyrosine-kinase, an enzyme involved in cellular changes of some cancer cells, especially chronic myeloid leukaemia. Generit name, imatinib. Trade name, glivec or gleevec.
Tamoxifen	A drug that combines with oestrogen receptors of cells thus "blocking" the attachment of oestrogen to the cells.
Telangectasia	A collection of distended capillaries in skin giving a red lacework pattern or "spidery" localised appearance to an area of skin.
Therapy	Treatment.
Tissue	A layer or group of cells of particular specialised types that together perform a special function.
Toxic	Poisonous.
Transcription Factor	A protein transferred from DNA to RNA that is responsible for the first step in manufacture of cellular proteins.
Trauma	Injury (e.g. broken bones) or response to surgery or sepsis.
Traumatised or Traumatized	Injured.

Tumour	A swelling or lump. Commonly used to describe a swelling caused by a growth of cells—a new growth or neoplasm that may be a cancer.
Ulcer	A deficiency or hole in a covering or lining such as a hole in lining of skin or a mucous membrane.
Ulcerative Colitis	An inflammatory condition of the large bowel characterised by small ulcers in the bowel lining and causing episodes of diarrhoea, often with blood loss.
Ultrasound	High frequency sound waves that cannot be heard by the human ear.
Uterus	The womb. The organ in the female pelvis in which a foetus develops.
Varicose Ulcer	An ulcer in the skin, usually on the lower leg, caused by poor circulation in the tissues due to long standing varicose veins.

Appendix

Table A.1 Worldwide incidence of more common cancers: male

	Brain/ nervous system	Thyroid	Non-Hodgkin lymphoma	Hodgkin disease	Leukaemia	Multiple myeloma
World	3.6	1.2	6.1	1.3	5.2	1.5
More developed countries	5.9	1.8	10.3	2.3	7.9	2.7
Less developed countries	2.8	1.0	4.3	1.0	3.9	0.9
Eastern Africa	0.7	1.6	7.9	2.1	3.9	0.9
Middle Africa	0.1	1.1	4.4	0.8	1.2	1.5
Northern Africa	2.5	0.8	4.8	2.0	4.3	0.8
Southern Africa	1.5	0.9	4.8	0.9	3.7	1.6
South Africa	*1.6*	*1.0*	*5.0*	*0.9*	*3.7*	*1.6*
Western Africa	0.4	0.7	7.3	1.7	2.4	0.9
Caribbean	3.4	0.8	4.9	2.0	6.6	2.7
Central America	4.5	1.2	5.2	2.0	6.3	2.2
South America	4.8	1.8	6.9	1.4	5.8	1.9
Argentina	*4.2*	*1.5*	*8.1*	*1.5*	*6.9*	*1.8*
Brazil	6.0	2.1	6.6	1.3	5.5	1.7
USA	**6.5**	**3.0**	**16.1**	**2.3**	**9.6**	**4.0**
Canada	6.8	2.3	14.6	2.7	10.4	4.3
Eastern Asia	3.5	0.8	3.7	0.3	4.6	0.8
China	*3.6*	*0.7*	*2.9*	*0.2*	*4.3*	*0.6*
Hong Kong	4.4	2.1	8.7	0.6	6.7	1.7
Japan	2.7	1.4	7.4	0.4	5.9	1.8
Korea	3.7	1.4	6.6	0.8	5.2	0.8
S.E. Asia	1.6	1.4	5.2	0.7	4.3	0.8
Indonesia	*1.4*	*1.2*	*6.0*	*0.7*	*4.4*	*1.3*
Malaysia	2.1	1.9	7.7	1.1	6.1	2.0
Philippines	2.5	2.5	4.9	0.7	6.0	0.8
Singapore	2.5	1.9	7.5	0.7	6.2	1.3
Thailand	1.9	1.1	3.7	0.6	3.3	0.3

(continued)

Table A.1 (continued)

	Brain/ nervous system	Thyroid	Non-Hodgkin lymphoma	Hodgkin disease	Leukaemia	Multiple myeloma
South Central Asia	2.4	1.0	3.4	1.3	3.0	0.9
India	*2.6*	*1.0*	*3.2*	*1.1*	*3.1*	*1.0*
Pakistan	3.4	1.2	5.1	2.8	3.4	0.9
Saudi Arabia	3.9	2.9	10.0	3.3	6.0	2.2
Turkey	3.8	0.8	5.7	1.3	6.5	0.9
United Arab Emirates	4.6	2.4	5.7	6.0	4.8	2.0
Eastern Europe	5.8	1.5	6.6	2.9	6.6	1.5
Russian Federation	5.7	1.5	6.0	2.7	6.1	1.4
Northern Europe	7.0	1.0	10.1	2.1	8.7	3.2
Denmark	*7.0*	*1.3*	*9.7*	*2.1*	*8.6*	*3.6*
Ireland	7.3	1.0	10.4	2.1	9.2	4.2
Norway	8.0	1.6	10.7	2.2	8.2	3.7
Sweden	11.1	1.7	10.6	2.0	10.5	3.5
UK	6.4	0.7	10.4	2.0	8.8	3.2
Southern Europe	6.8	1.2	9.2	2.5	8.0	2.8
Italy	*6.3*	*1.8*	*12.3*	*3.1*	*8.7*	*3.4*
Greece	10.6	0.8	5.6	4.9	8.8	2.3
Spain	6.5	0.5	8.3	1.6	8.0	2.6
Western Europe	6.5	1.7	11.1	2.9	8.9	3.2
France	*5.7*	*1.4*	*12.8*	*2.3*	*8.7*	*3.4*
Germany	7.0	2.0	10.5	3.0	9.2	3.0
Netherlands	6.2	1.0	10.7	2.1	8.5	4.2
Australia	**7.0**	**2.2**	**14.4**	**2.1**	**10.3**	**4.0**
New Zealand	**8.6**	**1.7**	**14.0**	**1.9**	**11.8**	**5.1**
Melanesia	0.4	1.3	8.0	0.7	3.8	0.2
Polynesia	2.3	4.6	8.4	1.1	7.6	2.0

Table A.1 (continued)

	Oral cavity	Naso-pharynx	Oro-pharynx	Oeso-phagus	Stomach	Colon/rectum
World	6.4	1.7	3.8	10.8	21.5	19.1
More developed countries	7.6	0.7	4.8	6.7	24.6	37.3
Less developed countries	6.0	2.0	3.5	12.8	19.9	9.9
Eastern Africa	5.9	1.6	2.6	10.4	7.1	7.2
Middle Africa	4.8	0.7	1.3	1.9	17.0	2.0
Northern Africa	3.5	2.8	1.0	2.7	5.6	6.5
Southern Africa	12.4	1.6	1.5	17.6	8.6	12.7
South Africa	*11.3*	*1.6*	*1.2*	*16.4*	*8.8*	*13.7*
Western Africa	2.4	0.4	0.4	1.1	5.4	4.3
Caribbean	7.7	0.8	3.9	6.7	14.5	15.5
Central America	3.8	0.4	2.0	3.1	18.6	9.5
South America	7.4	0.4	4.7	8.3	23.1	15.6
Argentina	*6.5*	*0.3*	*2.1*	*8.6*	*12.8*	*27.9*
Brazil	10.5	0.6	7.9	10.8	21.6	13.6
USA	**6.3**	**0.6**	**3.1**	**4.9**	**7.6**	**40.6**
Canada	**7.4**	**0.8**	**2.9**	**4.1**	**9.1**	**40.8**
Eastern Asia	1.7	2.6	0.6	21.8	42.6	17.8
China	*1.2*	*3.0*	*0.4*	*24.5*	*36.1*	*13.0*
Hong Kong	4.8	25.2	2.6	14.2	19.4	35.0
Japan	4.0	0.5	1.8	10.0	69.2	43.2
Korea	3.3	0.5	1.1	10.1	70.0	14.9
S.E. Asia	3.6	5.8	2.3	3.1	8.7	12.6
Indonesia	*1.5*	*5.7*	*0.7*	*0.6*	*3.5*	*11.9*
Malaysia	2.4	9.7	1.5	3.0	12.1	25.7
Philippines	5.8	6.4	2.3	2.5	9.2	18.1
Singapore	3.7	15.0	2.5	5.9	21.4	37.9
Thailand	5.3	3.5	3.3	3.7	4.9	10.3
South Central Asia	13.0	0.6	8.8	8.5	6.6	4.8
India	*12.8*	*0.5*	*9.6*	*7.6*	*5.7*	*4.7*
Pakistan	14.7	1.2	6.7	6.3	3.8	5.0
Western Asia	3.7	1.4	1.2	2.4	11.2	11.4
Saudi Arabia	3.7	3.4	1.2	3.9	6.6	7.7
Turkey	3.5	0.9	1.5	2.2	10.5	9.1
United Arab Emirates	2.9	2.8	1.0	2.8	6.1	9.4
Eastern Europe	7.8	0.7	5.3	7.2	34.1	32.9
Russian Federation	7.7	0.7	5.1	9.0	42.9	31.8
Northern Europe	5.0	0.4	2.2	7.4	12.7	34.7
Denmark	*7.7*	*0.3*	*3.4*	*6.4*	*8.4*	*38.8*

(continued)

Table A.1 (continued)

	Oral cavity	Naso-pharynx	Oro-pharynx	Oeso-phagus	Stomach	Colon/rectum
Ireland	5.9	0.6	2.8	8.6	12.9	44.2
Norway	5.8	0.3	2.2	3.2	11.6	40.0
Sweden	4.5	0.3	1.7	3.1	8.8	33.0
UK	4.4	0.4	1.9	8.9	12.4	35.4
Southern Europe	9.2	0.9	4.9	4.7	19.5	32.9
Italy	*6.7*	*0.9*	*3.8*	*4.0*	*19.9*	*35.3*
Greece	3.0	0.5	1.7	1.6	11.6	17.4
Spain	13.8	1.0	6.1	6.1	17.9	32.0
Western Europe	12.6	0.8	10.6	7.7	13.8	42.1
France	*14.9*	*0.7*	*19.2*	*11.9*	*11.1*	*39.8*
Germany	13.2	1.0	7.7	5.8	16.2	45.0
Netherlands	5.8	0.5	3.0	6.4	12.9	41.6
Australia	**13.6**	**0.6**	**3.2**	**5.2**	**9.6**	**49.9**
New Zealand	**4.6**	**0.7**	**2.0**	**5.4**	**10.9**	**55.3**
Melanesia	36.3	0.2	1.5	3.1	5.9	9.2
Polynesia	5.2	2.8	4.9	3.9	13.0	14.3

Table A.1 (continued)

	Larynx	Lung	Melanoma	Prostate	Testis	Bladder
World	5.5	34.9	2.2	21.2	1.6	10.0
More developed countries	7.7	55.6	6.7	46.7	5.0	18.9
Less developed countries	4.5	24.8	0.8	7.7	0.8	5.5
Eastern Africa	3.4	3.1	1.8	14.8	0.5	4.9
Middle Africa	2.0	5.7	3.0	25.4	0.1	2.5
Northern Africa	5.2	15.4	0.9	7.2	0.7	25.3
Southern Africa	6.4	23.8	6.0	41.1	0.7	12.1
South Africa	*5.7*	*25.5*	*6.4*	*42.8*	*0.7*	*13.4*
Western Africa	0.7	2.2	1.2	17.8	0.5	3.2
Caribbean	7.0	28.8	0.9	38.6	0.8	7.5
Central America	5.1	22.7	2.1	26.9	1.5	5.2
South America	7.3	25.3	3.1	28.5	2.2	8.6
Argentina	*8.5*	*40.8*	*4.1*	*29.4*	*4.3*	*14.7*
Brazil	9.3	25.0	3.5	28.7	1.6	8.5
USA	*5.3*	*58.7*	*13.3*	*104.3*	*4.0*	*23.4*
Canada	*5.0*	*55.1*	*8.2*	*83.9*	*3.9*	*17.9*
Eastern Asia	2.3	39.4	0.3	3.4	0.5	5.0
China	*1.7*	*38.5*	*0.2*	*1.7*	*0.4*	*3.9*
Hong Kong	7.8	74.7	1.0	7.6	1.3	14.3
Japan	3.2	40.3	0.4	11.1	1.3	9.2
Korea	10.0	31.1	0.3	4.2	0.6	9.5
S.E. Asia	3.8	27.8	0.4	7.1	0.8	4.0
Indonesia	*2.0*	*20.8*	*0.5*	*7.0*	*0.9*	*4.0*
Malaysia	3.6	35.6	0.4	11.7	1.1	6.0
Philippines	5.8	51.6	0.8	18.8	0.8	4.1
Singapore	5.4	47.5	0.4	13.8	1.1	7.1
Thailand	3.3	26.0	0.4	4.4	0.4	5.2
South Central Asia	7.1	11.6	0.4	4.3	0.7	4.2
India	*6.2*	*9.0*	*0.3*	*4.6*	*0.6*	*3.2*
Pakistan	8.5	20.1	0.2	5.6	0.7	8.8
Western Asia	8.1	31.2	1.3	9.1	1.6	12.7
Saudi Arabia	2.8	10.3	0.6	7.9	0.8	8.2
Turkey	10.2	40.1	1.0	6.9	1.9	11.6
United Arab Emirates	3.1	15.1	0.4	9.7	0.9	6.4
Eastern Europe	12.1	69.7	5.2	19.4	6.4	17.7
Russian Federation	13.0	74.9	5.4	15.9	6.4	16.4
Northern Europe	4.2	44.3	7.4	45.4	5.6	18.2
Denmark	*5.6*	*46.8*	*10.6*	*31.2*	*10.4*	*13.6*
Ireland	3.7	39.6	7.9	47.8	4.3	14.3

(continued)

Table A.1 (continued)

	Larynx	Lung	Melanoma	Prostate	Testis	Bladder
Norway	3.2	35.1	14.1	65.3	8.8	21.3
Sweden	2.1	21.4	12.6	70.0	6.2	17.9
UK	4.2	47.6	6.1	40.2	5.6	19.2
Southern Europe	11.7	58.8	3.8	23.9	4.6	24.6
Italy	*10.8*	*59.4*	*4.6*	*24.9*	*5.8*	*28.0*
Greece	6.9	55.8	1.9	20.2	3.7	22.5
Spain	14.1	53.2	2.8	24.2	3.8	28.4
Western Europe	8.2	53.2	7.0	54.9	7.3	20.0
France	*10.2*	*53.5*	*6.8*	*56.5*	*6.3*	*25.6*
Germany	7.3	50.3	6.5	53.6	8.9	18.0
Netherlands	5.7	62.0	9.4	55.9	4.9	15.5
Australia	*4.3*	*42.2*	*40.5*	*76.0*	*5.7*	*15.6*
New Zealand	*2.9*	*41.4*	*36.7*	*101.1*	*6.5*	*17.1*
Melanesia	3.3	4.7	5.1	4.6	0.8	2.0
Polynesia	2.0	38.4	5.8	35.4	2.6	6.3

The table shows the incidence of the more common cancers in different parts of the world and in major countries in these world regions. (Countries are italicised, regions not italicised.) They show the incidence per 100,000 people per annum. These figures are not the absolute incidence but have been age standardised to give a truer comparison because of different life expectancies of people in different parts of the world and in different countries

The table has been compiled from Globocan website. Specific download reference as follows: 09/01/2004, http://www-dep.iarc.fr/cgi-bin/exe/globom.exe

Table A.2 Worldwide incidence of more common cancers: female

	Bladder	Kidney	Brain/nervous system	Thyroid	Non Hodgkins lymphoma	Hodgkins lymphoma	Leukaemia	Multiple myeloma
World	2.4	2.3	2.5	3.0	4.0	0.8	3.7	1.1
More developed countries	4.1	4.6	4.1	4.4	6.6	1.8	5.4	1.1
Less developed countries	1.5	1.1	2.0	2.5	2.6	0.5	3.0	0.6
Eastern Africa	2.7	0.8	0.5	2.7	4.6	0.9	2.9	0.6
Middle Africa	0.5	0.7	0.1	2.1	7.8	0.3	1.0	2.2
Northern Africa	4.5	1.6	1.6	3.3	2.6	0.8	2.9	0.7
Southern Africa	3.5	1.4	0.9	1.9	2.9	0.5	2.1	1.0
South Africa	*3.7*	*1.4*	*1.0*	*2.0*	*3.0*	*0.5*	*2.2*	*1.1*
Western Africa	1.5	0.5	0.2	2.0	3.3	1.0	2.7	0.3
Caribbean	2.6	1.7	2.8	3.2	3.5	1.2	5.2	1.8
Central America	1.9	2.4	3.7	4.2	3.5	1.1	5.0	1.5
South America	2.8	2.7	3.7	3.5	4.7	0.9	4.5	1.5
Argentina	*2.6*	*3.7*	*2.9*	*2.6*	*5.0*	*0.9*	*4.6*	*1.3*
Brazil	*3.2*	*2.6*	*4.6*	*3.3*	*4.5*	*0.9*	*4.3*	*1.5*
USA	**5.4**	**6.0**	**4.4**	**6.2**	**10.9**	**2.0**	**6.3**	**2.9**
Canada	**4.6**	**5.8**	**4.8**	**6.8**	**10.5**	**2.2**	**6.8**	**3.0**
Eastern Asia	1.2	1.3	2.6	2.2	2.1	0.1	3.4	0.6
China	*1.0*	*1.0*	*2.8*	*1.6*	*1.5*	*0.1*	*3.3*	*0.3*
Hong Kong	4.6	2.3	3.4	7.3	6.4	0.3	4.8	1.7
Japan	2.0	2.5	2.0	4.8	4.2	0.2	3.8	1.4
Korea	1.5	1.7	2.8	5.5	3.5	0.4	3.5	0.5

(continued)

Table A.2 (continued)

	Bladder	Kidney	Brain/nervous system	Thyroid	Non Hodgkins lymphoma	Hodgkins lymphoma	Leukaemia	Multiple myeloma
S.E. Asia	1.1	1.3	1.0	4.0	3.1	0.3	3.4	0.5
Indonesia	*1.0*	*1.5*	*0.8*	*3.9*	*3.6*	*0.4*	*3.4*	*0.7*
Malaysia	*1.5*	*2.6*	*1.3*	*5.6*	*4.7*	*0.5*	*4.3*	*1.3*
Philippines	*1.3*	*2.0*	*1.8*	*8.2*	*3.3*	*0.4*	*5.4*	*0.7*
Singapore	*1.8*	*2.4*	*2.0*	*5.9*	*4.6*	*0.4*	*4.2*	*1.1*
Thailand	*1.3*	*0.7*	*1.4*	*3.2*	*2.4*	*0.3*	*2.7*	*0.3*
South Central Asia	1.1	0.6	1.5	2.3	2.0	0.6	2.2	0.5
India	0.7	0.5	1.6	1.9	1.7	0.5	2.1	0.6
Pakistan	*3.4*	*0.9*	*1.8*	*3.9*	*3.5*	*0.8*	*3.8*	*0.7*
Western Asia	2.4	1.8	2.9	3.1	4.5	1.8	3.9	1.1
Israel	5.6	5.5	4.3	8.1	11.1	2.9	5.5	2.2
Saudi Arabia	*1.9*	*1.8*	*2.4*	*7.7*	*7.3*	*2.0*	*4.5*	*1.3*
Turkey	*1.6*	*1.7*	*3.0*	*2.0*	*4.0*	*0.7*	*3.5*	*0.9*
United Arab Emirates	*1.8*	*1.9*	*2.6*	*7.3*	*4.5*	*3.6*	*4.5*	*1.1*
Eastern Europe	4.0	4.7	3.8	2.7	3.9	2.0	5.0	1.0
Russian Federation	*3.9*	*4.4*	*3.7*	*2.4*	*3.5*	*1.8*	*4.9*	*0.9*
Northern Europe	5.3	4.6	5.4	3.1	6.9	1.5	6.2	2.4
Denmark	4.2	5.2	5.8	3.1	7.0	1.7	6.3	2.3
Ireland	*4.4*	*4.0*	*5.0*	*1.6*	*7.9*	*2.1*	*6.3*	*3.0*
Norway	*5.9*	*5.9*	*6.6*	*3.9*	*7.6*	*1.4*	*6.0*	*2.4*
Sweden	5.4	5.7	11.3	3.4	7.8	1.7	8.1	2.5s
UK	6.0	3.8	4.4	2.4	7.0	1.4	6.1	2.4

Southern Europe	4.1	3.5	4.8	5.2	6.3	2.1	5.3	2.1
Italy	5.0	4.3	4.4	8.5	8.1	2.7	6.2	2.5
Greece	*4.2*	*2.8*	*7.1*	*3.0*	*3.3*	*4.0*	*5.5*	*1.5*
Spain	*3.3*	*2.7*	*5.0*	*2.8*	*6.3*	*1.4*	*4.9*	*2.0*
Western Europe	4.2	5.4	4.6	4.4	7.1	2.5	5.9	2.3
France	4.0	4.7	4.2	6.5	7.6	2.1	6.0	2.3
Germany	*4.4*	*5.9*	*4.8*	*3.7*	*6.7*	*2.8*	*6.0*	*2.2*
Netherlands	*3.5*	*5.2*	*4.5*	*2.5*	*7.7*	*1.6*	*5.1*	*2.7*
Australia	4.6	6.0	4.8	5.8	10.8	1.9	6.9	2.8
New Zealand	**4.7**	**4.9**	**5.5**	**3.9**	**11.1**	**1.6**	**8.7**	**3.4**
Melanesia	**0.5**	**0.9**	**0.2**	**4.2**	**4.8**	**0.4**	**2.8**	**0.1**
Polynesia	1.0	1.5	2.9	18.8	4.7	1.0	6.1	1.9

Table A.2 (continued)

	Oral cavity	Nasopharynx	Oropharynx	Oesophagus	Stomach	Colon/rectum	Liver	Pancreas
World	3.3	0.6	0.8	4.5	10.4	14.4	5.5	3.2
More developed countries	2.4	0.3	0.6	1.3	11.0	25.4	2.9	5.1
Less developed countries	3.7	0.8	0.8	6.2	10.0	7.9	6.8	2.1
Eastern Africa	6.0	0.9	0.4	5.1	6.7	4.9	6.0	1.6
Middle Africa	2.7	0.2	0.6	0.2	14.1	3.3	13.0	4.0
Northern Africa	1.7	1.2	0.3	1.8	3.3	5.2	2.7	1.1
Southern Africa	3.4	0.4	0.3	6.4	3.7	8.7	2.1	1.1
South Africa	*3.2*	*0.4*	*0.3*	*6.2*	*3.8*	*9.4*	*2.1*	*1.2*
Western Africa	1.5	0.1.	0.1	1.4	3.9	3.8	6.2	0.7
Caribbean	4.5	0.3	1.4	2.0	7.2	15.4	4.2	3.0
Central America	1.8	0.2	0.5	1.2	13.1	9.1	1.6	4.8
South America	2.4	0.2	0.7	2.5	11.7	14.3	3.7	4.2
Argentina	*1.7*	*0.1*	*0.3*	*2.5*	*5.4*	*18.9*	*3.3*	*5.9*
Brazil	*2.9*	*0.2*	*1.1*	*2.8*	*9.7*	*13.8*	*4.5*	*3.7*
USA	*3.7*	*0.2*	*0.7*	*1.4*	*3.6*	*30.7*	*1.7*	*6.3*
Canada	*2.6*	*0.3*	*0.8*	*1.3*	*4.2*	*29.8*	*1.1*	*5.9*
Eastern Asia	1.0	0.9	0.1	8.9	19.6	12.5	12.7	3.2
China	*0.9*	*1.1*	*0.1*	*10.9*	*17.5*	*9.8*	*13.3*	*2.6*
Hong Kong	2.7	9.7	0.4	3.2	10.1	28.9	9.8	3.0
Japan	1.7	0.1	0.2	1.6	28.6	25.3	8.1	5.7
Korea	1.0	0.2	0.2	1.0	25.7	10.3	11.6	3.7

S.E. Asia	2.6	2.2	0.7	1.3	4.8	10.0	5.7	1.6
Indonesia	*1.0*	*1.9*	*0.3*	*0.4*	*2.1*	*10.6*	*2.6*	*1.6*
Malaysia	1.8	3.1	0.4	1.1	6.7	21.0	3.7	2.7
Philippines	5.4	2.5	1.7	1.3	5.5	13.5	6.8	3.4
Singapore	1.9	5.1	0.3	1.5	11.8	30.3	4.9	3.2
Thailand	4.0	1.2	0.6	1.3	2.9	7.4	15.2	1.0
S Central Asia	8.6	0.3	2.0	6.3	3.5	3.7	1.5	0.8
India	*7.5*	*0.3*	*1.8*	*5.1*	*2.8*	*3.2*	*1.1*	*0.8*
Pakistan	14.7	0.9	2.6	6.3	2.8	5.1	3.6	0.9
Western Asia	2.1	0.5	0.5	1.4	6.1	8.3	2.1	2.1
Israel	*3.0*	*0.4*	*0.1*	*1.2*	*6.9*	*33.6*	*1.8*	*6.3*
Saudi Arabia	4.1	1.5	1.1	4.3	3.9	7.2	5.9	1.7
Turkey	1.9	0.3	0.5	0.9	5.6	5.3	1.0	1.2
United Arab Emirates	2.5	1.2	0.9	3.2	3.0	8.0	4.0	2.6
Eastern Europe	2.1	0.5	0.5	1.1	14.5	21.5	2.6	4.8
Russian Federation	*2.0*	*0.5*	*0.4*	*1.5*	*18.0*	*22.1*	*2.3*	*4.6*
Northern Europe	2.1	0.2	0.7	3.2	6.1	25.2	1.4	5.2
Denmark	*3.2*	*0.3*	*1.1*	*1.9*	*4.2*	*30.5*	*2.0*	*5.9*
Ireland	2.2	0.1	0.6	3.6	6.2	28.7	0.9	5.8
Norway	2.6	0.1	0.5	0.8	5.6	33.8	0.8	6.3
Sweden	2.7	0.1	0.5	0.9	4.7	24.6	2.4	5.3
UK	2.0	0.2	0.7	4.3	5.5	25.3	1.1	4.9
Southern Europe	1.6	0.2	0.4	0.7	9.7	22.0	3.5	4.7
Italy	*1.4*	*0.2*	*0.5*	*0.7*	*10.3*	*24.0*	*4.6*	*5.5*
Greece	1.0	0.2	0.3	0.4	6.4	13.6	4.6	3.9
Spain	1.7	0.3	0.3	0.6	8.5	21.0	2.4	3.5

(continued)

Table A.2 (continued)

	Oral cavity	Nasopharynx	Oropharynx	Oesophagus	Stomach	Colon/rectum	Liver	Pancreas
Western Europe	3.0	0.3	1.2	1.3	7.0	29.4	1.6	4.6
France	2.6	0.2	1.3	1.4	4.5	26.8	1.8	3.0
Germany	3.3	0.3	1.3	1.1	9.2	32.0	1.6	5.3
Netherlands	3.1	0.2	1.1	2.2	5.2	30.4	0.8	5.2
Australia	5.4	0.2	0.7	2.2	5.0	35.4	1.0	5.5
New Zealand	2.6	0.3	0.5	2.4	5.2	43.4	2.0	6.2
Melanesia	23.6	0.2	0.5	2.4	3.8	4.6	10.2	0.5
Polynesia	2.2	1.7	0.8	0.9	9.2	13.7	3.9	3.0

Table A.2 (continued)

	Larynx	Lung	Melanoma	Breast	Cervix/uterus	Body/uterus	Ovary
World	0.7	11.1	2.2	35.7	16.1	6.4	6.5
More developed countries	0.7	15.6	6.1	63.2	11.4	11.3	9.9
Less developed countries	0.6	6.8	0.7	23.1	18.7	3.9	4.9
Eastern Africa	0.5	2.1	3.3	20.2	44.3	3.4	9.0
Middle Africa	0.2	0.8	2.3	13.5	25.1	3.0	2.9
Northern Africa	0.7	2.8	0.7	28.3	16.8	2.2	3.2
Southern Africa	0.8	7.3	4.6	31.8	30.3	4.6	3.9
South Africa	*0.8*	*8.0*	*4.8*	*33.5*	*28.9*	*4.8*	*4.0*
Western Africa	0.1	0.4	1.3	24.8	20.3	1.6	3.1
Caribbean	1.3	9.7	0.7	33.8	35.8	8.6	5.6
Central America	1.0	8.4	1.6	36.2	40.3	15.8	7.0
South America	1.0	8.3	2.0	45.1	30.9	14.3	7.3
Argentina	*0.7*	*8.3*	*1.8*	*64.7*	*14.2*	*28.8*	*12.7*
Brazil	*1.1*	*8.9*	*2.2*	*46.4*	*31.3*	*12.9*	*6.8*
USA	*1.2*	*34.0*	*9.4*	*91.4*	*7.8*	*15.5*	*10.6*
Canada	*0.9*	*30.2*	*8.0*	*81.8*	*8.3*	*14.9*	*11.7*
Eastern Asia	0.3	15.0	0.2	18.1	6.4	2.4	3.7
China	*0.3*	*15.7*	*0.2*	*16.4*	*5.2*	*2.2*	*3.2*
Hong Kong	0.8	32.1	0.8	34.4	15.6	7.1	7.5
Japan	0.1	12.1	0.3	31.4	11.1	4.5	6.6
Korea	0.6	12.1	0.2	12.5	15.3	1.5	4.1
S.E. Asia	0.5	9.1	0.5	25.6	18.3	4.3	7.1

(continued)

Table A.2 (continued)

	Larynx	Lung	Melanoma	Breast	Cervix/uterus	Body/uterus	Ovary
Indonesia	*0.2*	*6.8*	*0.8*	*26.1*	*15.7*	*5.3*	*8.1*
Malaysia	0.3	12.9	0.8	41.9	12.0	7.7	11.4
Philippines	0.9	14.2	0.6	44.7	22.7	6.0	10.2
Singapore	0.4	18.9	0.5	47.1	14.9	8.2	11.1
Thailand	0.4	10.9	0.4	15.9	20.7	2.8	4.7
South Central Asia	1.0	2.3	0.4	22.2	26.5	2.2	5.2
India	*0.8*	*2.0*	*0.2*	*19.1*	*30.7*	*1.7*	*4.9*
Pakistan	1.5	2.8	0.8	50.1	6.5	5.8	9.8
Western Asia	0.9	4.8	1.2	27.9	4.8	4.9	5.9
Israel	*0.7*	*9.7*	*9.8*	*79.1*	*5.8*	*11.5*	*11.7*
Saudi Arabia	0.4	3.3	0.4	21.6	5.0	3.1	5.0
Turkey	0.6	4.0	0.9	20.4	3.9	4.0	6.2
United Arab Emirates	0.4	4.9	0.3	27.1	4.6	3.4	5.3
Eastern Europe	0.5	8.8	5.0	49.4	16.8	10.7	10.3
Russian Federation	0.4	7.6	4.7	48.8	13.6	10.1	9.3
Northern Europe	0.7	18.9	8.7	73.2	9.8	11.1	12.6
Denmark	*1.0*	*27.7*	*13.0*	*86.2*	*15.3*	*13.1*	*16.1*
Ireland	0.6	18.7	10.2	71.6	7.9	9.8	13.9
Norway	0.6	16.6	15.9	68.5	12.6	13.5	13.1
Sweden	0.3	12.1	13.3	81.0	9.4	15.2	11.9
UK	0.8	21.8	7.7	74.9	9.3	9.3	12.2

Southern Europe	0.5	8.0	4.6	56.2	10.2	13.8	8.7
Italy	*0.6*	*9.0*	*5.5*	*64.9*	*9.1*	*16.5*	*8.7*
Greece	*0.6*	*8.3*	*2.0*	*47.6*	*6.9*	*6.4*	*7.7*
Spain	*0.2*	*4.0*	*4.5*	*47.9*	*7.2*	*12.0*	*8.3*
Western Europe	0.8	10.7	8.1	78.2	10.4	10.9	11.1
France	*0.9*	*7.4*	*8.0*	*83.2*	*10.1*	*9.6*	*9.2*
Germany	*0.7*	*11.4*	*7.1*	*73.7*	*11.5*	*11.4*	*12.2*
Netherlands	*0.9*	*17.5*	*12.9*	*91.6*	*7.3*	*11.6*	*11.9*
Australia	*0.5*	*17.5*	*31.9*	*82.7*	*7.1*	*10.6*	*9.1*
New Zealand	*0.6*	*21.7*	*34.9*	*82.6*	*10.6*	*11.5*	*12.4*
Melanesia	0.9	2.9	3.1	21.7	43.8	7.1	7.1
Polynesia	0.2	14.2	2.1	55.2	29.0	15.3	3.8

The table shows the incidence of the more common cancers in different parts of the world and in major countries in these world regions. (Countries are italicised, regions not italicised.) They show the incidence per 100,000 people per annum. These figures are not the absolute incidence but have been age standardised to give a truer comparison because of different life expectancies of people in different parts of the world and in different countries

The table has been compiled from Globocan 2002 database. Specific download reference as follows: 09/01/2004, http://www-dep.iarc.fr/cgi-bin/exe/globof.exe?

Index

Printing: Krips bv, Meppel, The Netherlands
Binding: Stürtz, Würzburg, Germany